Graham Harvey won the BP Natural World Book Prize for *The Killing of the Countryside* in 1997. He is an agricultural graduate and has written on food and rural issues for a wide range of publications. A former script-writer on the long-running radio drama series *The Archers,* he is currently the programme's Agricultural Story Editor.

We Want Real Food:
The Local Food Lover's Bible

Graham Harvey

Robinson
London

Constable & Robinson Ltd
3 The Lanchesters
162 Fulham Palace Road
London W6 9ER
www.constablerobinson.com

First published in the UK by Constable,
an imprint of Constable & Robinson Ltd, 2006

This fully revised and updated edition
published by Robinson, 2008

A copy of the British Library Cataloguing in Publication
Data is available from the British Library

ISBN: 978-1-84529-545-5

Printed and bound in the EU

1 3 5 7 9 10 8 6 4 2

Contents

Preface

If there's one word that sums up Britain's attitude to healthy eating it's 'confused'. And it's hardly surprising. Scarcely a day goes by without some new piece of research showing a particular food to be either super-healthy or guaranteed to take years off your life. Sometimes it's the very same item.

On food labels the term 'healthy' seems to apply to pretty well everything. Processed foods are labelled 'healthy' because the manufacturer has halved the salt and sugar content or cut back the level of fat. But isn't there more to the health-giving properties of food than this?

What about the sum total of the nutrients it contains – the minerals, vitamins, antioxidants, phytonutrients and the rest? Surely it's these that make a food healthy – or not. Yet it's these the labels seldom tell us anything about.

The same is true of fresh foods. Food guides may tell you that carrots are good for you, but not all carrots are the same. Depending on the way they're grown – and the soil they're grown in – some will have far more health-giving nutrients than others. If you're interested in health you need to make sure you're eating the good ones and not the 'fakes'.

This book will give you the facts you need to choose the truly healthy foods, the ones packed full of nutrients. It'll also tell you how to find them at a retailer near you. Though celebrity chefs like to hype up nutrient-dense foods as rare and precious jewels, they're pretty much everywhere if you know what you're looking for. And they don't have to be expensive.

So turn your back on the muddle and prepare to embark on a new exploration of healthy eating. You may get a few surprises along the way, but you'll also get a better idea of what's genuinely good for you and what isn't. Healthy, nutrient-rich foods aren't for the lucky few. They're the birthright of everyone. Good hunting.

1

Foods Aren't What They Used To Be

The technology that has done most to debase British foods is now almost a century old and it owes much of its dominance to the exigencies of war. Five years before the outbreak of the First World War, three of Germany's top chemical engineers made the journey from Ludwigshafen to the southern city of Karlsruhe to observe a momentous laboratory experiment.

It wasn't an arduous journey. All three worked for the company BASF – *Badische Anilin und Soda-Fabrik* – just sixty kilometres to the north. Even so, it would take something special to bring scientists of this seniority to the small lab in the physical chemistry department of Karlsruhe's technical university. At the time, BASF was the most powerful chemical company in the world.

In the lab the experimental apparatus had been set up on a bench. It was a compact and skilfully crafted piece of equipment made up of metal vessels, small-bore tubing and pressure gauges. Intrigued, the engineers inspected it carefully, though they had serious doubts that it could ever be made to work.

Its designer, a brilliant research scientist called Fritz Haber, had been emphatic. His process could harness the virtually limitless supply of the element nitrogen present in the earth's atmosphere. In doing so it would free the world from famine, the scourge that had stalked mankind from the dawn of history.

At the heart of Haber's apparatus was an iron tube containing a nickel heating coil. Inside the tube a mixture of the two gases nitrogen and hydrogen would be introduced under pressure and heated to more than five hundred degrees centigrade. In the presence of a suitable metal catalyst, the gases could be made to react, claimed Haber, forming the pungent white gas ammonia. What's more, the reaction would take place at a rate that made it a real commercial undertaking.

For BASF this was a prize beyond measure. Ammonia was easily converted to a soluble salt such as ammonium sulphate, a valuable nitrogen fertilizer. The company that found a way of producing it in quantity, and at a reasonable price, was on the road to riches.

Food shortages remained a real worry in early twentieth-century Europe, particularly for countries like Germany and Britain, where industrialization had been accompanied by rapid population growth. Farmers of the time relied mainly on organic wastes and legume crops such as clover or beans to return nitrogen to their soils, and so maintain fertility.

There was also a thriving international trade in Chilean sodium nitrate, mined from the vast natural deposits on the arid plateau between the Andes mountains and the Pacific Coastal Range. This had followed an earlier boom in the mid-nineteenth century for guano, the nitrogen-rich deposits of seabird droppings from islands off the Peruvian coast.

By the turn of the century the guano deposits had been largely exhausted, and it was clear that the nitrate-containing *caliche* would soon run out, perhaps in as little as twenty years. 'We are drawing on the earth's capital, and our drafts will not perpetually be honoured,' the chemist Sir William Crookes had warned in his presidential address to the British Association meeting in Bristol in 1898.

During the second half of the nineteenth century pioneer farmers had ploughed up vast tracts of the world's natural grassland to grow wheat for the industrial cities. South America, Australia, and Russia had all yielded virgin grasslands to the plough.

The greatest transformation of all had taken place on America's Great Plains, and on the prairie lands of Canada. In a few short decades the ancient prairie grass-lands – haunt of vast bison herds and hunting ground of Native Americans – had been replaced, from horizon to horizon, by industrial wheat.

For a number of years following the ploughing up of old grassland, crops produce good yields. They are sustained by the natural soil fertility built up under the turf. But after a series of wheat crops the land will eventually become exhausted. Unless some new form of fertilizer is made available in large quantities, the prairies, the steppes and the pampas will have to go back to grass.

In his Bristol address, Crookes set out the threat with the impeccable logic of nineteenth century science. In the next century larger populations would need more wheat, he warned in sonorous tones. Yet there were few virgin territories left to be exploited. If the industrial world were not to go hungry, today's wheat lands would have to be induced to produce more.

It was Crookes who drew the scientists' attention to the vast reserves of nitrogen present in the earth's atmosphere. Here was a way to feed the industrial masses. The 'fixation' of atmospheric nitrogen was essential to the progress of civilization.

This was a chemist's solution. Crookes concluded his address: 'It is the chemist who must come to the rescue... It is through the laboratory that starvation may ultimately be turned into plenty.'

Eleven years later the British scientist's challenge was about to be fulfilled in a laboratory in Karlsruhe. That it should be happening in Germany was no great surprise. At the time, the German chemical industry led the world. It was bound to be at the forefront of any new technical development.

There was another reason why Germany had a vital interest in cracking this particular nut. Antagonism between Britain and Germany was running high. To German military strategists it was clear that in any future conflict the Royal Navy would quickly block imports of Chilean nitrate, jeopardizing the nation's food supply.

It would also threaten her military might. For nitrates were not just a valuable fertilizer, they were an essential raw material in the manufacture of explosives. Without Chilean nitrate Germany would have been unable to fight a protracted war. The conversion of ammonia to nitric acid, and then to nitrates, were straightforward chemical processes. A limitless supply of ammonia derived from atmospheric nitrogen would add immeasurably to German military strength.

These were the imperatives that brought the three BASF scientists to Karlsruhe on that warm July day in 1909. It was a journey they made more in hope than in expectation. One of them, Carl Bosch, had already made a detailed study of ammonia synthesis. On joining the company as a young scientist his first assignment had been to investigate the work of an earlier chemist who claimed to have produced ammonia from its elements. The claim turned out to have been mistaken.

While cautiously backing Haber's experiments, BASF had hedged its bets. The company had already invested in a Norwegian system for producing nitrogen compounds by passing electric sparks through air. This was a highly energy-intensive process. It could only make economic sense in a country with plentiful supplies of low-cost electricity, as in Norway. Even so, the company thought it a more promising development than the super-heating of gases under pressure.

If Fritz Haber entertained any such doubts about his process, no one would have guessed it on that July day. He confidently pointed out the finer details of the laboratory apparatus. It included a number of innovative features. Research involving extreme temperatures and pressures threw up immense difficulties for scientists.

Many of those encountered by Haber were solved by his talented English assistant, Robert Le Rossignol. Among the features designed by the Englishman were specialized valves to control the flow of pressurized gases and a double-acting steel pump for circulating them.

For all its fancy design features, the apparatus almost failed on a simple engineering fault. One of the bolts in the high-pressure system sprang a leak during last-minute tightening. Producing a replacement delayed the experiment by several hours. Not until the afternoon was Haber able to open up the gas inlets and switch on the pump. By this time Carl Bosch was on his way back to a meeting in Ludwigshafen.

The two company men who remained were rewarded for their patience. Within minutes the first synthetic ammonia – now in liquid form – was beginning to rise in the water gauge. One of the two BASF engineers, Alwin Mittasch, turned to Haber and clasped his hand. He sensed this was an historic moment. And so it turned out to be.

Today, most of the food we eat is grown with the aid of Fritz Haber's nitrogen. Around 40 per cent of the nitrogen in our bodies is derived, not from the natural fertility processes of the soil, but from super-heated gases in a steel chamber somewhere in Texas, China or Ukraine. It has fulfilled the chemist's dream of making food plentiful and cheap, at least in the industrial countries.

But there's a dark side to the small, crystalline hailstones that agribusiness companies promote with such relish. They have become destroyers of family farms and rural communities. They pollute the seas and waterways. Worst of all, they have spoiled the foods of the countryside so they no longer promote good health.

Nitrogen fertilizers are a product of nineteenth-century industrial thinking. As a means of acquiring railways, roads and consumer goods it has proved to be highly effective, but when let loose on the complex ecosystem of the soil it has taken us to the brink of disaster.

Once while on holiday in the Black Forest I made a short detour to Karlsruhe University. I wanted to find the building where Haber had carried out his historic experiment, if it still existed. It occurred to me there might even be some sort of museum with the original apparatus on permanent display.

I found the building easily enough. It looked no different from the pictures taken in the early 1900s. There was no science going on any more. The sign on the wall declared that it was now the Department of Architecture. I asked a couple of staff members about Haber's apparatus, but they couldn't tell me much.

Walking back through the old campus, I came across a piece of industrial art. On a stone pedestal had been placed what looked like an enormous metal cylinder, rather like the boiler of an old steam locomotive placed on its end. Then it dawned on me. I'd seen something like it in old photographs. This was the scaled-up production version of Haber's 'furnace' – now called a converter. The date on the accompanying plaque was 1919. The development of large-scale ammonia synthesis was as much a triumph of engineering as of science.

After Haber's remarkable discovery, BASF put Carl Bosch in charge of developing the experimental process for full-scale production. He did it with a speed that was little short of extraordinary. The original bench-top converter had been just seventy-five centimetres tall. Four years later an eight-metre high converter was producing more than four tonnes of ammonia a day in the first commercial plant at Oppau, near Ludwigshafen.

In another four years the company opened its second plant near the village of Leuna, on the river Saale in Saxony. This one was capable of producing more than a hundred thousand tonnes of ammonia a year.

By this time both factories were producing nitrates for Germany's war effort. Without them the Second Reich might well have collapsed within months of the start of the First World War. It was only a steady supply of ammonia from the Haber-Bosch process that prevented the country from running out of munitions early in 1915.

Fritz Haber spent the war making another distinctive contribution to Germany's struggle. Following his success with ammonia synthesis, he had been invited to become director of the new Institute for Physical Chemistry, part of the Kaiser-Wilhelm Institute in Dahlem, near Berlin. When war broke out, he turned the entire institute over to the development of poison gas. In the spring of 1915 he himself supervised the first gas attack of the war, releasing chlorine against French troops at Ypres.

At the end of the war he went briefly into hiding in Switzerland for fear of Allied reprisals. Gas warfare was prohibited under the Hague Conventions. But far from being indicted for war crimes, he was honoured with the Nobel chemistry prize for his work on ammonia synthesis. It was a controversial award. Many scientists objected to the Swedish Academy's choice of 'the inventor of gas warfare'.

In his acceptance speech Haber declared: 'Nitrogen fertilization of the soil brings new nutritive riches to mankind. The chemical industry comes to the aid of the farmer who, in the good earth, changes stones into bread.'

Born in 1868 in Breslau, Prussia, Haber belonged to that eminent school of scientific rationalists who emerged in the late nineteenth century. Physics and chemistry were the dominant sciences. Haber combined the two with his interest in physical chemistry and, like most German scientists of his day, he made no distinction between science and engineering. To him the job of the scientist was to provide practical solutions to society's problems. He was equally happy working on the efficiency of steam turbines, the thermodynamics of bunsen flames, or the extraction of gold from seawater. His role was to serve humanity and, in time of war, to serve his country.

Nitrogen fertilizer is a product of that culture, of a nineteenth-century industrial mindset. From the moment the first ammonia dripped from the condenser in that Karlsruhe laboratory, industrialists around the world have been lining up to take it out into the countryside.

With the coming of peace in 1918, any hope BASF had of keeping the ammonia secret to themselves was quickly doused. Under the terms of the Versailles Treaty, the company was obliged to license construction of an ammonia plant in France. Within a short time companies in Italy and the United States were building their own versions of the Haber-Bosch process, based on what they knew about the basic principles.

In Britain, the chemical company Brunner Mond had been producing ammonium nitrate by a variety of methods and it was determined not to be left out of the race. During the war the company had worked closely with the Ministry of Munitions, running two Cheshire plants which produced ammonium nitrate by crystallization from sodium nitrate and ammonium sulphate.

In 1918, the government drew up plans to build a larger plant producing ammonium nitrate by the Haber process. A large site was purchased at Billingham near Stockton-on-Tees, but following the Armistice it was sold on to Brunner Mond to develop.[1] The government also passed on all the details it had of the Haber-Bosch process, but crucial details remained a mystery. What were the operating pressures chosen by the German company? What catalysts were they using?

A team of Brunner Mond chemists was despatched to the Rhineland to study the processes used in the Oppau plant. They were accompanied by the assistant director of the government's explosive supply department, H. A. Humphrey. Under the Armistice agreement German companies were supposed to disclose their industrial secrets. Even so, the Brunner Mond board knew that without government backing the mission would not succeed.

At Oppau, BASF managers were outraged at the spying mission and did all they could to disrupt the visit. Production was brought to a halt, dials were hastily painted over, and access ladders removed.

The 'spies' were banned from taking photographs or making notes. Whenever they walked into a production area, the staff would stop working and stare at the unwelcome visitors. Each night the British chemists would return to their hotel rooms and make notes and sketches from memory.

After a little over a month they thought they'd found out all they could. As they prepared to leave Germany, their baggage, including their report, was locked overnight in a railway wagon and placed under armed guard. This didn't stop a thief, or patriot, cutting through the floor of the wagon and plundering its contents.

Fearing such an incident, one of the team, a Brunner Mond engineer called Captain A. H. Cowap, had kept his notes and sketches with him. Back in Britain they were enough to fill in many of the missing process details. For years afterwards the Oppau mission was referred to in the company boardroom as 'the burglary'.[2]

Thanks to this early industrial espionage, the Billingham ammonia plant was finally completed in 1923. Three years later Brunner Mond merged with Nobel Industries and two other chemical companies to form Imperial Chemical Industries (ICI). Its first chairman, Sir Alfred Mond, later Lord Melchett, saw it as his mission to spread artificial fertilizers, not only across Britain, but throughout the Empire. Crucial to the enterprise would be propaganda.

Two run-down farms were bought near Maidenhead in Berkshire, one of which was called Jealott's Hill. They would become the company's research centre, along the lines of Rothamsted, the widely-respected Hertfordshire research station which had been founded by an earlier fertilizer manufacturer, John Bennet Lawes. Jealott's Hill was to be the proving ground of the new nitrogen fertilizers. It would undertake serious scientific research to back up the marketing effort.

To give the company's research some credibility, an eminent scientist was needed to take charge. Mond persuaded Sir Frederick Keeble, Professor of Botany at Oxford, to become head of 'fertilizer research and propaganda'. He seems to have been well up to the task. After only four years research, he declared that the station had 'established beyond all question' how fertilizers could be used to increase food production and boost the fertility of farmland.[3]

Agriculture in the early thirties was still sunk in recession. Keeble correctly identified the cause. Then, as now, farming stood exposed to global economic forces. New methods of transport meant that even perishable foods could be brought to Britain cheaply and efficiently. At the same time, vast tracts of fertile, uncultivated land were being brought under the plough. British farmers were unable to compete.

Keeble had the solution. If farmers were to prosper in these stricken times, the fertility of the land, both arable and grass, would have to be raised. Only then would it produce more food; only then would it provide a decent profit for the farmer. And there was one obvious way of raising fertility quickly, through the liberal use of fertilizers.

Keeble was particularly keen to see livestock farmers applying the new nitrogen fertilizer to their grasses.

> Nitrogen and mineral plant foods make grassland earlier, and more resistant to drought. They lengthen seasonal production, and convert the natural periodic exuberance into steadier growth. They increase the quality of grass as well as the quantity, and add to its health-giving properties. They give strength to the better grasses, encourage them to drive out the poorer, and so lead to permanent improvement of the grassland itself.[4]

Farmers weren't impressed. At the time, they were applying a tiny amount of nitrogen fertilizer to their wheat crops, just five pounds to the acre. Hardly any went on grassland. Instead most farmers chose to rely on the fertility-building properties of clover. Despite the exhortations of Keeble and his colleagues, they had no intention of spending what little cash they could spare on chemicals.

With cheap grain pouring into UK ports from the American prairies, the response of many farmers was to get out of grain and put their fields down to pasture. Milk, poultry, vegetables, beef and sheep meat all did well between the wars. Farmers found they could survive the recession perfectly well without ICI's fertilizers.

With unsold stocks piling up outside the Billingham factory, the company had no option but to shut down a large part of the plant. The budget for Jealott's Hill research station was cut by half and shortly afterwards Keeble retired, a disillusioned man. Propaganda had failed. ICI had set out to become the farmer's friend. Unfortunately the farmer hadn't wanted to play.

The company had to find another way to spread the new chemical culture across the countryside of Britain. Instead of appealing direct to farmers, the decision was made to concentrate on influencing government. If policy-makers could be made to see that chemical fertilizers were in the national interest, then they would do the marketing. The new strategy was given a shot in the arm by the outbreak of war.

Shortly before the war ICI's chief agricultural advisor, William Gavin, had joined the Ministry of Agriculture. So the company already had its man on the inside. He and his former ICI colleagues began pressing the government to adopt a set of radical farming measures, 'in the national interest'. The main measures involved putting a lot of nitrogen fertilizer on grassland.

Research at Jealott's Hill had shown that an early application of nitrogen stimulated pastures to put on a spurt of growth in the spring, so extending the grazing season. Other experiments had shown that silage, fermented grass, was a more reliable form of winter fodder than hay, the crop most farmers relied on. Needless to say, silage-making required far heavier inputs of nitrogen fertilizer than haymaking.

In the spring of 1940, the company mounted a vigorous lobbying campaign. They wanted the government to set national targets of a million acres of early grazing, and two million acres of silage. The extra grass would lead to enormous savings in imported cattle feed, they claimed, reducing the pressure on a merchant fleet that was daily running the gauntlet of Atlantic U-boats. What the company failed to stress was that the programme would require up to two hundred thousand tons of ammonium sulphate fertilizer.

At the start of the war the government was unconvinced. ICI chairman Sir Harry McGowan went as far as rebuking the agriculture minister, Reginald Dorman-Smith, in *The Times* for failing to set a clear farming policy. When Winston Churchill formed his government in May 1940, the new minister, R. S. Hudson, seemed more compliant.

He announced a campaign for a million tons of silage. It was to be run by the 'War Ags', the county committees that now controlled farming. They would rely heavily on help and support from ICI, the minister announced.

The following year Hudson approached the ICI chairman – 'My dear Harry' – for help with a wider campaign of grassland improvement to run alongside the silage programme. He appealed for the help of company staff to train and work with the government advisors. McGowan promised to help 'in every possible way'.

In the House of Lords the government's spokesman on agriculture, the Duke of Norfolk, was forced to deny connivance with the powerful chemical industry. He added:

'There is no evidence that a balanced use of fertilizers has a harmful effect on soil, crops or man.' Nor, he candidly admitted, did it do any harm to ICI's profits.[5]

The company's plan to change the farming culture had worked like a dream. Before the government took on its emergency wartime powers, farmers showed they were uninterested in nitrogen fertilizers, particularly for use on grass. Once the war started they had no choice but to comply. The 'War Ags' had absolute powers to control the way farms were managed. They could even throw families off their own land if they didn't do what they were told.

Not surprisingly, farmers started making more use of chemical fertilizers. The threat of invasion had set Britain on the path to industrial farming. ICI's own wartime campaign had been a textbook example of how to manipulate the British political system.

In peacetime, the unholy alliance went from strength to strength. The post-war Labour government introduced guaranteed prices for all the major farm commodities. For the fertilizer manufacturers this was a triumph. The state was contracting to pay farmers for whatever they could deliver. The message was clear. It was output that mattered, not quality.

This was exactly what Keeble had been calling for in 1930. Forget traditional methods, he had urged farmers. There was profit to be made by using chemical fertilizers to give a quick boost to production. At the time farmers had been sceptical. Now the government was introducing the price guarantees to make it happen.

And in case there should be any confusion about the government's intentions, the new price guarantees were backed by special subsidies on fertilizers. The politicians and the chemical manufacturers were now on the same mission.

The state-run National Agricultural Advisory Service (NAAS), which replaced the county 'War Ags,' swamped the countryside with meetings, farm demonstrations and discussion groups, all promoting fertilizers, especially nitrogen fertilizers. The chemical companies, most notably ICI, were doing the same thing. Many farmers believed that NAAS, the government advisory service, was simply a division of ICI. Others thought ICI was part of the government.[6]

The company was more than happy with the confusion. Endorsement by the official advisory service lent authority to the sales pitch. An advisory booklet for dairy farmers, jointly published with the government-funded Grassland Research Institute, had cover and illustrations printed in familiar 'ICI blue'. A popular saying with farmers was that the best grass seed came out of 'the blue bag' – the ICI fertilizer bag.

All these events took place fifty or more years ago. Yet the stranglehold of the chemical industry on the production of everyday foods is as tight as ever. Fritz Haber's breakthrough came out of the science of the nineteenth and early twentieth centuries, the age of industrial chemistry. In the rest of the economy it's a science that has been in steep decline. After all this is the age of microelectronics and biotechnology.

As Colin Tudge puts it in *So Shall We Reap*: 'In agriculture, though not in most of the rest of the world's economy, the glory days of industrial chemistry continue, confident and insouciant as ever.'[7] The farmers who once refused to put Haber's nitrogen on their pastures now throw it down at the rate of more than two hundred kilograms to the hectare. Wheat growers on some of the world's best soils now find it necessary to use the world's highest rates of fertilizer nitrogen.

Generations of British farmers have grown up believing it's impossible to grow a decent crop without a bag full of chemicals and half a dozen pesticide sprays. Organic farming is seen as odd, chemical farming as the norm. It's as if agriculture had no history before 1940. This is how effectively a handful of politicians and industrialists succeeded in changing rural culture.

Even as the fertilizer manufacturers were getting their hands on the levers of power, Sir Albert Howard was warning of the catastrophe that would follow. In *England and the Farmer* he forecast that the widespread use of artificial fertilizers would be condemned by history as 'one of the greatest misfortunes to have befallen agriculture and mankind'.[8] The crops they grew were poorly nourished, so they had little resistance to disease. Nor would the animals and people that ate them.

Despite the warnings, Europe's farm policymakers repeated the mistake of Britain's post-war government. They, too, put inflated prices at the heart of farm policy. For more than fifty years Europe's farmers have been paid handsomely to maximize production with the aid of Haber's nitrogen. Much of the tax paid by Europe's citizens to support agriculture ended up swelling the profits of chemical companies.

Subsidies encourage farmers to produce more, which leads to higher prices for chemicals, seed, fertilizers, land and all the other inputs and resources they use. Only about a quarter of the subsidy ends up in the pockets of farmers, and then only the big operators.[9] The rest is paid out by farmers to supplier companies, such as those providing fertilizers and pesticides, and in higher rents and land charges.

Only in 2005 were production subsidies finally scrapped, too late to protect the health of generations of Europeans.

Today, nitrogen fertilizers have become an international commodity, traded, like oil, around the globe. A large part of the world's synthetic ammonia capacity is owned or controlled by energy companies. Because the process is so energy-intensive, most ammonia plants are situated in regions rich in natural gas, such as Siberia, Central Asia, the Middle East and the southern United States.

Ammonia synthesis now supplies about half the nitrogen used in crop production around the world. The biggest expansion came during the sixties and seventies with the development of short-strawed, high-yielding varieties of wheat and rice. Many of the 'dwarf' varieties were bred by seed companies owned by chemical manufacturers. They had the great advantage of requiring large amounts of chemical nitrogen.

Norman Borlaug, architect of the 'Green Revolution', said that 'if the high-yielding wheat and rice varieties are the catalysts that have ignited the revolution, chemical fertilizer is the fuel that has powered its forward thrust'.

While the revolution has boosted the world supply of edible protein and energy, the crops it produces are depleted in minerals and anti-oxidants. Industrial agriculture is designed to produce large amounts of second-rate foods. It's these that dominate world markets, driving down prices and making it impossible for traditional farmers to compete. In rich countries and in poor, family farms are driven out of business by Haber's nitrogen.

When Sir Frederick Keeble was enthusiastically promoting ICI fertilizers in 1930, he promised farmers that the new chemicals would become their passport to a better future. Fertilizers would lift their output, he assured them, and secure them a better income.

In reality, the very opposite is true. Chemical companies have put them on a treadmill, forcing them to produce more and more to stay afloat. Colin Tudge sees the Haber-Bosch process as a highly significant step on the path to industrial farming.

> Before Haber and Bosch, fertility had mostly been a matter for farmers themselves... Farmers decided whether to grow clover, and how to balance stock against crops. Now the single greatest input (apart from water and sunshine and air) came courtesy of the fertilizer factory. Food processing and distribution were already well on the road to industrialization by the start of the twentieth century, but the production itself was not. After Haber and Bosch, the entire food supply chain had been brought within the purlieus of industry; and in particular, the chemical industry was firmly on board.[10]

Geographer Vaclav Smil believes the world's dependence on Haber's nitrogen is absolute and irreversible. Without them, he says, there's no way of maintaining high yields from most of the world's farmland. They now provide up to 80 per cent of the nitrogen used to grow the main food grains such as rice, maize and wheat.

In his book *Enriching the Earth*, a review of the achievements of Haber and Bosch, he estimates that 40 per cent of the current world population is alive only because of ammonia synthesis.[11] The dependence is greatest in China, where political mismanagement of agriculture under the regime of Mao Tse Tung led to the worst famine in human history.

Following the opening up of China to world trade, the country placed orders for thirteen of the world's most modern plants for synthesizing ammonia and converting it to urea for fertilizer. In 1979, China became the world's largest user of nitrogen fertilizer, and a decade later it became the world's largest producer. Today, two-thirds of the nitrogen in China comes from Fritz Haber's furnace.

The United States is also a large user and producer of fertilizer nitrogen. But while China relies on it to keep its population alive, the USA uses it to keep its people eating huge amounts of steak and its farmers exporting vast amounts of food. About 70 per cent of US grain production is fed to livestock.

The world pays a high price for its acceptance of cheap food produced from synthetic ammonia. Quite apart from the health burden, there's a heavy environmental cost. Only half the nitrogen fertilizer spread on the world's farmland gets taken up in crops. The other half escapes to the wider environment, where it frequently plays havoc with natural ecosystems. Much of it damages soil structure, leading to disease in crops and the disruption of microbial activity.

Nitrates leaching from farmland pollute rivers, streams and lakes across the globe. By the early nineties more than one in ten of Europe's rivers had nitrate levels above the official maximum contaminant limit. High nitrate levels have been found in water wells throughout the American Midwest for more than twenty years.

Nitrogen enrichment of streams, lakes and estuaries encourages the growth of algae. When they decompose they take oxygen from solution, leading to the death of many aquatic species. The worst-affected offshore area in North America is in the Gulf of Mexico. Every spring eutrophication by nitrates produces a huge toxic zone which drives away fish and kills many bottom-feeding species.

The nitrogen fertilizer industry now puts into the world's life systems as much reactive nitrogen – nitrogen that is chemically active, unlike nitrogen gas in the atmosphere – as all the earth's natural processes. Human interference in the global nitrogen cycle is now at a far higher level than for either the carbon or sulphur cycles.

Vaclav Smil's claim that without Haber's ammonia much of the world would go hungry has been seized upon by advocates of a global, industrial food system. Here's the choice, they claim. We either accept today's chemically grown commodity crops or many of us starve. Yet on Britain's deep, inherently fertile soils this is a false premise. There's plenty of evidence that well-managed soils can produce copious amounts of healthy food without chemical fertilizers.

2

Why We Like Sweet Things

It started with a bunch of organic bananas. I bought them in a wholefood store. They hadn't looked particularly promising – a sort of washed-out grey in colour, but I felt sure they'd ripen once I got them home.

A week later they were starting to get soft, though the skin had turned even greyer. I peeled one and took a bite. It wasn't that it tasted bad. Quite the opposite. There was no discernible taste of any kind. Not so much as the merest hint of sweetness. I might as well have been eating damp cardboard.

It's a common enough experience in modern Britain. We're all acquainted with the tasteless carrot, the bland piece of broccoli, the apple devoid of any tang. I used to believe it didn't matter much. Why worry about the taste, I thought, so long as it's doing you good. These days I know better.

Flavour is our first measure of quality – an early primer on the nutrient status of a food. It's produced by dozens – perhaps hundreds – of aromatic compounds. Plant cells are essentially small chemical factories turning out organic compounds by the thousand.

Some contribute to what we experience as taste. Others act as *phytonutrients*, playing a direct role in the maintenance of human health, often in ways we don't fully understand. Flavour in a fruit or vegetable is an indication that the cells are doing their job – that they're well supplied with trace elements and are producing their full complement of plant compounds.

For man, the hunter-gatherer, flavour was crucial. A sweet taste, for example, denoted ripeness in fruits and berries, a sign that they were rich in health-giving antioxidants. For early man there was an evolutionary advantage in developing a sweet tooth. It was a means of selecting healthy foods.

Today's fresh foods rarely taste good; in fact many of them taste of very little at all. Nor do they contain the levels of vitamins, trace elements and phytonutrients you'd have found in traditionally-grown foods. A revolution in the way they're produced has depleted them of the very things that once promoted good health. Our staple foods have been 'dumbed down'.

Typical of these lost nutrients are a group of cancer-fighting compounds called *salvestrols*. They occur in a number of green vegetables including cabbage and broccoli; in red fruits such as strawberries, blackcurrants and red grapes; and in culinary herbs such as parsley and basil. Inside cancer cells the salvestrols activate an enzyme which causes cancer cells to die.

But modern methods of growing food – including the use of chemical fungicides on crops – have dramatically reduced the level of salvestrols in everyday diets. A typical five-a-day diet now provides only 10 per cent of the amount of these compounds needed to keep cancer at bay.[1]

In parallel with the 'dumbing down' of everyday, staple foods, Britain has seen a steep increase in chronic diseases. Degenerative conditions such as heart disease, arthritis, diabetes and asthma are reaching epidemic proportions. No fewer than one in three of us will be struck down with cancer at some stage in our lives. Mental illness, too, is rife – everything from depression to dementia.

Although we seemed to be genetically programmed for a life of 100 years or more, few of us will die of old age. We're far more likely to have our lives cut short by the 'diseases of civilization' and the chances are that our later years will be spoiled by chronic infirmity.

It seems scarcely credible that our food could be responsible for such a catastrophe. Yet it has struck at a time when many of our basic, everyday foods have been subtly changed. The foods we eat today – including many 'fresh foods' – are poorer in nutrients than those enjoyed by the countless generations which went before.

Britain – like other western countries – is forty years or so into a mass experiment in human nutrition. We're all eating basic foods that have been stripped of the antioxidants, trace elements and essential fatty acids that once promoted good health. Can it be coincidence that our body maintenance systems are breaking down in middle age or earlier?

Some nutritionists argue that agriculture can never produce truly healthy food. Human beings evolved as hunter-gatherers. The foods they selected from the animals and plants around them were perfectly matched to their nutritional needs. So long as they were not hit by some environmental catastrophe, the natural foods that surrounded them were likely to contain the nutrients to keep them healthy. They were, after all, part of the natural order.

The emergence of agriculture put human beings outside nature. It allowed them to build up food surpluses, which in turn led to the development of cities and civilizations. But there was a price to be paid. The foods produced by farmers could never quite match the nutritional qualities that human beings had evolved to extract from natural foods.

Nitrogen compounds – the products of a worldwide chemical industry – are the powerhouse that drives modern farming. It's those small, white pellets – or prills as the manufacturers like to call them – that have degraded our everyday foods. Farmers use them because they stimulate extra growth, and in an economic climate that rewards output and pays little regard to quality it makes good sense.

But high output comes at a cost. In nature there's a phenomenon known as the dilution effect. While you can stimulate a crop to produce more per acre, the total nutrients produced are more or less fixed. All you get is more grains containing fewer trace elements or vitamins. In the same way a cow can be goaded into producing higher yields, but the resulting milk will contain fewer health-protecting vitamins per litre. The principal result of chemically-driven agriculture is dumbed-down foods.

Nitrate fertilizers promote ill-health. They weaken plants by stimulating excess growth of sappy tissue with thin cell walls. Crops grown this way are more prone to disease, which is why they need constant spraying with pesticides to keep them standing. And when fed to livestock, they make animals sick. Hence the need for routine antibiotics. It should come as no surprise that they contribute to human illness, too.

The steady erosion of agriculture has been a tragedy for Britain. For much of their history the British used to be rather good at farming. As far back as Roman times these islands off the north-west coast of Europe were regularly exporting wheat back to the mainland. They had been blessed with deep, fertile soils – a legacy of the post-glacial forest – and a mild, moist climate that was superb for growing a wide range of crops.

In the late eighteenth century the island farmers developed a revolutionary cropping system that practically doubled the output of food. It was a clever way of alternating cereals with livestock-feeding crops, especially root crops and nitrogen-fixing clover.

In Victorian times British farming was known and admired across the world. Our great breeds of cattle – the Hereford, the Shorthorn, the Aberdeen Angus and the Ayrshire – were sought after everywhere. These were livestock that thrived on pastures, which is hardly a surprise since grass is the natural food of ruminant animals. Wherever there was grassland – which covers around one-quarter of the world's land surface – these great breeds flourished, producing healthy meat and milk for their peoples.

Modern research has shown that foods produced from grass-fed animals are rich in many of the nutrients that protect against disease. They include fat-soluble vitamins such as A, D and E, protective fats including omega-3s, and the powerful anti-cancer agent known as conjugated linoleic acid, or CLA.

In 1996, former world motor racing champion Jody Scheckter bought Laverstoke Park, a large agricultural estate near Basingstoke, in Hampshire. He had one simple aim – to grow the healthiest, finest-tasting food possible without compromise. To achieve it he has made use of the latest research on health and nutrition, much of it from the United States, Germany, Holland and South Africa. But he also went back to literature produced a century ago.

Ten years on, his system for producing truly healthy food owes more to traditional farming than modern agribusiness.[2] His dairy cows are not the fashionable, high-yielding Holsteins but traditional, slow-growing Jerseys. They graze pastures containing 30 or more different herbs, grasses and clovers, a mixed turf not unlike that of the Neolithic farmers 6,000 years ago.

The beef cattle are traditional breeds, too – the Aberdeen Angus and the traditional Hereford. Sheep include the old Hebridean, the Lleyn and the Polled Dorset breeds. It's as if the farming revolution of the past fifty years had never taken place.

For Scheckter there's one guiding principle – good health starts below ground. A healthy soil produces healthy grass which in turn produces healthy animals. And healthy meat and milk make for healthy people.

'We believe in improving health through the food we eat,' he says, 'not by relying on medicines and other chemicals. This applies equally to soils, our crops and our animals. And, of course, it carries through to people. But because there's such a ready availability of medicines and cure-alls, it's a philosophy that has been forgotten both in farming and in the way we live our lives today.'

On a bright December morning I joined Scheckter for a drive round his estate. I wanted to see for myself this unique experiment in human nutrition. It was soon apparent that no expense has been spared in the quest for healthy food.

The farm even has its own state-of-the-art abattoir. 'Where's the sense in producing the finest beef, then spoiling it with a stressful truck journey to slaughter?' said Scheckter.

There's another remarkable feature about this farm in the rolling Hampshire countryside. Although the tractors and machinery are clearly twenty-first century, the landscape of herb-rich pastures and traditional livestock breeds could easily be a century older. When the search criteria are food, health and taste, today's high-yielding crops and livestock don't even register.

The principles of sound agriculture hardly change from generation to generation. Why should they? The human body has scarcely altered since the Stone Age. The foods required to keep it in good working order are no different from those of our hunter-gatherer ancestors.

The first requirement for wholesome, nutrient-rich crops is a fertile soil. It's the same for livestock. When it comes to raising cattle for healthy beef or dairy products, all you need is a field or two of good grassland – grown on a fertile soil.

Whenever I take the train north, I pass a series of intensive vegetable fields strung out alongside the railway. In the summer months it's mostly planted up with salads or veg, laser-straight lines of cabbages, carrots or iceberg lettuces. From the train you can see the tramlines, the spaced tractor wheel marks that show the pesticide sprayer is frequently taken through the crop.

In the winter the ground is bare. There's not a weed to be seen. When the weather's wet, great pools of water lie on the surface, unable to drain away. The bare ground in between has crusted over, making it impossible for air to penetrate into the soil spaces and supply the myriad life forms that could give the land heart and help to grow healthy plants.

Even from the train you can see this land is sick. So drenched has it been in sprays and chemical fertilizers that its normal function has virtually broken down. The robust crumb structure which allows water and air to pass through the top layers has disappeared. Beneficial organisms like earthworms will have suffocated – to thrive they need well aerated soils with open channels and pore space.[3] Deep below the surface processes of putrefaction will be taking place. The only way vegetable plants can be induced to grow here is with constant spraying with pesticides otherwise they will inevitably succumb to disease.

Who will buy these vegetables, I wonder. They'll have been washed and packed for a supermarket somewhere. Perhaps it'll be some harassed young mum keen to do the best she can for her uninterested youngsters. She'll cajole them into trying a carrot or a floret or two of broccoli with their chicken dinosaurs. It'll do them good, she'll promise.

But she'll be wrong. Judging from the abused and miserable soil that grew them it's hard to imagine they'll produce any sort of nourishment. The tragedy is that with a season or two of care and attention those fields beside the railway tracks could begin growing the sort of food that would make her kids strong.

Robert Plumb is a soil doctor. His mission is to revitalize sick and ailing farmland, ruined by years of assault by chemical fertilizers. He started his career in the fertilizer business. For a time he ran his own blending business, supplying nitrates and other chemical fertilizers to farmers.

Twenty years on he's had a change of heart. He's convinced the constant use of chemicals has brought many soils to the verge of collapse, threatening public health. His company – Independent Soil Services – now advises worried farmers on how best to restore their damaged fields to health. That's the only way they can be made to grow good food again.

I met up with Plumb in a potato field in the Welsh Marches. The crop looked dense and green in the bright sunshine of an August morning. There was no sign of blight, the great scourge of potatoes that had been the cause of the Irish famine. I assumed the field had been sprayed with fungicide, a precautionary measure taken by most non-organic growers to protect their investment.

But the crop hadn't been sprayed, Plumb assured me. There was no need. It stayed healthy because it was growing on a fertile soil.

Four years earlier it was a different story. A crop like this would have been impossible to grow, Plumb explained. The land had been so damaged by endless applications of nitrogen fertilizer, its structure had completely broken down. With yields plummeting, the desperate farmer had sought specialist help. Plumb prescribed soil supplements to replace depleted minerals, particularly calcium. He also recommended organic compounds to reinvigorate the teeming mass of soil microorganisms, which are the key to soil fertility.

Today, the farmer has cut back dramatically on sprays and chemical fertilizers. At the same time he is growing better crops than he has for years.

I walked with Plumb into the potatoes for a closer look. An hour earlier there had been a heavy shower, and our trousers were quickly drenched. Even so our boots remained remarkably free of mud, as Plumb was keen to point out.

'If we'd walked across this field a couple of years back we'd be carrying half a stone of soil on our boots by now,' he said. 'The soil structure was shot to hell. Even after a light shower you'd get pools of standing water. The ground was so compacted it couldn't drain away.

'Now there's a structure to the soil. There are plenty of air spaces, so the water can drain away. This means the plant roots can reach down to get the nutrients they need. This land is alive again. For the first time in years it's producing good, healthy food.'

Today the fields around us are filled with fantastic machines. There are tractors big enough to develop five hundred horsepower at the flick of a switch. Modern forage harvesters can chomp their way through a field full of shoulder-high maize in less time than it took a gang of us to load up a single trailer-load of hay when I started working on farms.

Combines are now so smart they can monitor their precise geographical position by satellite as they move through the crop, then record the grain yield of every square metre in a field the size of Heathrow Airport. But what use is this technology when it gathers second-rate foods from land that's worn out?

There's no machine yet that can add an extra microgram of iron to a wheat grain, no machine that'll boost the level of cancer-fighting vitamins in cows' milk. The only useful measure of a farming system is how well it feeds the people. On this basis the new agricultural revolution and the nitrogen fertilizers that power it have been an unmitigated disaster.

How could such a catastrophe have befallen British food? Much of the damage can be attributed to political mismanagement. When Britain joined the European Common Market in 1973 it introduced a series of farm subsidies that were to have far-reaching consequences for the health of the nation. One of the first effects was that large numbers of lowland farmers abandoned their traditional rotations, got rid of their cattle and sheep, and reinvented themselves as commodity grain growers.

It promised an easier life and the cereal subsidies were generous. Unfortunately, it's a system that can be maintained only with heavy inputs of chemical fertilizers and pesticides.

In a speech to the 2006 Royal Show, Rural Affairs Minister David Miliband coined the phrase 'one planet farming'. His goals for agriculture included the building of 'a profitable, innovative and competitive industry meeting the needs of consumers'. The chances of the government ever attaining this goal are negligible.

The biggest single step politicians could take to raise food standards would be to stop underpinning industrial grain production with public subsidies. But years of fruitless talks aimed at cutting farm subsidies through the World Trade Organization have shown this isn't going to happen quickly. If we want to return to healthy, nutrient-dense food produced by proper farming, we're going to have to find it for ourselves. And given the current mythology about food, this may not be easy

Walk round any up-market food store and you're likely to be deluged with food stories. You'll see them on display boards, point-of-sale leaflets and on the product packaging: a few well-chosen lines telling the story of the food and the people who produced it. There may well be a picture of a smiling farming family in some suitable agrarian setting, perhaps surrounded by a bunch of contented pigs or curious cattle.

The words are likely to be sprinkled with comforting phrases such as 'high welfare standards' and 'freedom to roam'. On a tour round my local superstore I found references to pigs in 'cosy straw yards' and 'happy cows grazing freely in pastures rich in lush green grass, clover and other wild plants'.

In *The Omnivore's Dilemma*, US writer Michael Pollan refers to this emerging literary form as 'supermarket pastoral'.[4] Shopping at a wholefood store has become a little like browsing in a bookshop, he muses. This 'seductive literary form, beguiling enough to survive in the face of a great many discomfiting facts' is, he suspects, a response to some of our deepest, oldest longings. It's not that we simply want safe food. We long for a closer connection with the earth and the domesticated animals we've long depended on.

'Supermarket pastoral' reveals something else: the depth of our confusion about what constitutes healthy food. In Edwardian Britain there seems to have been a general consensus on the subject. While the industrial bakers, sugar refiners and margarine manufacturers had begun to erode it at the edges, the core belief remained intact. No one seriously departed from the idea that good food was for the most part grown naturally, and eaten whole and unprocessed. At that time terms like 'naturally-grown', 'organic' and 'wholefood' had no meaning. Food was food.

From those early beginnings the food fabricators have succeeded in demolishing the entire body of food knowledge that once passed from generation to generation.

Today we're confronted by a bewildering array of product choices with no firm tenets to guide us through them. Little wonder that we feel in need of food stories. The question is can we believe them? If it's healthy food we're looking for the answer's probably 'No.'

For many, healthy food has come to mean 'organic'. The organic movement – spearheaded by the Soil Association – began as a resistance campaign against the steady industrialization of our food. Today those same industrial forces have begun to embrace organic food itself. Supermarket price pressure is shifting organic production from the small mixed farms that can produce genuinely healthy foods to large, mechanized outfits that can't.

While the principles of organic production are sound enough, the mere presence of an organic label is no guarantee that a food will be rich in health-protecting nutrients. A field converted to organic crops after 20 years in intensive chemical production is unlikely to have a good balance of trace elements no matter how much manure is thrown on. Under the rules, organically-managed dairy cows need only receive 60 per cent of their rations in the form of forage. In terms of nutrient content, the milk of non-organic cows getting 80 per cent of their nutrition by grazing fresh, herb-rich pastures will beat the organic version hands down.

Supermarket food stories provide, at best, a stilted version of the truth. Organic labels may steer us away from the poorest, most contaminated foods but are no guarantee of quality. If we're after truly healthy food we're going to have to get better acquainted with the farm it comes from. It means finding out a little about the production process of the foods we eat. In short, we'll need to adopt something of the hunter-gatherer spirit of our Stone Age forebears.

While the agricultural industry is geared to turning out large amounts of energy, protein and fat relatively cheaply, as a means of producing the nutrient-dense foods our bodies crave, it has been a failure. Healthy foods come from crops grown on fertile, biologically-active soils and from animals fed on their natural diets. Only a return to foods like these will restore the nation to health. The good news is it's still out there if you look for it. And finding it may even save you money.

A couple of years ago I was amazed to discover that some of the best beef in the world was being produced on a farm just a couple of miles from where I live. The farmer kept a small herd of Devon cattle, the breed whose chestnut red colour earned them the popular name of 'Red Rubies'. They're one of Britain's traditional breeds – now relatively scarce – that date back to a time when the quality of meat mattered more than the profit they made for the wholesaler.

I met the farmer at an agricultural show in Dorset. He was winning just about every award in sight with his champion stock bull. Two days later he showed me round his farm, a patchwork of meadows and pastures, all of them full of wild flowers and herbs.

Here was the ideal formula for healthy beef, a slow-growing native breed grazing on species-rich grassland unspoiled by chemical fertilizer. In a Hampstead restaurant it would have been worth a fortune. Yet the farmer was selling his finished cattle through the local livestock market where the buyers – well-briefed on the requirements of the supermarkets – rated them a poor second to the large, grain-fed Continental breeds.

I asked him if he ever sold privately. He told me he occasionally had a beast back from the abattoir to sell as freezer packs to friends. I asked him to add my name and number to his order book. He told me that though he used no chemical fertilizers or sprays, his farm wasn't actually registered organic. For small farmers like him the cost of registration was prohibitive. I assured him that to me his non-organic status did not matter at all. His beef was better than organic.

By going direct to the producer I now buy this superb food for the price I'd pay in the supermarket for second-rate, grain-fed beef. Yet at this price the farmer makes far more than when he sells into the conventional food chain. Everybody wins, except, of course, supermarket shareholders.

Today, we're accustomed to good food being expensive; in fact, we expect it. Organic food in the supermarket must carry a premium price tag. Everything at the farmers' market must be reassuringly pricey, or we start to worry that we're not getting the real thing. Celebrity chefs reinforce the idea with their tales of farmers as heroes and good foods as rare and precious jewels.

In reality, high prices have more to do with the distortions of modern marketing than with true production costs. The healthiest foods come from farming systems that emulate nature. These aren't dependent on costly chemicals or fertilizers, nor do they require expensive livestock buildings. Sold direct to the consumer – and with no powerful wholesalers and retailers taking a sizeable cut – healthy foods should be affordable to most people.

The truth is there's good quality, affordable food to be found all over Britain. In a world of large-scale, commodity agriculture my local Devon beef producer might seem an anachronism. But there are farmers like that across the country, many of them unknown and unsung. While tracking them may take some effort, it'll be richly rewarded.

3

The Importance Of Minerals

One of the most remarkable studies on the link between food and health was carried out by an American dentist, now hardly remembered. In the early years of the twentieth century Weston A. Price ran a thriving dental practice in the industrial city of Cleveland, Ohio. Then in the early thirties he gave it all up. He and his wife set out on a series of epic journeys to some of the most remote places on the planet.

Price's idea was to visit peoples untouched by 'civilization' – peoples reputed to display remarkable health, and to enjoy long lives, untroubled by sickness and disease. He wanted to find out whether the stories were true. And if they were, he wanted to know what foods these peoples ate.

He published his exhaustive findings in 1939.[1] But in those tumultuous times no one took a great deal of notice, either in the USA or in Britain. This was a tragedy.

To live long and healthy lives, Price discovered, human beings needed the natural foods of the countryside, including animal products with their full complement of saturated fats.

By the time Price embarked on his travels, he had reached the very pinnacle of his profession. He had taught at American dental schools, written textbooks, and directed a classic study on the role of root canals in promoting disease.[2] But his overriding interest was in nutrition and its effect on human health.

At the time the people of Cleveland were abandoning their traditional diets in favour of the new, manufactured foods – white bread, margarine, pasteurized milk and refined white sugar. Price saw the results daily in his surgery. Most of his adult patients had rampant tooth decay, often accompanied by degenerative diseases such as arthritis, osteoporosis, diabetes and chronic fatigue.

The health of younger patients was even more worrying. Their teeth were often crowded and crooked. Many had facial deformities such as 'overbites' and narrow, pinched faces with no well-defined cheekbones. The same children frequently suffered from other health complaints with names that sound all too familiar today: allergies, recurring infections, anaemia, asthma and behavioural difficulties. All these had been rare when Price started in practice around the turn of the century.

One of the more serious infectious diseases of the day was tuberculosis, widely known as the 'White Scourge'. Price observed that children were increasingly afflicted by the disease. And among the most vulnerable youngsters were those with bad teeth. That's when he hit on the idea of travelling to the most remote parts of the world where the inhabitants had not yet been touched by civilization. He gave up his practice, and – in company with his wife – set out on the journeys of discovery that were to preoccupy him for the next ten years.

The couple's first visit was to a valley high in the Swiss Alps. Until the building of an eleven-mile-long railway tunnel a few years earlier, the Loetschental Valley in the Bernese Oberland had been virtually isolated from the outside world. There Price was astonished to find children tough enough to walk barefoot in freezing mountain streams without ill effects. These children seldom caught colds, and infections were virtually unknown. No case of tuberculosis had ever been seen among the valley community, though the people had been exposed to the bacillus. The children's teeth and gums were in perfect condition, Price discovered, with no sign of dental decay.

The people of this Swiss valley lived mainly on unpasteurized milk and dairy products from their own cows as they grazed on the steep mountain pastures. But the diets of other communities visited by the American couple were very different.

On the Isle of Lewis off the north-west coast of Scotland the local people ate few dairy products. They lived mainly on cod and other seafoods, especially shellfish. These were supplemented with oatmeal. On the thin island soils oats were the only grain that could be grown. A prized local dish – considered especially beneficial for growing children and pregnant women – was cod's head stuffed with oats and mashed fish liver.

Price also visited Inuit, or Eskimo, people whose diet was almost wholly made up of animal products. These included fish, walrus, seal and other marine mammals. During the brief summer months the people would gather nuts, berries and a few grasses. These provided small diversions in a diet made up overwhelmingly of animal products, including large amounts of blubber.

Of the African peoples he visited, Price found the Dinkas of Sudan to be the most healthy. They ate a combination of fermented grains and fish, together with small amounts of red meat, vegetables and fruit. By contrast, cattle-herding tribes like the Masai ate no plants at all. They lived exclusively on beef, raw milk, offal meats, and – in times of drought – blood.

The Cleveland couple visited tribes of hunter-gatherers in northern Canada, the Florida Everglades, the Amazon rainforest and Australia. These people consumed game meats of all types, especially offal, but they supplemented them with a variety of whole grains, vegetables and fruits.

Wherever he went Price found these remote peoples to be in good health. The foods they ate were, without exception, natural and unprocessed. There were no preservatives, colourings or additives; no refined oils or hydrogenated fats; no processed foods such as white flour or skimmed milk. Nor was there added sugar, though a number of peoples ate naturally sweet foods such as honey or maple syrup. All the foods were grown or raised on fertile soils, uncontaminated with pesticides or chemical fertilizers. Milk and dairy products were always consumed in their raw or unpasteurized state.

Wherever he went Price took photographs of the locals. By the time he'd finished his journeys he had amassed no fewer than eighteen thousand of them. Some were later published in his classic book, *Nutrition and Physical Degeneration*. Today it serves as a remarkable social record of healthy, well-nourished people, with broad facial structures which allowed full development of the dental arch.

Nutrition researcher Sally Fallon – founder of the Weston A. Price Foundation in Washington – says of the book: 'No one can look at the handsome photographs of so-called primitive people – faces that are broad, well-formed and noble – without realizing that there's something very wrong with the development of modern children.

'In every isolated region he visited, Price found tribes or villages where virtually every individual exhibited genuine physical perfection. In such groups tooth decay was rare, and dental crowding and occlusions – the kind of problems that keep American orthodontists in yachts and vacation homes – non-existent.

'Price took photograph after photograph of beautiful smiles, and noted that the natives were invariably cheerful and optimistic. Such people were characterized by "splendid physical development" and an almost complete absence of disease, even those living in physical environments that were extremely harsh.'

As well as taking photographs, Price collected samples of local food wherever he travelled. Carefully preserving them, he brought them back to Cleveland. He wanted to find out whether such diverse natural diets had any common attributes that might account for the robust good health of those remote peoples.

In his laboratory, he made detailed analyses of each sample, calculating its total complement of nutrients. From the full set of figures he was able to calculate the nutrient intake of each community. The results amazed him. They showed that these health-giving diets contained at least four times the level of minerals and water-soluble vitamins – vitamins C and B-complex – than the average American diet of his day. And they contained no less than ten times the levels of fat-soluble vitamins, including vitamins A and D, together with a new nutrient he called 'activator X'.

Price considered these fat-soluble vitamins to be the key component of healthy diets. He called them 'activators', or 'catalysts', because the assimilation of all other nutrients in the diet – protein, minerals and water-soluble vitamins – depended on them. Price wrote:

> It is possible to starve for minerals that are abundant in the foods eaten because they cannot be utilized without an adequate quantity of the fat-soluble activators. The amounts [of nutrients] utilized depend directly on the presence of other substances, particularly the fat-soluble vitamins. It is at this point probably that the greatest breakdown in our modern diet takes place, namely in the ingestion and utilization of adequate amounts of the special activating substances, including the vitamins, needed for rendering the minerals in the food available to the human system.

Price's 'activator X', a powerful catalyst to mineral absorption, occurred in foods considered sacred in many primitive societies: liver and other offal meats, fish-liver oils, fish eggs, and butter from cows grazing on rapidly-growing spring and autumn grass. These vital foods are mostly missing from the modern British diet. At a time when many of these foods have fallen from favour, the toll of degenerative diseases has risen inexorably.

Here was the reason for the legendary health and stamina of these remote peoples. Their staple foods – whether from the sea or from the land – were highly mineralized and rich in antioxidants. And here was the reason for the rising ill health in Price's city of Cleveland. The people's diets had been debased by the substitution of industrial foods for the natural foods of the countryside.

In his book, Price cites many examples of the link between minerals in the soil and human health. He writes of a glacier which, during the last ice age, covered one-half of the state of Ohio. It occupied an area west of a line starting east of the city of Cleveland and extending diagonally across the state to Cincinnati.

At the time he was writing, human degenerative conditions were higher in areas south and east of this line than in areas that had been covered by the glacier thousands of years before. For example, infant mortality was 50 per cent higher in the non-glacial areas than in the glaciated parts of the state. According to Price, this was the result of the poorer mineralization of soils in non-glaciated areas.

Price also studied the American Heart Association's figures for death rates from heart disease across the United States during the 15 years leading up to the Second World War. He found that in some regions they were higher by more than 50 per cent, the rises being greatest in areas that had been under human occupation for the longest period – New England, the states bordering the Great Lakes, and the Pacific Coast states. Through demineralization these soils had gradually lost their capacity for maintaining human and animal health.

'This is one of the evils that has accompanied our progress in modernization,' wrote Price. 'We do not realize how much modern human beings are handicapped and injured since they learned how to modify nature's foods.'

The damage has increased immeasurably since Price's time. Today's fresh produce has little in common with the nutrient-rich foods of pre-industrial societies. Years of chemical farming and soil mismanagement have robbed them of health-giving minerals and antioxidants. In the fresh produce sections of every neighbourhood supermarket, the shelves are packed with fruits and vegetables from around the globe. All are bright and colourful. The choice seems bewildering. But if all are depleted in nutrients it is no choice at all.

There are two easy ways to measure the nutrient content of fresh foods. First you can taste them. Foods that seem bland and flavourless are almost certain to be low in essential minerals. Plants produce thousands of compounds that aren't essential for the vital life processes of the cell, but which give each plant species its own unique characteristics. It's these 'secondary metabolites' which give colour and fragrance to flowers, for example. They're also responsible for the tastes and textures of fruit and vegetables.

Minerals are essential for the cell processes that produce this battery of chemical compounds, so it's not surprising that fresh foods that have strong flavours and fragrances should be well-endowed with essential minerals. But for people who don't quite trust their taste buds, there's another, less subjective way to find out if a food's any good or not. It's called the Brix refractometer.

Professor A. F. W. Brix was a nineteenth-century German chemist who will be forever revered by the world's wine-growers.[3] Brix devised a way of measuring the quality of grape juice using a hydrometer, an instrument that measures the density of liquids. His ingenious device enabled Europe's wine-makers to assess the potential of a grape juice before going to the expense of fermenting and bottling it.

Today the chemist's name is used as a measure of the quality of fresh produce. The Brix number of a plant juice refers to its concentration of sugars, principally, but also vitamins, minerals, amino acids, proteins, plant hormones and other solids. But it's closely correlated with the plant's mineral content, so it's a good guide to food quality.

For example, a sour-tasting grape grown on an exhausted and overworked soil is likely to give a Brix reading of eight or less. But a full-flavoured grape grown on rich, fertile soil will give a reading of twenty-four or even higher. And what's true of grapes applies equally to other food plants. A Brix number is a measure of the real food value of the fresh produce in modern supermarkets.

My hand-held Brix refractometer arrived by post in a neat package bearing the name of the supply company in San Pedro, California. It had cost me about thirty pounds sterling. Both my wife and I reckoned it was a small price to pay for the means to establish the quality of our foods.

The device looks a bit like a short telescope. At one end there's an eyepiece, at the other a small prism. It measures the quality of a plant juice by the degree light is bent – or refracted – when passing through it. The denser the liquid, the more the light is refracted.

Thankfully it's easy to use. First you have to extract a few drops of juice from the item under test. I did this with the aid of a kitchen garlic press. Then with a glass eye-dropper, you have to transfer a drop or two onto the prism, and flatten it with the glass cover-plate. After that it's simply a matter of looking through the eyepiece and reading off the Brix number from a calibrated scale.

Using the Brix refractometer to first measure the quality of a home-grown apple, I set out to test the integrity of our local supermarkets. I visited the three biggest stores – Tesco, Sainsbury's and Morrisons. In total I bought twenty-five fruit and vegetable items, both UK-grown and imported. I took them home and analysed them that same day.

Where the items were in packs, I tested two or three pieces from each. Usually the readings were similar, but two pears – purchased loose from the same supermarket box – scored 'poor' and 'excellent', even though they looked exactly the same. If nothing else, this aberrant result demonstrates the huge variation in nutritional quality that can occur in items of similar appearance.

My results are grouped under four quality headings – poor, average, good and excellent, as suggested by Carey Reams, who used the Brix refractometer to test the quality of fruit juices in the 1960s. Based in Orlando, Florida, Reams worked chiefly with citrus growers, though he provided a consultancy service for a wide range of crops.

The Reams chart ranks fresh foods from poor to excellent according to the refractive indices of their juices. Foods scoring 'excellent' are most likely to be rich in minerals and antioxidants. They are also the foods that taste good. Of almost a hundred pieces of fruit and vegetable tested in my survey, only one – a pear – came out as 'excellent'. No less than 70 per cent fell into the 'poor' or 'average' categories. These are foods which, according to Reams, are too low in nutrients to promote good, long-term health.

Undoubtedly the best foods – those scoring 'excellent' on the Reams chart – are the ones most likely to deliver both sound nutrition and a good flavour. As I discovered, those rated as 'good' can also be tasty, and probably supply an acceptable level of nutrition. But foods rated as 'average' or 'poor' are hardly worth eating.

According to my small-scale survey more than two-thirds of the fresh produce sold in our local supermarkets on that March day was substandard. Though the big retailers make a show of their support for government 'healthy eating' campaigns, the foods they supply are often deficient in the very qualities that make them special.

As I carried out my quality survey I sampled every item tested. Though opinions on flavour are necessarily subjective, to me there was no question. Foods that produced a low Brix reading tasted dire. Take the pack of Moroccan strawberries, for example. They were on sale at a reduced price in Tesco. On the Reams scale they ranked as 'poor'. They tasted watery and bland. Eating them was an unpleasant experience. By contrast, a tray of American-grown Pink Lady apples – on sale in the same store – tasted sweet and delicious. The refractometer reading put them in the 'good' category.

My survey also confirmed that the term 'organic' provides no absolute guarantee of nutritious food. A tray of organically-grown Spanish strawberries from Sainsbury's came out as 'poor' on the Brix chart, the same category as Tesco's conventionally-grown crop.

A bag of Israeli organic oranges from Tesco were ranked as only 'average', as were the store's organically-grown carrots from Scotland. A box of organic tomatoes – grown in Spain – was classed as 'poor'. A pack of conventionally-grown carrots from Morrisons fell into the 'average' category, while UK-grown organic carrots from the same store were ranked as 'poor'.

Organic crops are produced without pesticide sprays or chemical fertilizers. But this doesn't mean the soils they're grown in will contain the right balance of minerals and trace elements to grow a healthy crop,

It used to be assumed by scientists that soil provided all the elements plants needed to grow sturdy and strong. The crop simply took up those minerals it needed. This is now known to be untrue. Some agricultural soils have long-term, structural imbalances in trace elements. Sandy or peaty soils, for example, may be deficient in copper. Manganese and boron deficiencies often occur in soils that contain large amounts of chalk or limestone.

Many more soils have had their normal mineral balance destroyed by decades of chemical farming. A change to organic methods doesn't automatically make them capable of growing healthy, well-mineralized crops.

A good supply of minerals is vital for the health of human beings – as it is for all living organisms. Life on Earth developed in the Pre-Cambrian Sea, a rich primeval soup containing the full complement of ninety or so minerals. All were incorporated in the single-cell organisms from which plants and animals evolved.

Ancient soils were so rich in minerals that trees were capable of growing up to ten metres in a single year. In the late Jurassic period the mighty thunder lizard – *Apatosaurus* – was the size of a tennis court and weighed twenty-five tons. Yet it consumed its vegetarian diet through a mouth no bigger than that of a horse. Nutritionists estimate that to sustain such a vast animal, the plant life of the period must have contained thirty times the mineral levels of today's vegetation.

For good health, human beings need seven minerals in relatively large amounts.[4] These are calcium, chloride, magnesium, phosphorous, potassium, sodium and sulphur. These are the so-called macro-minerals. In addition, the body needs a number of essential trace elements. Though they are required in only minute amounts, they are vital to the normal functioning of key metabolic processes. Important trace elements include boron, copper, chromium, germanium, selenium, iodine, zinc, molybdenum, silicon, manganese, iron and vanadium. The number known to be essential to life now exceeds thirty, though the exact role of many of them is not fully understood.

A fertile soil can provide the plant with all of them but to do so it needs to be well mineralized. It also needs a healthy structure with plenty of biological activity. Plants cannot efficiently extract trace elements from the tiny rock fragments that make up the mineral fraction of soils, though acids secreted by their roots can help to make them available.

Plants rely heavily on microscopic bacteria or fungi to release essential minerals from rock particles. Having been incorporated into microbial protoplasm, these trace elements are then circulated within the subterranean food chain until released in a form the plant can use. Without a large population of microbes, soils are physically unable to supply the plant with nutrients, even when chemical analysis may show them to be present.

This is why a rich, fertile soil is the only sure route to good health in the population living from it. This is not a new idea. As early as the 1930s an Alabama physician called Charles Northern was speaking out against the poorly-mineralized foods that many Americans were eating.

Northern specialized in biochemistry and nutritional medicine. But he gave up general practice to study ways of improving the nutritional value of foods by restoring the mineral balance of overworked soils. His claim was that human health depended on a good supply of minerals. So the best way to build a healthy population was first to build a healthy, fertile soil.

In 1936, Northern's views were presented as testimony to a Congressional investigation into US farm practices. He said: 'The more I studied nutritional problems and the effects of mineral deficiencies upon disease, the more plainly I saw that here lay the most direct approach to better health.

'We know that vitamins are complex chemical substances which are indispensable to nutrition... Disorder and disease result from any vitamin deficiency. It is not commonly realized, however, that vitamins control the body's appropriation of minerals, and that in the absence of minerals they have no function to perform.

'Lacking vitamins, the system can make some use of minerals. But lacking minerals, vitamins are useless.'

Northern was simply echoing the words of Nobel Prize-winner Alexus Carrel a quarter of a century earlier: 'Minerals in the soil control the metabolism in plants, animals and man. All life will either be healthy or unhealthy according to the fertility of the soil.'

Minerals are in our foods today because of events that took place more than ten thousand years ago, at the end of the last ice age. As the glaciers retreated they exposed the

fine dust produced by the grinding action of ice on the
rocks below. This mineral-rich dust was spread by the
wind across the surface of the planet, remineralizing soils
and producing a burst of biological activity.

Three thousand years after glaciation, soils across the
Earth's land surface reached an average depth of almost
two metres. Today the average soil depth is just twelve
centimetres. In the mineral-enriched soils, trees could
grow to massive proportions. In the primeval forest of
post-glacial Europe, trees grew trunks that measured
twenty-three metres to the first branch.[5]

The legendary 'giant elk' of Ireland – *Megaloceros gigan-
teus* – stood two metres tall at the shoulders, the male carrying a set of antlers spanning three metres from tip to tip.[6]
In reality it was no elk but a deer. Nor was it confined to
Ireland. In the late Pleistocene epoch it ranged widely
throughout northern Europe and Asia. Each year the male
would shed its antlers, growing in their place an even
bigger set. To support such a huge physiological demand,
the vegetation eaten by the animal must have contained
high concentrations of calcium and other minerals – the
gift of a fertile, mineral-rich soil.[7]

Over the past 5,000 years the glacial minerals have been
steadily washed from the soil. This is a natural process of
demineralization, brought about chiefly by the action of
rainwater on soil. But over the past four decades the whole
process has been cranked up by the rise of chemical
farming.

Traditional farming methods aimed to retain minerals
in the topsoil. By returning plant and animal wastes to the
land, communities were able to slow mineral loss – or even
stop it altogether. Farmers would also add natural mineral

fertilizers to the land. The aim was to boost levels of trace elements, or to improve soil structure so minerals could be more easily taken up by plants.

One of the earliest forms of fertilizer used by British farmers was marl – a soft, clay soil rich in calcium. Later they began spreading chalk or ground limestone to the land. In the first half of the twentieth century, basic slag – a by-product of steel making – became a popular fertilizer. Besides calcium and phosphorus, it added a large number of trace elements to the soil, including magnesium, iron, zinc and copper.

The era of chemical farming put an end to these traditional materials. Farmers came to rely on manufactured inorganic chemicals to stimulate the growth of their crops. Far from enhancing fertility, the new chemical fertilizers hastened the loss of trace elements from soil, or so damaged its structure that they were no longer accessible to plants. As the mineral content of soils fell, so did their levels in everyday foods.

Fortunately there are remedies. The country road from Pitlochry to Strathardle in Perthshire takes you through some of the most desolate and barren countryside in Scotland. Winding through Glen Brerachen, it follows the river between the high peaks of Ben Vrackie and Creag Dhubh on the southern slopes of the Grampian Mountains.

A less promising place to grow good crops would be hard to imagine. This glen was once covered in forest. Now the land is exposed to the full might of the Scottish winter. With many of its nutrients washed away, the soil has grown acid and sour. Coarse upland grasses clothe the hillside that once grew good potato crops.

But a remarkable couple – Cameron and Moira Thomson – have made this desert bloom again. They've found a way to grow superb vegetables – large cabbages and onions, while their greenhouses and polytunnels grow crops of tomatoes, cucumbers, sweetcorn, squashes, courgettes and marrows.

The secret of the Thomsons' gardening success is simple – so simple that it's hard to grasp the importance of what they've done. There among the heathers and the tussocky grasses they have recreated a fertile soil. And in doing so they've proved it's a good soil – not chemicals – that grows healthy crops.

As you walk up the farm lane from the little car park at Ceanghline, Straloch Farm, Enochdhu, you know you're witnessing something remarkable. Even on a rainy day the terraced gardens stand out like oases in the desert. Amid the drab green of the upland grassland, they are filled with tall, brightly-coloured flowers and healthy-looking vegetables.

The soil they're growing in is dark and slightly gritty to the touch. The Thomsons mix it themselves before spreading it onto their garden terraces. It's made from fine rock dust hauled from a nearby quarry, and compost made from green waste by Dundee City Council. Together the two ingredients produce ideal conditions for healthy crop growth. The dust – from the volcanic rock basalt – supplies minerals that rainfall and chemical farming have stripped out of many soils. Compost provides organic matter for microbial activity, the prerequisite of a fertile soil.

With their rock dust and compost mix, the Thomsons have produced an 'instant soil' – fertility on tap. And they've done it by copying nature. They have effectively reproduced post-glacial conditions on their worn-out twenty-first century hillside. They have shown that on a soil rich in minerals, and well endowed with organic matter, it's possible to grow large, healthy crops without the arsenal of chemical fertilizers and pesticides used by commercial farmers today.

If soil minerals can produce a good harvest high on a barren Scottish hillside, they'll transform the health and yields of crops across the country, say the couple. And this in turn will lead to a healthier, happier population.

'For years people have dismissed us as cranks,' says Cameron. 'How can it be possible to change the world simply by spreading a bit of rock dust on the ground? But it's nature's way, and it works.

'The life on this planet is sustained by the minerals in the soil. When they're gradually lost through natural leaching or intensive chemical farming, things start to go wrong. That's the reason we're so unhealthy – why the whole food chain is unhealthy. But if we're prepared to take account of nature we can quickly get things back on track. This way we can be healthy again.'

The Thomsons discovered the benefits of rock dust when, by chance, they listened to a radio review of a book by two American authors, John Hamaker and Don Weaver. Titled *The Survival of Civilisation*, the book proposed the re-mineralization of farms and gardens with fine rock dust as a way of combating global warming. Spreading rock dust on the land would produce an upsurge in biological activity, the writers argued. As the silicate rock weathered, carbon dioxide would be taken from the atmosphere and 'locked up' by the formation of calcium and magnesium carbonates. At the same time the release of trace elements would produce bigger and healthier crops.

To Cameron and Moira the idea came as a revelation. Cameron visited a number of quarries before choosing dust containing a broad spectrum of soil minerals. He then had no less than twenty tons of it ploughed into the quarter-acre garden the couple then occupied. To provide the necessary organic matter they grew 'green manure' crops of radish and vetch, digging them in by hand. Once the ground had been prepared, they began growing fruit and vegetables on the freshly 'mineralized' plot.

The results were immediate. The Thomsons began harvesting unusually big cabbages and cauliflowers, together with gooseberries, plums and blackcurrants that were full of flavour. No fertilizers or chemicals were used, and the crops never needed watering, such was the moisture-holding capacity of the reinvigorated soil.

So spectacular were the results that a sympathetic landowner offered them – rent free – seven acres below the crag face of Creag Dhubh, high in the Perthshire hills. That's where they opened their Sustainable Ecological Earth Regeneration centre – the SEER centre. And it's where rock dust has made the worn-out soils of this Scottish glen bloom again.

Cameron and Moira Thomson believe rock dust – a quarry waste – may be about to seed a cultural revolution. Spread across the farmland of Britain it could – at a stroke – raise the level of trace elements in everyday foods. And just as quickly it could start to bring down the frightening incidence of degenerative disease.

The Thomsons' rock dust is now being marketed through garden centres across Britain. And through the Soil Mineralization Forum, it's the subject of a major research programme. At the same time farmers, growers and gardeners in many parts of the country are trying out the material on their crops. They're hoping the dust of rocks hundreds of millions of years old will begin to undo the damage done by a few decades of short-sighted chemical farming.

The Minerals You Need

Boron

Ignored until recently by nutritionists, boron is now thought to work with the minerals calcium and magnesium in the building of strong bones. The mineral is found in almost every kind of fruit and vegetable. Dried fruits such as dried apricots and prunes are especially rich in boron.

Calcium

Essential for normal function of the heart, blood-clotting system and acid-alkaline balance. Promotes healthy skin, bone and teeth, plus normal nerve and muscular action. Deficiency symptoms include muscle tremors, insomnia, nervousness, joint pain, high blood pressure and tooth decay. Good sources include milk, cheese, beans, broccoli and bread.

Chloride

This non-metallic element is widely dispersed around the body in ionic form, in balance with sodium or potassium. It helps to maintain the acid-alkaline balance of blood and the passage of fluids across cell membranes. Essential to brain growth and function, it is needed for the production of hydrochloric acid required for protein digestion. It also regulates the production of amylase, the enzyme used for carbohydrate digestion. The most important source of chloride is salt.

Chromium

Essential for heart function and in the balancing of blood sugar. Helps protect DNA. Deficiency symptoms include sweating, hunger, drowsiness and thirst. Can lead to addiction to sweet foods. Good sources include liver, meat, nuts, shellfish, beans, wholegrains and brewer's yeast.

Copper

Required for healthy growth and for liver, brain and muscle function. Also required for the regulation of blood cholesterol and for enzyme systems involved in anti-oxidant protection. Deficiency symptoms include conditions such as Crohn's or coeliac disease. Other symptoms include heart muscle weakness, anaemia, fluid retention and raised blood cholesterol. Excess levels can be toxic. Anyone on a whole food diet is unlikely to be deficient.

Germanium

In its organic form has been found to enhance the immune system and protect against a number of degenerative diseases including cancer, heart disease, diabetes and senility. Trace levels of the element are found in most foods but rich sources are garlic, ginseng, aloe vera and comfrey. The role of germanium in human nutrition is still controversial and more research is needed to improve our understanding.

Iodine

Vital for the production of thyroid hormones, which control metabolic rate, conversion of food to energy and the maintenance of body temperature. Deficiency symptoms include underactive or swollen thyroid gland, fatigue, weight gain, muscle weakness and susceptibility to cold. Iodine is found in iodized salt, fish, milk, bread, meat and eggs.

Iron

As a component of haemoglobin, iron transports oxygen and carbon dioxide to and from cells. It is also essential for enzyme systems involved in energy production. Deficiency symptoms include anaemia, fatigue, listlessness, poor appetite and nausea. Sources include beef, liver, chicken, baked beans, chick peas and brown rice.

Magnesium

Strengthens bones and teeth and aids muscle function. Required for cardiac and nervous systems. Important for energy production and many enzyme systems. Deficiency symptoms include muscle spasms, insomnia, nervousness, high blood pressure, heart palpitations, hyperactivity, depression and fits. It can be found in beans, muesli, sardines, bread, Brussels sprouts and brown rice.

Manganese

Aids the formation of bones, cartilage and nerve tissue. Vital to a number of enzyme systems including those conferring immunity. Also stabilizes blood sugar, promotes healthy DNA, aids reproduction and red blood cell synthesis. Required for brain function and insulin production. Deficiency symptoms include muscle twitching, growing pains in children, dizziness, fits and joint pain. Sources include tropical fruits, nuts, seeds and wholegrains.

Molybdenum

Aids the removal of protein breakdown products, and strengthens teeth. Helps detoxify the body of free radicals. Deficiency symptoms rarely seen except where copper or sulphate interfere with its utilization. They may include anaemia, tooth decay, impotence, irregular pulse and hyperventilation. Tomatoes, wheatgerm, pork, lamb, lentils and beans provide molybdenum.

Phosphorus

A structural component of bones and teeth. Vital to normal metabolism, energy production and acidity regulation. Required for optimum athletic performance. Unlikely to be deficient because it is present in most foods. Signs of deficiency can include loss of appetite, susceptibility to infection, anaemia, muscle weakness, bone and joint pain, nervous system changes.

Potassium

Aids the flow of nutrients between cells, promotes healthy muscles and nerves. Important for insulin secretion and normal metabolism. Maintains heart function and gut movement. Deficiency symptoms include irregular heartbeat, muscle weakness, pins and needles, nausea, vomiting, diarrhoea and low blood pressure. It is found in bananas, watercress, mushrooms, courgettes, cabbage, cauliflower and pumpkin.

Selenium

An important antioxidant, selenium is required for efficient immune function and protection against cancer and infections. Also important for normal cell growth and the regulation of thyroid hormone production. Low selenium intake greatly increases the risk of many cancers. Deficiency is also associated with premature ageing, cataracts, high blood pressure and frequent infections. The best sources are herrings, tuna, oysters, cod, beef, liver, cottage cheese and chicken.

Silicon

Though silicon is the most abundant element in the earth's crust, this element is present in the body in only tiny amounts. Silica – the oxidized form of silicon – has a beneficial effect on hair, skin and nails. It has also been found to help in the treatment of a number of disorders including ulcers, gastritis, varicose veins, bronchitis and gum disorders.

Sodium

Maintains the body's water balance. Aids nerve function and muscle action, as well as helping move nutrients into cells. Deficiency symptoms include dizziness, heat exhaustion, low blood pressure, mental apathy, muscle cramps, nausea, vomiting and headaches. Sodium is found in most foods.

Sulphur

A non-metallic mineral found in all plant and animal cells. Sulphur is needed for the formation of the protein collagen and is linked with protein in the amino acids cysteine, taurine and methionine. It helps the liver secrete bile, improves mental functioning and maintains healthy hair, nails and skin. Broccoli, Brussels sprouts, eggs, milk and other animal products are sources of sulphur.

Vanadium

Needed for cell metabolism and the building of bones and teeth. It also plays a role in growth and reproduction and helps control cholesterol levels in the blood. Vanadium may be beneficial in the treatment of some mental disorders. Deficiency is linked to cardiovascular and kidney disease. Good sources include buckwheat, grains and olives.

Zinc

A component of many enzyme systems as well as DNA and RNA. Vital for growth and healing. Controls hormones and promotes brain function and a healthy nervous system. Aids bone and teeth formation. Deficiency symptoms include diminished sense of smell and taste, frequent infections, acne, low fertility, skin pallor, depression and appetite loss. Beneficial levels of zinc are found in red meat, fish, nuts, seeds and oysters.

Sources

Patrick Holford, *New Optimum Nutrition Bible*, Piatkus, 2004; Dr Sarah Brewer, *The Daily Telegraph Encyclopedia of Vitamins, Minerals and Herbal Supplements*, Constable & Robinson, 2002; Dr Michael Sharon, *Complete Nutrition*, Carlton Books, 2005.

4

What's Wrong With Farming

Most of us think of western agriculture as a success story. Today's farmers feed twice as many people as they did before the Second World War. With sophisticated machinery and the latest farm chemicals they produce vast amounts of food with an ever-dwindling labour force. Never in the nation's history has so much wheat poured into the grain silos; never have so many bulk milk tankers lumbered up and down the motorways delivering 'the white stuff' to processing dairies.

Yet, amid all this plenty, people are suffering ever more sickness. The conditions that afflict us today are not the great infectious diseases of old – cholera, typhoid, diphtheria and tuberculosis. Instead we're succumbing to what the health authorities term 'the diseases of civilization'; diseases that result not from invasion by pathogenic organisms, but from a collapse in the body's own support systems.

The names of today's illnesses are frighteningly familiar: coronary heart disease, cancer, diabetes, arthritis, osteoporosis, Alzheimer's and depression. Hardly anyone in western society remains untouched by them. In Britain – as in the United States – one in three of us will develop cancer. Half the population are likely to suffer from heart disease during their lifetime, and one-third of the population will develop an allergy.

Learning disabilities such as dyslexia and hyperactivity now blight the lives of tens of thousands of youngsters. At the other end of life, nine out of ten people will suffer the pain of arthritis by the time they reach sixty.

Despite this grim litany, health statistics show we are continuing to live longer. What the figures don't reveal is the massive increase in intervention medicine it takes to keep us going. Multiple-bypass surgery, chemotherapy and an avalanche of therapeutic drugs are prolonging our lives. But they don't protect us from years of pain and disability.

In his book *Health Defence*, medical pharmacologist Paul Clayton describes the majority of seemingly healthy adults as 'the pre-ill'. Their bodies contain the seeds of diseases that will eventually lay them low and may even kill them. Unseen, an artery is starting to silt up; bones are thinning; brain cells are dying. In time they will lead to heart attack, bone fractures and dementia.

Partially hydrogenated vegetable oils – in which extra hydrogen atoms have been inserted into fat molecules at high temperature and pressure – contain trans fats. These have been linked to steep rises in heart disease and obesity and are thought to trigger diabetes, Alzheimer's and a range of nerve ailments. Yet for more than half a century the food manufacturers have been including them in thousands of products from cakes and breakfast cereals to so-called 'heart-friendly' margarines.

Manufactured soups and sauces contain hydrolyzed protein and monosodium glutamate (MSG) to trick the taste-buds into thinking they're getting real meat instead of cheap grains and legumes. Processed sauces are essentially made up of MSG, water, thickeners, emulsifiers and artificial colours, a cocktail that delivers no nutrition and a sizeable dose of toxicity.

High fructose corn syrup (HFCS), a sweetener beloved of the food industry for its cheapness of manufacture, is today found in everything from bread and pasta to so-called health products such as protein bars; from soft drinks and fruit juices to beer. When the element copper is deficient in the diet, as it is in the diets of many children, HFCS can damage both the hearts and the livers of young males.[1]

In their ceaseless drive for profit industrial food manufacturers remove natural ingredients and replace them with cheaper substitutes, often at the risk of consumer health. They have commandeered the food system while robbing foods of their nutrients. Sadly, farmers, who might be expected to champion real food, have followed them down the industrial route.

It would be hard to imagine a healthier environment than the small Perthshire town of Aberfeldy. With its handsome, stone-built commercial centre it stands alongside the sparkling River Tay amid a countryside of pasture land and oak woods. On both sides of the valley the hills rise steeply to the crags and moors of the southern highlands.

It would seem the ideal place to bring up children. Here, surely, youngsters can grow up robust and happy, with the expectation of long, active lives. But clean air and crystal-clear lochs are no protection against the diseases of civilization. This little town has its full share of human misery.

Until he retired in the early 1980s, Walter Yellowlees had been a doctor in the town for almost thirty years. He first qualified during the Second World War and signed up in the Army Medical Corps. As a medical officer with the Cameron Highlanders he had witnessed some of the bloodiest battles of the war. When hostilities ended he joined the small rural practice at Aberfeldy. There he witnessed a different kind of tragedy.

The upper Tay Valley he found in those early post-war years still supported a scattering of small, family farms. Most were mixed farms, their tenants combining stock-rearing with a traditional form of crop rotation. The whole system was aimed at maintaining, and sometimes improving, the natural fertility of the soil.

But by the time he retired the small farms had mostly gone. So had the practice of mixed farming. The new lairds of the Tay Valley were large, specialist farmers. Their fields had become monocultures, worked by sophisticated machines and goaded into ever higher levels of production by heavy dressings of chemical fertilizer.

With the new farming came a fresh crop of degenerative diseases. Coronary heart disease – virtually unknown before the 1920s – began striking people who in other ways seemed perfectly fit. Clean air and hard physical work offered little protection. Heart disease was as likely to strike the shepherd or gamekeeper in the tranquil Highland glen as the stressed commuter caught up in the rush and din of the city. And along with heart disease came a host of gastrointestinal conditions, from constipation to peptic ulcers and bowel cancer.

The young GP quickly formed his own view on the cause of all this misery – the steady erosion of the ancestral

Scottish diet. In the mid-nineteenth century most rural Scots enjoyed robust good health, often well into old age. Their foods were the foods of the Scottish countryside produced by a farming system still dedicated to fertile soils.

Among the staple dietary items were oatmeal, potatoes, turnips, kale, cheese, butter, milk and ale. On these locally-grown and nourishing foods country people stayed healthy, often living to great ages. Historical records for the parish of Fortingall, to the west of Aberfeldy, showed that in the final decade of the eighteenth century there were a good number of octogenarians, a handful of people in their nineties, and even a few who were over 100.

The rot began with the introduction of the railway in 1867. Trains brought in cheap processed foods: sugar, margarine, and white flour, stripped of its nutrient-rich bran. The traditional Scottish high tea metamorphosed into a feast of starch and sugar – scones, jam, cakes and biscuits. The dangers of such foods were spelled out by one of Yellowlees's great mentors, Surgeon Captain T. L. Cleave, in his book *The Saccharine Disease*.[2]

From his rural practice Yellowlees became an outspoken critic of industrial foods. When the human body became overloaded with refined carbohydrates, he argued, conditions like diabetes, coronary disease, ulcers and colon cancer were the likely consequences

But there was powerful opposition to the theory. Medical chiefs on both sides of the Atlantic had latched on to an opposing idea, one that linked heart disease and many cancers to saturated fats, especially animal fats.

Traditional foods like beef, butter, eggs and whole milk began to be stigmatized. The powerful margarine industry weighed in with well-funded campaigns promoting low-fat spreads in place of butter. To Yellowlees the case was bogus. Were we really to believe that traditional foods, prized over the centuries for their health-giving qualities, had suddenly become the cause of catastrophic death and disability?

In 1978 – with the argument raging – he was invited to deliver the annual James MacKenzie Lecture to the College of General Practitioners. He called his lecture 'Ill fares the land'. In it he dismissed what he called 'the dogma of animal fat'. Instead he restated his belief that traditional foods grown on fertile soils would protect against the great disease scourges of the age.

He concluded: 'The new epidemics of degenerative disease are not inevitable, nor is their cause mysterious. They are nature's language telling eloquently of our failure to understand the supreme importance of her laws.'

His GP audience listened with polite scepticism. When he sat down the applause was courteous rather than appreciative. But he remained undeterred. Nearly thirty years later he holds to his view as strongly as ever. And the scepticism of his medical colleagues has at last begun to melt away.

Yellowlees saw the disaster unfolding in his daily dealings with patients amid the Perthshire hills. He later wrote about them in his book, *A Doctor in the Wilderness*. It is the story of a tragedy.

In his James MacKenzie lecture Yellowlees reported on the cancer incidence in his rural partnership practice of three-and-a-half thousand people. Over a three-year period there had been fifty-one new cases, many of which were of bowel cancer.[3] He also looked at the ailments that kept working males off work. The most common cause was bronchitis, followed by diseases of the circulatory system, heart disease and angina. The third most common causes of sick leave were arthritis and rheumatism.

At a time of unparalleled living standards and technological advance in medicine, Yellowlees believed he was witnessing human decay on a massive scale; decay of teeth, arteries, bowels and joints.

Today, the upper Tay Valley remains a tranquil and beautiful place. Doctor Yellowlees took me on an introductory tour of the local countryside. We drove along the main road to Ballinuig as it snaked its way through oak woods and past open fields running down to the gleaming river.

Most of the land was laid down to grass. Gone were the fields of oats that had provided generations of Scots with nourishment. Gone, too, were the fresh vegetables that had helped to make cancer and heart disease rare conditions. Nor was there any sign of the famous red-and-white Ayrshire cows.

The fields were now in a monoculture of industrial grasses, heavily dosed with chemical fertilizers. Rather than produce food for the local community the farms of the Tay Valley are now in the business of producing cheap raw materials for the food manufacturing industry. The concentration of food retailing in the hands of a few major multiples, with their centralized distribution points, has also created a demand for bulk, year-round supplies of uniform produce.

As we drove around the quiet Perthshire countryside we talked about an earlier medical pioneer who had explored the links between food and health. Sir Robert McCarrison, a doctor in the Indian Medical Service during the early 1900s, made his name for research into diseases caused by nutrient deficiencies.

For a time he served in India's North-West Frontier region. There he was struck by the robust health and vitality of local communities, particularly a hill people called the Hunzas, who lived in the Karakoram Range of the Himalayas, between Pakistan, Afghanistan, China and India. They seemed to suffer none of the afflictions of industrial nations; there was no cancer, no heart disease, no diabetes, not even tooth decay. Most remained in vibrant health throughout their long lives. By contrast the peoples of southern India suffered high mortality rates.

Later in his career McCarrison proved that the health of the northern Hunza people was due, not to any accident of genetics, but to good food. As India's director of nutrition research he set up an experiment in which a colony of rats was fed on foods typical of the northern hill people. A second group was given foods like those of the south.

The Hunzas were expert farmers. They needed to be. Land was scarce in this hilly region of India. Their food was mostly grown on high, terraced gardens. All waste materials were carefully composted and returned to the land. As a result their soils remained fertile and healthy even though they were expected to produce large amounts of food.

Most carbohydrates in the Hunza diet were in the form of wholegrain cereals. People ate no sugar or refined flour. Their protein came mainly from milk and dairy products such as butter and cheese. They ate a little meat, about one meal a week. This basic ration was supplemented with a variety of fruits and vegetables, many of which were eaten raw.

There was another, hidden benefit of their foods. The Hunza people irrigated their highland terraced gardens with the cream-coloured water from glacial streams. It was a rich source of minerals, released from the volcanic dust that had been held for millennia in the ice.

Here was a major reason for the legendary health and stamina of the Hunzas. Like the remote communities visited by the dentist Weston A. Price in the 1930s, their foods were enriched with high levels of essential trace elements.

This was the diet McCarrison fed to his little colony of laboratory rats. On it they remained vigorous and active from each generation to the next. But the group fed on a diet typical of poor people in the south of the country – in which polished rice was the main ingredient – failed to thrive. Their physique was poor and they quickly developed respiratory infections and intestinal conditions. Similar ailments appeared in rats fed on diets typical of poor people in Britain at the time: white bread, margarine, jam, tinned meat, boiled potatoes and sweet tea.

In 1936, McCarrison presented his findings in his Cantor Lectures before the Royal Society of Arts. They were later published in his book *Nutrition and Health*.[4] He expected an excited response from the medical profession. But the findings were largely ignored. Physicians were too preoccupied with disease and its treatment to pay much attention to this clue to prevention. A revolutionary group of drugs called the sulphonamides had burst onto the scene.[5] The way ahead seemed to lie with new, miracle drugs and innovative surgical techniques. The health benefits of good food seemed dull by comparison.

Within a few years the post-war Labour government began planning its most ambitious project, a free health service for the nation. The health reformers might easily have taken McCarrison's advice and made sound nutrition and disease prevention the basis of the new service. Instead they designed it around the treatment of illness.

Following the discovery of penicillin during the war a stream of new compounds flowed from the pharmaceutical industry. The anti-microbial streptomycin promised an end to the scourge of tuberculosis, particularly when used along with para-amino salicylic acid or PAS, a compound closely related to aspirin. It was quickly followed by tranquillizers, anticoagulants, the anti-inflammatory hormone, cortisone, and drugs to reduce high blood pressure. There seemed little that the new wonder compounds couldn't achieve.

In *The Rise and Fall of Modern Medicine*, James Le Fanu observes that the therapeutic revolution of the post-war years was not ignited by a major scientific insight.[6] Through the discovery of the sulphonamides, penicillin and cortisone, doctors and scientists had come to realize they didn't need any deep understanding of the diseases they were attempting to combat. Synthetic chemistry blindly and randomly would deliver the remedies that had eluded them for centuries. It was a period of supreme optimism.

In the Scottish Highlands, Yellowlees wrote that both doctors and patients had become 'dazzled by these bright, gleaming swords'. They were blinded to one simple fact: that many crippling diseases need never have been the scourges they later became. Decent housing and good nutrition could have held them in check.

It's one of the ironies of post-war Britain that even as the policymakers were planning their bold new health service, another branch of Whitehall was preparing to debase the nation's food. It was the 1947 Agriculture Act that drove farmers down the road of chemical production and turned them from growers of food into producers of raw materials for the food manufacturing industry.

Sixty years later the disease statistics still head obdurately upward. Between 1971 and the early 1990s, the numbers of newly diagnosed cancer cases went up by 45 per cent for men and by 55 per cent for women.[7] While deaths from coronary heart disease (CHD) have begun falling, non-fatal heart disease itself continues to afflict a growing number of people. Today, the disease accounts for one third of premature deaths in men and one quarter of premature deaths in women.[8] At the same time more than two million people in the UK face life with CHD.

Between 1991 and 2004 the UK incidence of diabetes rose by 65 per cent for men and 25 per cent for women. The number of people with the condition, which frequently leads to heart disease, is expected to reach three million by 2010. Osteoporosis is now the cause of bone fractures in one third of women and one fifth of men over fifty.[9]

In the meantime, health spending soars. In 1973, UK spending on the NHS and private health totalled £3.2 billion, equal to 4.4 per cent of the country's gross domestic product (GDP).[10] By 2004, health spending had risen to £98 billion, accounting for 8.5 per cent of GDP.

Watching the tragedy unfolding, Yellowlees and a group of like-minded doctors and dentists got together to found the McCarrison Society in 1966. All were members of the Soil Association, which promotes organic farming. Their aim was to open the eyes of health professionals to the role of nutrition in protecting health. Despite a series of well-supported conferences at Oxford University, the medical and dental professions remained unimpressed.

It's sometimes hard to comprehend the pace and scale of the revolution that has overtaken the countryside. For almost fifty years the people of Britain, like those in other industrial countries, have been the unwitting subjects of a mass experiment on diet.

Long before the introduction of modern nitrate fertilizers, farmers knew that nitrogen compounds could induce a sudden flush of plant growth. Many were using sodium nitrate from Chile or ammonium salts recovered from gasworks or coking ovens.

One nineteenth-century pioneer of chemical agriculture wrote to a farming journal after treating his sheep pasture. He admitted he'd been unaware 'that agricultural products raised with heavy dressings of nitrogenous manure are always of inferior quality and unwholesome for livestock'.

If ammonia, which is extremely soluble, be presented in excess when compared with the other elements of their growth, the result is that sap is circulated through the plant of too stimulating character. This produces in the vegetable organisms results similar to those too often observed in the human subject who imbibes too much soluble matter of a stimulating kind – high colour and vigorous vitality, but with a tendency to premature decay. In short, plants so treated are on the high road to gout.

Most modern farmers routinely manage their crops this way. Year after year they spread the little white granules of chemical fertilizer, particularly nitrogen in the form of ammonium nitrate or urea. They produce a flush of leafy growth. But it's an unhealthy form of growth with an imbalance of minerals and cell walls that are unusually thin.

The plant is weakened and prone to disease. That's why farmers are forever spraying their crops with fungicides. It's good business for the chemical industry. But as a way of growing healthy food it's flawed.

5

Essential Nutrients For Good Health

Looking across the lush grassland of David Stevens' west Wales farm it would be hard to imagine a healthier place to produce milk. The pasture fields shelve gently southwards to merge into a pastoral landscape of intense green. In winter the prevailing westerlies bring mild temperatures and soft rain from the Atlantic. The ideal place to grow grass and rear healthy cows, you'd think. But you'd be wrong.

When David Stevens took over the family farm all was far from well at Coed y Brain, Kidwelly. The cows seemed constantly nervous and on edge. Many were infertile and lameness in the herds was rife. Worst of all, calving had become a nightmare. Almost daily David would be called upon to deal with some kind of emergency, everything from malpresentations to retained afterbirths. The calves – when they were born alive – were frequently ailing. Some died within half an hour or so of birth. Many more simply failed to thrive, seeming to have no vigour or zest for life.

Throughout the epidemic of disease David looked to his vet for help. On the vet's recommendations he went through the arsenal of modern medicines and drugs including antibiotics, but none seemed to restore the animals to health. Then a neighbour told him about a specialist in trace elements, Danny Goodwin-Jones, who seemed to know a good deal about sickness in farm livestock.

In desperation David called in Goodwin-Jones and his company, Trace Element Services. They recommended that he should have his soils analysed for a number of key minerals. The results showed that molybdenum levels were high while copper, zinc and cobalt were all in short supply. The company arranged for the fields to be spread with a mineral supplement that would eliminate the deficiencies.

The results were spectacular. Within days David began to see improvements in the health of his animals. The cows grew quieter and more contented while their coats shone as never before. The incidence of lameness dropped dramatically and herd fertility steadily improved. Difficult calvings became rare and, best of all, the calves stopped dying. Within a few weeks of the soil treatment cows were giving birth unaided to healthy, vigorous calves.

David estimates that by simply restoring essential minerals to his soils he cut calf losses from a crippling 60 per cent to virtually zero. So nutritious has his mineral-rich grassland become that the cows now produce one fifth more milk on half the level of purchased, high-energy 'concentrate' feed. At the same time the incidence of lameness and mastitis in the herd has fallen by no less than 90 per cent.

For David, who admits to having been sceptical at the start of the soil treatment, the results have been little short of miraculous. Soil mineralization has tripled his farm profit, he estimates, and ensured a better future on the farm for his young son Robert. He might have added that the soil treatment will have provided the unknown consumers of his milk with a healthier product.

Meat and dairy products from livestock deprived of the minerals they need are likely to be themselves depleted. Trace elements such as cobalt and zinc are as vital to the health and well-being of humans as they are to the health of farm livestock. The soil conditions that induce mineral deficiencies in food animals have the same effect on the people who eat the products.

But the risk to human health goes far beyond a simple trace element deficiency. Minerals are key players in a wide range of metabolic processes in farm animals. The element zinc, for example, is essential for the maintenance of fertility, for the normal functioning of the immune system, for protein metabolism and for bone growth.

When this and other essential elements are in short supply, food animals no longer produce the full complement of compounds that will later safeguard human health – vitamins, antioxidants and protective fats.

In the yard at Coed y Brain I talked to David Stevens about the health crisis that almost cost him his farm. It's now more than ten years since he discovered the importance of a fertile, well-mineralized soil in keeping his cattle healthy and productive. Regular soil testing for trace elements is now a routine part of his management, a practice that ensures the milk he sends to his dairy company contains the full range of nutrients needed for human health.

But at the dairy his milk is mixed with that of dozens of other dairy farmers, few of whom have their soils tested. The ailments that once posed such a threat to David Stevens' herd – infertility, lameness and mastitis – are endemic among Britain's dairy herds. How much is this general malaise of livestock contributing to the infertility and chronic ill-health currently afflicting the human population?

David Stevens remains cynical about the role the vets played – or didn't play – in the control of his herd health crisis. They offered him a range of expensive pharmaceutical drugs and supplements, none of which did the job. But he recalls that they were totally uninterested in the possibility that the answer might lie in an imbalance of soil minerals.

Their reaction, though disappointing, is hardly a surprise. Like human medicine, veterinary medicine is largely based on drugs. Today's veterinary practices make a good deal of their income from supplying expensive, branded medicines and they don't have the motivation to look for disease prevention rather than disease treatment.

Since David Stevens began routinely balancing the trace elements in his soil his spending on vets' bills and animal medicines has dropped by half.

The most nutritious foods are likely to come from farms where the vet seldom calls. I recently met a Leicestershire farmer who had set up what he intended to be a low-cost beef enterprise. He'd established a herd of Longhorn cattle, a traditional breed that thrives on natural grassland and produces superb meat.

The animals stay so healthy on their herb-rich pastures that on the rare occasions the local veterinary firm has to be called in to deal with an accident such as a fracture, the duty vet invariably gets lost and has to phone for directions.

That's the kind of farm to buy your meat from. The farmer calculates his annual veterinary costs – covering vets' fees and medicines – at a paltry £3 per animal, an extraordinarily low figure. The irony is that the quality of the beef is so high supermarkets compete for the limited supply. They know that in-store this 'low-cost beef' will sell at a premium.

The health-promoting properties of mineral-rich pastures were once well known. More than sixty years ago the French biochemist Andre Voisin suggested that observations on grazing animals provided the best guide to the condition of the soil and its ability to provide healthy food for people.[1]

Voisin taught at the French national veterinary school and held an honorary doctorate from the University of Bonn. But at heart he remained a farmer. A laureate member of the Academy of Agriculture, his main interest was the way soil management affected the health of people who ate the food.

He considered grass to be the telltale indicator of the state of a nation's soil and its ability to keep people healthy. Voisin became convinced that studies on grazing animals were the best guide to the condition of a soil and its ability to produce healthy food for people. The key intermediary was grass. Human beings got their food from a variety of sources across the world, so it was difficult to link disease with any particular soil. But the mineral balance in grass was linked directly to the health and mineral status of the soil it grew on. It was like a 'biochemical snapshot' of the soil below. And it had a profound effect on the animal grazing on that grass.

It was Voisin who made the startling proposal that chemical disorder in the soil could lead inexorably to disorder in the human cell. He was able to show that cancer was less common in areas where the soil was *calcareous* –

lime rich – in character. He also showed that chemical fertilizers could lead to copper deficiency, and that the breakdown of normal copper metabolism in the human body might result in cancer.

Working with farm animals he found that copper deficiency in the heavily pregnant ewe was the cause of a nervous disease called sway-back in the lamb. Sway-back develops after breakdown of the *myelin* sheath, the white insulating tissue that surrounds particular nerves. Voisin established that the degenerative process began in the foetus and was the result of copper deficiency in the soil. Simply spraying pastures with a copper solution would prevent the disease.

At the time his books were published in the 1950s no one took much notice of such bizarre ideas. The medical profession was firmly in thrall to the medical physicists. The future lay in new medicines and technology. Who was this farmer to suggest that doctors go out into the fields for answers to some of the twentieth-century's most intractable diseases? The idea seemed preposterous. But with health budgets now devouring ever more of the national wealth the logic of this clear-thinking Frenchman has begun to look compelling.

It was time to meet the trace element guru, Danny Goodwin-Jones. I caught up with him at the end of a long, bone-shaking track that wound its way down a beautiful green valley. As I pulled up outside his handsome farmhouse he stepped from the porch to greet me, a tall, ebullient figure whose energy and enthusiasm belied his seventy-plus years.

We gazed across the valley to where a small flock of sheep nibbled at the lush pasture.

'Not mine I'm afraid,' he said, anticipating the question. 'I don't have time for that sort of thing any more.' We went into the house to talk about the things he does have time for.

As it happens he has spent a good deal of his life farming. He was born and brought up on a dairy farm near Welshpool at a time when most farms were organic. After a long army career he retired at the rank of colonel and bought a small farm in west Wales. This was in the mid-1970s. He was looking forward to the challenge of a new career rearing livestock.

But the second time around farming was not as he had remembered it. His sheep fell ill and died. His prized Welsh Black cattle failed to thrive. Vets advised him 'to feed his livestock better' without explaining exactly what that meant. Nothing he tried would make the animals flourish. By the time he had reached the desperate decision to sell up, his financial reserves were practically exhausted.

But Goodwin-Jones was not the sort of man to walk away from a defeat. He would not accept that he'd been a bad farmer, and he was determined to uncover the cause of so many ailments among his stock. Then a friend, a retired agricultural advisor, suggested that a deficiency of the mineral cobalt might have been to blame. It was an element he had never even heard of. But the chance remark sparked an intense study into the role of soil minerals in animal health. Now he runs a thriving business advising worried farmers up and down the country how to cure the sickness in their livestock.

We sat at the kitchen table and looked through sheaves of thank you letters he had received over the years from relieved farmers. There was the Cornish sheep farmer whose flock had staggered from one health crisis to the next. Ewes had died by the dozen for years and barely one in ten lambs ever reached finishing weight. At any one time almost half the flock was suffering from lameness. Though sick with worry the farmer had to endure constant complaints from passing walkers concerned about the condition of one or other of the animals.

Soil analysis revealed an imbalance of minerals, quickly corrected by soil treatment. The effect on flock health was immediate. Ewe losses fell to a fraction of their former level. Foot rot and lameness virtually disappeared. In the year following soil treatment 95 per cent of lambs were sold 'fat' off the farm.

A Welsh dairy farmer wrote that mastitis cases in his herd had been cut by three-quarters following the application of minerals to his soil, while the incidence of lameness had halved. Another dairy farmer reported 'a dramatic improvement in stock of all ages' following the treatment of his land with trace elements. He expressed his 'heartfelt thanks' for the advice that had transformed the financial fortunes of his farm and probably saved the business.

Goodwin-Jones is convinced that impaired immunity – the result of faulty nutrition – plays a part in epidemics amongst farm animals. The latest disease scourge to afflict the nation's cattle is bovine tuberculosis. Farmers blame badgers for spreading the disease to their stock; badger groups blame the reckless movement of cattle. But according to Goodwin-Jones, this disease, too, is the result of degraded soils and reduced fertility.

He sees both cattle and badgers as victims of soils depleted in selenium and other trace elements. Cattle feed on grass low in essential minerals; badgers dig for worms and grub about in the same pastures. Both end up with impaired immunity, leaving them defenceless whenever they come up against the ubiquitous TB bacillus.

Supporting evidence dates as far back as the sixties. At the University of Pennsylvania Max Lurie demonstrated the role of thyroid hormones in mobilizing mammalian resistance to the TB bacillus.[2] More recently, dairy chemist Helen Fullerton showed that to function efficiently the thyroid depends on a number of trace elements, including selenium, copper, cobalt, zinc and iodine.[3]

According to Fullerton many of the areas of Britain and Ireland where the eradication of bovine TB is proving so intractable have soils derived from red sandstone, granite or limestone where trace elements are often deficient or unavailable to plants. If the trace elements removed by modern, intensive farming were restored to the soil, she argued, both cattle and badgers would acquire a natural immunity to TB.

I suggested to Goodwin-Jones that since livestock were paying the price for impoverished soils, there must be a good chance that human beings were also affected? He had no doubts.

'Just take a look at the health statistics,' he said. 'Even with all the drugs and fancy procedures, people are becoming sick prematurely. It's what we've done to our food and our soil. Not that you'd ever get the medical profession to acknowledge it. They've got too much invested in treating illness to accept such a simple and obvious solution.'

The French biochemist Andre Voisin also thought it extraordinary that doctors and medical scientists around the world scarcely gave a thought to the foods being eaten by their patients. He told the story of a tribe of native

Americans among whom cancer was extremely rare. The Navajo lived on a reserve straddling the states of Arizona, Utah, Colorado and New Mexico.

Doctors working in the local hospitals observed that cancer rates among the eighty thousand or so population were unusually low. They suspected that some special feature of the Navajo diet might be the cause, and a team of scientists was drafted in from several states to investigate. After months of exhaustive study the researchers published their results. They concluded that the Navajo diet was hardly any different from that of other sections of the population. Low cancer rates were probably due to some unknown genetic characteristic of the tribe.

But when Voisin read the report he found the scientists had ignored one vital factor. They had made no reference to the nature of the soil, nor to Navajo cultivation methods. The tribe held strongly to the belief that they had been formed from the 'dust' of their soil. And they were in the habit of adding a little of it to their maize flour.

They would burn cedar branches and mix the resulting ash with their flour. They were, in effect, adding a mineral supplement to their food. Dieticians might prescribe any number of special foods, wrote Voisin, but unless they took account of the soils the foods had been grown on their results were meaningless.

The consequences of this neglect of our soils have been apparent for years to those who took the trouble to look.

In 1940, the Medical Research Council published the results of a survey into the nutrient content of many everyday foods. The authors were a doctor, R. A. McCance, and a nutritionist, E. M. Widdowson. Their studies were continued over the next fifty-one years and were eventually taken over by the Ministry of Agriculture. During this period a total of five reports were published of the McCance and Widdowson results.

Known as *The Composition of Foods*, the dusty reports show how mineral levels in many everyday items have fallen during a period of intensive chemical farming. The finding was made by David Thomas, a geologist who later trained as a nutritionist. He discovered that between 1940 and 1991 vegetables had on average lost 24 per cent of their magnesium, 46 per cent of their calcium, 27 per cent of their iron and no less than 76 per cent of their copper.[4]

The results for two main dietary staples were even worse. Carrots lost 75 per cent of their magnesium, 48 per cent of their calcium, 46 per cent of their iron and 75 per cent of their copper. The traditional 'spud' lost 30 per cent of its magnesium, 35 per cent of its calcium, 45 per cent of its iron and 47 per cent of its copper.

According to Thomas you'd have needed to eat ten tomatoes in 1991 to get the amount of copper a single tomato would have supplied in 1940.

The results for other produce were scarcely more comforting. Among seventeen varieties of fruit the contents of both magnesium and calcium were 16 per cent lower in 1991 than they had been in 1940. The zinc content was down by 27 per cent, the iron content by 24 per cent and the copper content by 20 per cent.

Even meat showed a fall in mineral levels. In a range of ten popular cuts the iron content fell by 54 per cent and the copper content by 24 per cent.

During the period of these changes other aspects of the British diet have undergone a seismic shift. There's been a dramatic switch to processed and fast foods. The raw materials they're made from are often contaminated with weedkillers, pesticides, antibiotics and hormones.

David Thomas finds the results alarming. He says: 'Physiologically it would be hard to overestimate the importance of minerals and trace elements. They often act as the catalyst for other nutrients the body uses to maintain good health. It is improbable that we can function at our optimum on a physical, mental and emotional level if the foods we have available are deficient.'

The exact role of minerals in human nutrition is still unclear. The long neglect of nutrition by orthodox medicine has left big gaps in the scientific knowledge. There's not even any agreement about which of the ninety or so trace elements found in nature can be considered 'essential' for human health. Some nutritionists believe that every living cell, whether in microbe, plant, animal or human being, requires all ninety minerals to operate efficiently.

What is clear is that, along with the familiar elements such as iron, calcium, and potassium, the human body needs a number of less well-known minerals such as boron, cobalt and germanium. These elements are required in tiny amounts. But without them – and the vitamins which often work in tandem with them – the body's support systems begin to break down.

Trace elements such as magnesium, zinc, iron and selenium are all essential to the normal functioning of the human immune system. But the fresh foods we now eat contain, on average, 50 per cent less than the foods of fifty years ago.

Chemical fertilizers have stripped many of these vital nutrients from the soil or blocked their uptake by plants. More are removed from crops during processing.

The element selenium is a classic example. In Britain, average intake of selenium is just thirty-five micrograms a day. The recommended rate for health is between one hundred and fifty and two hundred micrograms.

Selenium plays a key role in the human immune system. Low blood selenium levels have been linked to heart disease[5] and most cancers.[6] Yet virtually everyone in Britain – unless they're taking mineral supplements – are likely to have low blood selenium levels. This is because most UK soils are poor in the element, as are the soils in much of Europe. The widespread use of high-nitrogen fertilizers has made matters worse by blocking its uptake in plants.

GP Mark Draper is convinced that a sizeable section of the UK population suffers from type-two malnutrition, in that they are deficient in essential micronutrients. The major nutrients such as protein, carbohydrates, and fats are present in abundance – sometimes in excess – but people no longer get the essential minerals they need. The elements iron, zinc and selenium are the ones most likely to be in short supply.

The problem is exacerbated by the decline in average energy intakes. People engaged in hard physical work can easily utilize four thousand calories a day.[7] That's the kind of intake that was common in Britain fifty years ago. Today, with our largely sedentary lives, most people have calorie intakes of half that or less. That means their intake of micronutrients is also halved. When the foods themselves have been depleted of minerals, vitamins and phytochemicals by intensive farming or processing, many people are likely to go short.

According to Draper, common signs of micronutrient deficiency are recurrent infections, the sort of everyday ailments that fill doctors' waiting-rooms with patients seeking prescriptions for antibiotics. But there can be far more severe consequences for health. For the unborn child a deficiency in one or more essential trace elements can lead to developmental difficulties later in the child's life. There's an increased risk of conditions such as dyslexia, Asperger's syndrome and dyspraxia.

In adults, micronutrient deficiency may be the cause of chronic fatigue and reduced immunity. In the elderly it leads to the common degenerative conditions like osteoporosis, Alzheimer's, cancer and cardiovascular disease. In Britain, the world's fourth largest economy – where food is cheap and plentiful – five out of six people over sixty suffer from one or more degenerative conditions.

'In the midst of all this plenty we're seeing an epidemic of these diseases,' says Draper. 'Conditions you'd expect to see only in the elderly are occurring in younger people. And all for the want of a few minerals.'

The ideal solution would be a return to well-grown wholefoods, he believes. But where these are not available the only alternative is a good food supplement to replace the micronutrients missing from the diet. For the past seven years he has worked as a consultant to food supplement company Cytoplan.

His first experience of mineral supplements came while working as a young GP in the West Indies. He discovered that many of the youngsters queuing up at his surgery for antibiotics to treat minor respiratory infections were, in fact, deficient in iron. He prescribed an iron supplement, and within six weeks the number of youngsters attending his surgery each day fell from an average of twenty to just two.

Trace element deficiencies don't just affect physical health. They're also implicated in a range of emotional and behavioural disorders. In a celebrated study at Aylesbury young offenders centre in Buckinghamshire, youngsters were offered dietary supplements containing minerals, vitamins and essential fatty acids.[8] At the start of the trial more than half the youngsters were found to have low intakes of zinc, while three-quarters had low intakes of magnesium and almost all of them were deficient in selenium.

During the nine months of the trial young offenders on the dietary supplement committed a quarter fewer offences than those in a group given dummy pills. The greatest reduction was in the number of serious offences, which fell by 40 per cent.

In his book *Rare Earth's Forbidden Cures*, Joel D. Wallach cites examples of teenage violence which he believes could have been averted by proper nutrition. He argues that the chief cause of violence among young males is an 'explosive' mixture of testosterone, mineral deficiencies and an excess of sugar. The remedy, he says, is a diet free of sugar and supplemented with minerals – including copper, chromium, vanadium and lithium – vitamins, amino acids and essential fatty acids.

Deficiencies of calcium, iron, magnesium, zinc and copper all play a part in the onset of depression. Mineral and vitamin supplements have also been found to reduce rage and mood swings in children with psychiatric disorders. Poor food from degraded soils is the likely cause of many of the behavioural problems that blight the lives of thousands of youngsters.

It's not only in western countries that people are suffering the ill-effects of degraded soils. The West has exported its industrial farming methods around the world, including many developing countries. Even in countries where food intake has increased, diseases linked to mineral and vitamin deficiencies remain common or have gone up.[9]

The United Nations estimates that no fewer than two billion people worldwide are suffering from iron deficiency anaemia, a condition that undermines their physical and mental health.[10] Iodine deficiency is the greatest preventable cause of brain damage and mental retardation worldwide, and is estimated to affect more than seven hundred million people, most of them in less developed countries.

In his book, *Soil, Grass and Cancer*, first published in 1959, Andre Voisin wrote:

> We should meditate on the words of Ash Wednesday: 'Man, remember you are dust and that you will return to dust.' This is not merely a religious and philosophical doctrine but a great scientific truth. It should be engraved above the entrance to every faculty of medicine in the world. We might then remember that our cells are made up of mineral elements which are to be found in the soils of Normandy, Yorkshire and Australia. If these 'dusts' have been wrongly assembled in plant, animal or human cells the result will be imperfect functioning.[11]

It's a view endorsed by Danny Goodwin-Jones. Restoring minerals to Britain's worn-out soils would benefit everyone, he says: consumers, farmers and retailers. Meat from remineralized soils doesn't just taste better, it has a longer shelf life. Salt-marsh lamb, for example, tastes so good it commands a premium price. This is because the fattening lambs eat salt-marsh plant species containing high levels of minerals, the result of their regular dousing in seawater.

New research has revealed that salt-marsh lamb contains higher levels of vitamin E and healthy omega-3 fats than lamb raised on chemically-fertilized agricultural grasses.[12] And because of its extra antioxidants it keeps better in store. The research shows that the same health benefits are associated with lamb raised on moorland and heathland too. These 'unimproved' grasslands have not been damaged by chemical fertilizers. The herbs and deep-rooting plants they contain boost the mineral nutrition of grazing animals.

The results show how easily all meat could be made more healthy. It's simply a matter of restoring the mineral balance of damaged soils and seeding them with pastures containing a range of grasses, clovers, herbs and deep-rooting plants. Goodwin-Jones explains: 'Where I live in Wales we make sure the lamb we buy comes from unimproved mountain grazings. This simply means ordinary, mixed-species grassland that hasn't been mucked about with chemical fertilizers.

'It's lamb that tastes better and, I believe, is a lot healthier. If we got our soils right this healthy meat would be available to everyone at an affordable price.'

6

White Bread Is Bad For You

One of the busiest stalls in our local farmers' market is run by a community bakery selling what it calls 'hand-crafted, artisan breads'. Their aim, according to the sales leaflet, is 'to make something different, combining health and quality'.

The ingredient list looks impressive enough. It includes spring water, sunflower seeds, linseed, and sea salt with its full spectrum of trace elements. And there's certainly something different about the product range. Two of the most popular loaves are sourdoughs, yeast-free bread made by the traditional process of slow fermentation using the natural leaven of the grain. This is a time-consuming process, one that's rarely undertaken by profit-minded commercial bakers.

But this delicious bread, which often has customers queuing down the street, is made by people who aren't all that interested in profit. The Common Loaf Bakery is run by a small religious community from a farm high on the Blackdown Hills in Devon. For them making healthy, nutritious bread is part of their joyful service to God.

The most remarkable thing about their bread, apart from its superb flavour, is that none of it is made from wheat. Instead the community have chosen to make all their loaves from either stoneground rye flour or from stoneground spelt, an ancient grain from the wheat family *Triticum*.

When the aim is to make truly healthy bread, modern, hybrid wheats of the sort grown on arable farms up and down the country are no longer good enough. 'Packed with wholewheat goodness,' says the slogan on the supermarket cereal box. And so it could be. Grown in a fertile, well-nourished soil, wholegrain wheat is rich in B vitamins and in vitamin E. It's also well endowed with trace elements, including calcium, magnesium and iron, together with a number of disease-fighting phytonutrients and antioxidants. Well-grown wheat has more of them than many fruits and vegetables. But today's wheat is not well-grown.

Modern wheat is the product of nineteenth-century industrialism. It was conceived in the age of the Titanic, and developed on the American plains. Today it is traded as a global raw material for edible products that have little in common with real food.

Driving through Britain's 'big wheat country' in early summer you could almost believe you were crossing the prairies. In every direction the bright green crops stretch away across the boundless plain. The short, sturdy plants are packed tightly together. If there are any wild flowers to be seen, they're likely to be growing on the roadside verges. Out on the farmland there's precious little room for them, except under some EU-funded conservation scheme. For this is a landscape dedicated to production.

For the facts about modern wheat production there's no better place to start than the annual Cereals Event in East

Anglia. I follow the signs and park in the show car park, one enormous field. A small township of marquees, awnings, banners and flags has sprung up in the middle of an arable prairie.

I stroll among the crowded trade stands. This year's crop of new farm machines looks bigger than ever. There are giant combines, each capable of swallowing up dozens of acres of wheat in a single day, while ranks of heavy-duty cultivators stand ready to stir up and shatter the soil in preparation for the next crop.

New crop varieties are much in evidence, too. The plant breeding companies are constantly introducing new hybrids that promise a little more yield or better bread-making qualities. The new high performers have names like Einstein, Gladiator, Smuggler and Nijinsky.

But the real stars of the Big Wheat Fest are chemicals, the fertilizers and pesticides that underpin crop growing across the western world. Most of the demonstration plots are devoted to them. And the largest, plushest trade stands belong to the companies that market them.

I join a small group of farmers walking around the demonstration plots, small-scale wheat crops grown to show off a new variety or the effects of the latest fungicide. Beside one plot of dense, weed-free plants there's a sign listing the chemicals that have gone on to them.

Here's what the go-ahead farmer of the twenty-first century puts on the wheat that will go into our 'healthy' breakfast cereals or the 'nourishing' daily loaf. The pro-gramme begins in the autumn when the wheat plants are still very small. First they're sprayed with a mixture of weed-killers – the chemicals isoproturon and pendimethalin – together with a pyrethroid insecticide – lambda-cyhalothrin.

The following spring, at the start of stem growth, they're sprayed with a mixture containing two fungicides, propiconazole and chlorothalonil, to keep the plants free of fungal diseases. Also in the spray mix is a plant growth hormone called chlormequat, though the chemical companies prefer to refer to these compounds as growth 'regulators'.

As the plants grow taller they're sprayed with a further fungicide mixture, this time containing the chemicals azoxystrobin, chlorothalonil, and tetraconazole. Along with the fungicides is a blend of growth hormones: trinexapac-ethyl, chlormequat again, choline chloride, and imazaquin.

During the stage of rapid stem growth another trio of fungicides is applied – tebuconazole, azoxystrobin and chlorothalonil. A final dose of fungicide, metconazole, is sprayed on as the flag leaf emerges. It's this large leaf at the top of the stem that will supply much of the carbohydrate to fill the swelling grains. If it's smothered in fungal disease, the pesticide specialists warn, the final grain yield will be much reduced.

While the wheat plants are being bombarded with chemicals they're also receiving large amounts of chemical fertilizer, particularly nitrogen. It's the lush, 'watery' foliage stimulated by the chemical nitrogen that makes the plant susceptible to disease. Hence the need for an endless sequence of fungicide sprays.

This is the kind of spray programme that's followed by thousands of farmers in Britain. The cost in seed and chemicals adds up to £100 an acre more than the value of a ton of wheat at today's high prices. Without subsidies few farmers would have started growing the crop this way.

I turn to a farmer standing next to me. He's wearing a bright check shirt and a baseball cap bearing the logo of an American tractor company.

'Just think what you'd save if you didn't use any of this stuff,' I say in a jocular sort of way. He looks at me as if I needed sectioning under the Mental Health Act. 'If you didn't use 'em you wouldn't get a bloody crop at all,' he mutters, and walks off to inspect the new varieties.

As it happens he's wrong. Wheat was feeding entire civilizations thousands of years before fungicides were dreamt of. This was the grain found in earthenware jars by archaeologists opening up the tombs of the Egyptian Pharaohs. In ancient Greece, Hippocrates, the father of medicine, once recommended stoneground flour for its beneficial effects on the digestion.

When I first got interested in farming in the mid-1960s wheat was grown by what today would be called low-input methods. The farmer I worked for grew mostly spring-sown varieties. The place wasn't entirely chemical-free – a little nitrogen fertilizer went 'down the spout' with the seed when it was drilled in March.

But once the crop had been sown and rolled in there wasn't much else to do. In those days there were no fungicides to protect against disease. Nor were they needed. The farmer simply shut the gate and walked away until harvest time, apart from the occasional visit to see how the crop was progressing.

Yields varied, of course, just as they do now. In a good year we might harvest two or two and a half tons of grain to the acre. Today, yields are more than twice as big. But there's far less profit in it for the farmer. The extra income is swallowed up in the cost of chemicals. And at the end of it consumers get a degraded product.

Residues from pesticides turn up routinely in today's bread. In 2003, no fewer than 56 of 72 samples tested by the UK Pesticide Residues Committee – the government's official watchdog – were found to be contaminated.[1] The four most common contaminants were chlormequat, the growth hormone; glyphosate, a non-selective weedkiller; malathion and pirimiphos-methyl, both insecticides.

The three chemicals found at the highest levels in bread were subjected to risk assessments by the Residues Committee. They concluded that 'there was no concern for human health'. Not all experts agree.

The weedkiller glyphosate, which is widely used in the production of wheat and other crops, is marketed by its manufacturers as largely benign. They describe the pesticide products containing the chemical as of 'low toxicity'. In fact these products are acutely toxic to animals, including human beings. The symptoms include eye and skin irritation, headache, nausea, numbness, raised blood pressure and heart palpitations.[2]

In California studies on occupational risks showed glyphosate-containing weedkillers to be the third most commonly reported cause of pesticide illness among agricultural workers.[3] While many of the reports concerned 'irritant effects', mostly to the eyes and skin, a survey of one hundred reports found that over half of them involved more serious effects including burning of eyes or skin, blurred vision, skin peeling, nausea, headache, vomiting, diarrhoea, chest pain, dizziness, numbness, burning of the genitals and wheezing.[4]

Exposure to malathion, an organo-phosphate insecticide, produces a range of symptoms including headache, nausea, burning eyes and breathing difficulties.[5] In laboratory studies it has given rise to genetic changes in mice.

According to the United States Environmental Protection Agency there is 'suggestive evidence' that the chemical causes cancer.[6] Later studies have provided firmer evidence. A commercial malathion insecticide product caused breast cancer in laboratory animals.[7]

The government's so-called risk assessment is a desk study taking account of the known toxicity of a chemical compound and the theoretical intake of people eating the bread. It pretty well rules out any catastrophic, short-term threat to health. No one's going to collapse after eating from a contaminated loaf. But it cannot measure the long-term risk of consuming small amounts of different chemicals over many years.

Yet this is the kind of chemical cocktail consumed daily by almost everyone who eats bread. Current safety tests are carried out on each chemical in isolation. But there's evidence that a combination of two or three pesticides at low levels can be many times more harmful than the individual chemicals acting alone.

Dr Vyvyan Howard, a pathologist specializing in the effect of toxins on human development, says a true test of pesticide safety would mean testing them in all possible combinations. Since this would be impossible it makes sense to minimize human exposure to these chemicals.[8]

In Canada, the Ontario College of Family Physicians – a voluntary, non-profit-making association of doctors – has carried out a comprehensive review of research into pesticide hazards. As a result they have recommended that people reduce their exposure to these chemicals 'wherever possible'.[9]

In their study the Canadian doctors found 'positive associations' between pesticide exposure and a number of cancers, including those of the brain, prostate, kidney and pancreas. They also discovered a 'remarkable consistency' in research linking pesticide exposure to damage of the nervous system. Occupational exposure to agrochemicals might also be associated with reproductive damage, including birth defects, foetal death and retarded growth in the uterus.

Dr Margaret Sanborn, one of the report's authors, concluded: 'Many of the health problems linked with pesticide use are serious and difficult to treat. So we are advocating reducing exposure to pesticides and prevention of harm as the best approach.'

The link between crop health and human vitality is far from new. It's an idea developed by a scientist working a century ago. Sir Albert Howard spent much of his early career in India, eventually becoming director of the Institute of Plant Industry in the state of Indore. One of his first jobs in the country was to improve crop-growing on the research station at Pusa, in Bengal.

He soon discovered there wasn't much he could teach the locals about good food. He was struck immediately by the vibrant health of the crops grown by Bengali farmers. He decided to try out their methods on the crops grown at the research station.

As he became more skilled so the incidence of crop disease steadily fell. Within a few years he had learned how to grow healthy, disease-free crops. He was convinced that fertile soils – rich in humus from the breakdown of plant and animal wastes – were essential for the growing of healthy foods. He later wrote that plants were nourished in two ways.[10] First they absorbed through their roots small quantities of nitrate, phosphate and potash salts from solution in the soil. But they also relied on the symbiotic relationship with mycorrhiza – thread-like soil fungi – for many other nutrients.

Only when plants were nourished in this double way were they able to take up adequate levels of trace elements. And only then could they resist disease and produce high quality foods for both animals and human beings, wrote Howard. In marked contrast, crops grown with chemical fertilizers were only partially nourished. Chemical farming destroyed soil humus and severed the link with mycorrhiza. This meant that crop plants were no longer resistant to disease. Nor were their products able to protect human health as well as foods from well-nourished plants.

More than sixty years after Howard issued his dire warning, it is now largely forgotten. It's difficult to grasp the scale and pace of the revolution that has overtaken the business of growing wheat for our daily bread.

On the Thames Valley farm where I worked in the sixties, crops were still sown into fertile soils, soils enriched by plant and animal residues from the grass 'ley' that always preceded wheat. As the land warmed up in spring, soil microorganisms got to work on these residues, breaking them down and releasing minerals in the form plants could use them.

Mycorrhizae flourished in these soils, helping crops to extract the nutrients they needed. Wheat plants generally stayed healthy without the need for fungicide sprays. The natural living processes of the soil produced the conditions in which they could thrive.

Forty years on, that system of farming looks as ancient as the bullock cart. Modern wheat growing is chiefly a matter of selecting the appropriate chemical and spraying it on at the right time. So profligate are wheat growers with their pesticides that they're producing new super-races of weeds and diseases that are immune to them. Weedkiller-resistant forms of blackgrass, wild oats and common chick-weed are widespread. So are fungicide-resistant strains of the crop diseases mildew, septoria and yellow rust.

In the face of this threat of their own making the chemical companies urge farmers to use a range of fungicides with differing modes of action. In their bid to outsmart the disease organisms the manufacturers even supply ready-made chemical mixtures.

What no one suggests is a return to growing crops on fertile soils. The countryside is now run by a generation of farmers who are convinced that chemical agriculture is the only way to grow crops for profit.

But the chemical onslaught didn't arise because of some immutable law of progress. It is a legacy of political mismanagement. And it was largely funded by the tax-payer.

In 1973, when Britain joined the European Union – or the Common Market as it was – we became bound by the rules and regulations of the Common Agricultural Policy. Farmers were at once paid inflated prices for most agricultural products. For wheat this artificial market was supported by border taxes on imports and generous subsidies on exports, allowing European surpluses to be dumped on world markets.

In this protected climate farmers could afford to ditch their time-honoured practice of mixed farming. One of the benefits of having both livestock and cash crops on the farm was that it provided a measure of protection against a fall in the price of any particular commodity. When the wheat price tumbled there were always sales of milk, beef or lamb to offset the loss. And when the price of lamb or beef was low, the chances were that cereal prices would be on the way up. 'Down horn, up corn' went the old farming adage.

With high prices guaranteed by Brussels, farmers no longer needed a range of different enterprises to give them financial stability. Looking after animals every day of the year was demanding, so many chose to get rid of their livestock and reinvent themselves as specialist wheat growers.

It was likely to be costly in machinery and chemicals. And without cattle and sheep to maintain fertility, plant nutrients would have to be bought in as fertilizers. But with generous EU subsidies the UK wheat area doubled to five million acres after 1973.

In this new super-heated farm economy the chemical companies have been quick to seize their opportunity. In this they were ably assisted by the plant breeders who have delivered a host of varieties that need chemicals to thrive.

In Mexico, Norman Borlaug developed a clutch of short-strawed wheats from a Japanese variety. It was a breeding programme that would lead to the Green Revolution and win him the Nobel Prize. Some of the new breeding material was crossed with a variety called Cappelle Desprez, a wheat that was once widely grown in Britain. From this cross a team at Cambridge developed a family of semi-dwarf varieties, the first of which was called Hobbit.

These new short-strawed wheats had a greatly improved 'standing power' – they were far less likely to fall over or 'lodge'. This meant the farmer could safely put on far higher levels of nitrogen fertilizer without the risk of damage.

Compared with traditional tall wheats the short-strawed varieties directed a higher proportion of sugars into the seed head or 'ear' of the plant. In this way they were capable of producing dramatically higher yields, but to achieve it they needed high inputs of chemical nitrogen. At a stroke an ancient grain had been made a hostage to the multinational chemical industry.

'Thirty years of progress,' says the headline above a special feature in the weekly farming tabloid *Farmers Guardian*. The feature, sponsored by Monsanto, makers of the top-selling weedkiller Roundup, celebrates the wheat-growing revolution that has marked Britain's first three decades of EU membership.

It is a revolution that has brought few benefits for consumers. In a generation it has demolished the safe and stable pattern of mixed farming that delivered wholesome, nutrient-rich grain. It has given them instead wasteful surpluses of a degraded product, depleted of nutrients and laced with pesticide residues.

It's a system of farming that has its origins on the other side of the Atlantic, in the heartland of the United States. Modern intensive wheat production was nurtured by European settlers on the vast American prairies.

Wheat-growing is part of the American dream. As Americans began to populate the vast territory west of the Mississippi – lands that had been acquired from France in the early nineteenth century – the 'wilderness' at America's heart became productive through the hard work and fortitude of the homesteaders. That is the legend.

In reality this land wasn't a wilderness at all. It was a highly productive, grassland ecosystem supporting a wealth of life forms, among them the vast herds of bison.

For a brief period, the Europeans respected this living producer of plenty.[11]

But from the mid-nineteenth century the white settlers began to destroy this great natural production system. They ripped up the ancient turf with their steel ploughs and planted the new Turkey Red wheat which was tough enough to withstand the harsh prairie climate.

For a few decades they harvested bumper crops, nourished as they were by a thousand years of accumulated fertility. Grain poured from these untouched soils and was exported across the world, bringing ruin to many a British farmer. By the 1930s it was all over. The prairies died in a billowing, black dust cloud that rolled across the nation's heartland, turning day into night. Robbed of its life-giving organic matter the soil simply blew away in the dust bowls of the West.

Today the prairie lands still grow crops – mostly corn, wheat and soya – but only because they are constantly dosed with chemical fertilizers and pesticides, and because the US government is prepared to spend billions of dollars annually on irrigation and subsidies. Two-thirds of the grain is then fed to the cattle that have replaced the bison slaughtered by the settlers.

American-style grain growing is the enemy of traditional agriculture. It is an extractive industry, a mining of the soil; an exploitation of an ancient storehouse of fertility using industrial tools – hybrid seeds, pesticides and fertilizers. It's also a 'lame-duck industry', wholly dependent on public subsidies for its continuing survival. Yet this is the model of grain growing that the USA has exported to the world.

A handful of food grains – wheat, maize and rice – produced this way now dominate world diets in what has been called 'the green revolution'. Their production relies on heavy inputs of fertilizer and pesticides, generating big profits for the chemical companies and machinery manufacturers.

There is no doubt that the 'miracle seeds' – the compact, fertilizer-dependent crop varieties of the 1960s and 1970s – fed millions who might otherwise have gone hungry. But a United Nations report estimates that two billion people around the world now suffer from 'hidden hunger' – vitamin and mineral deficiencies that undermine their physical and mental health. The essential nutrients that have fallen to critically low levels include iron, zinc, iodine, vitamin A and folic acid. As a remedy the UN is proposing a whole range of 'fortified foods' such as soy sauce with added zinc, salt with extra iron, and cooking oil fortified with vitamin A.

Modern chemical wheat production is designed to produce surpluses and drive down prices. Under its ruthless rules only the biggest farmers can make a profit, while small farmers and farm-workers are driven from the land.

In Britain 'big wheat' has cost the jobs of thousands of farm staff as farms have grown bigger and their owners have relied on large machines. It's the advance of intensive wheat growing that has pushed families from the countryside, emptying village schools and closing village shops. And the damage continues because consumers are willing to put up with degraded food.

For more than twenty-five years the EU has maintained a chronic surplus of cereals, despite paying farmers to keep thousands of acres out of production. Up to half of this grain mountain is used to feed livestock, making it uneconomical to feed cattle on their natural, all-grass diet.

Cheap, chemically-grown grains from Europe and the US flow around the world putting traditional farmers out of business and destroying real food. Sadly there's little sign that the politicians, having unleashed the power of rampant agribusiness, can put the genie back in the bottle.

Referring to the American maize crop, Michael Pollan writes of 'a plague of cheap corn.'[12] US government farm programmes – once designed to limit production and support farmers' prices – were quietly rejigged during the Nixon administration to increase production and drive down prices, he says. Instead of supporting farmers, the government began supporting corn at the expense of farmers. Corn – already the recipient of a biological subsidy in the form of synthetic nitrates – would now receive an economic subsidy too, ensuring its final triumph over the land and the food system.

What is true of American maize applies equally to wheat in Europe and elsewhere. The capacity of the 'big wheat' industry to put small farmers out of business has been described as a kind of 'warfare' by Vandana Shiva, who trained as a quantum physicist but now campaigns for traditional farming in her native India. Industrial agriculture, she says, has become a war against ecosystems.[13] She challenges the 'myth' that the industrial growing of grains is more productive than traditional, ecological agriculture based on a range of different crops. Traditional farming systems evolved because more food could be harvested from an area planted with a mixture of crops than from the same area growing separate patches of monoculture.

The alternative approach to intensive grain growing has been demonstrated by Takao Furuno, a farmer in southern Japan, and author of *The Power of Duck*. He was determined not to grow rice in a conventional monoculture, with its dependence on pesticides and fertilizers. Instead of the industrial paradigm he took an ecological approach, introducing fish and ducks into his paddy fields. First he planted his rice seedlings into the flooded paddies. He then introduced a gaggle of ducklings which started feeding on the insects that would normally attack young rice plants. Next he brought in loaches, edible fish that are easily cultivated and produce tasty meat. He also planted azolla, a nitrogen-fixing herb that's usually thought of as a weed.

In Furuno's paddy fields the ducks feed on insects, and – like the loaches – on the azolla weed. Since it is continuously grazed the weed never becomes dominant enough to compete with the rice. At the same time it supplies nitrogen to the crop. Along with the droppings from the ducks and fish, the rice gets all the nutrients it needs.

Around his paddy fields Furuno has integrated vegetable, wheat and fig crops. Without fertilizers or pesticides he harvests rice crops that are up to half as big again as industrial rice-growing systems. His six-acre farm produces a gross income slightly higher than the average six hundred-acre rice farm in Texas.[14]

This ecological approach to high-yield farming can be applied equally well to wheat. French ecologist and farmer Marc Bonfils developed a system of wheat growing that produced spectacular yields without fertilizers or pesticides.[15] Instead he made full use of the strength and vigour of the ancient wheat plant before it was weakened by modern plant breeders trying to shorten the straw. He also utilized the natural fertility-building power of clover plants to provide the nutrients, particularly nitrates, for a healthy grain crop.

Today's wheat growers plant their hybrid seeds in early autumn for harvesting in summer the following year. They have to sow the seeds densely. Soil temperatures begin to fall soon after sowing and widely-spaced plants wouldn't have time to develop a thick crop before the onset of winter.

By the time the frosts begin, modern crops are still struggling to put down decent root systems. That's why large amounts of chemical nitrogen have to be applied the following spring if the still-frail crop is to produce a decent harvest. And because spring growth is 'forced' with nitrogen fertilizer, the plants must be bombarded with pesticides to keep them alive.

Marc Bonfils took a radically different approach. He discovered through research that ancient wheat varieties were remarkably strong and robust. They had the capacity to grow dozens of side shoots producing wheat 'bushes' instead of the single stems that characterize chemically-grown crops. These bushes were able to put down huge root systems, but to do so they had to be planted far earlier in the year.

On the Bonfils system, winter wheat is sown in early summer – just a few days after the solstice in June. By the start of winter the plants have developed numerous side shoots and extensive root systems. When the soil warms up in the following spring they're ready to produce masses of seed heads.

In another radical feature the seeds are sown into a low-growing clover crop. It's the natural action of soil microbes at the clover roots that produces the nitrogen the growing wheat plants need. Well nourished in a fertile soil, the crop stays healthy without the need of pesticides. And at harvest – which is two weeks earlier than with chemically-grown crops – it produces a bigger yield than the modern dwarf hybrids.

The Bonfils system is ignored by the farming establishment. Not surprisingly the agrochemical manufacturers – who dominate the industry – see it as a threat. Developed on a larger scale it could provide health-giving wheat grains, free of pesticide residues and rich in essential vitamins and minerals.

Impoverished foods have long been the legacy of chemical wheat growing. Around the time the American homesteaders were ripping up the prairie grassland, a parallel revolution was taking place in the flour-milling business. A group of commercial millers in Minnesota installed a new French device called the purifier, which separated flour from the coarser parts of the grain.

This was quickly followed by the roller mill, a high-speed machine in which the traditional millstones were replaced with steel rollers. Within two decades the new milling process had made the old-style gristmill obsolete. The business of milling was transformed from a small-scale local enterprise to a factory process turning out thousands of tons of white flour.

In Britain, the new-style mills were built at ports so they could process imported American wheat. Until then the local grist-mill had been a key part of the rural economy. Almost overnight they were made uneconomical. Milling had become an industrial process. The local baker, obtaining his flour from the country mill, was replaced by the 'plant baker', the large-scale manufacturer of white bread.

A century ago the writer William Edgar hailed the milling revolution as a great advance for civilization. In *The Story of a Grain of Wheat* he celebrates the close of 'the era of black bread, coarse and dirty, fit only for strong teeth and the digestive apparatus of a rugged outdoor man'. Gone, at last, were 'the black bread times, when the flour of all save the very rich was dark and filled with impurities'.[16]

The belief that white bread was somehow superior has become a dominant idea in the industrial world. The wrestlers and athletes of ancient Greece may have insisted on coarse, wheat bread to maintain their power and strength. But in the modern world we're all convinced that white flour is a far finer food.

When wheat was ground between stones in traditional gristmills, the flour retained all the nutrients of the original grain. Modern roller mills reject all but the starchy endosperm of the grain. The bran and wheatgerm are lost, along with many of the minerals, vitamins and essential fatty acids.

The resulting white flour contains only a small fraction of the original nutrients. To compensate, the plant bakers are required to 'enrich' or 'fortify' white bread with a number of added nutrients. It's hardly an equal trade.

During processing millers remove up to 80 per cent of the nutrients in the original grain. These include the minerals calcium, zinc, copper, iron, magnesium, manganese, potassium, phosphorus and selenium; the B vitamins niacin, riboflavin, thiamine and pyridoxin; and vitamin E. In return the millers add calcium, iron, thiamine and niacin.

In her book *Nourishing Traditions*, nutritionist Sally Fallon debunks the idea of 'fortification'.[17] It adds a handful of synthetic vitamins and minerals to white flour after dozens of essential nutrients have been removed or destroyed. Some of the added nutrients may even be harmful. There's evidence that excess iron from fortified flour can cause tissue damage, and other studies link excess or toxic iron to heart disease. Vitamins B1 and B2 – added to grains without vitamin B6 – lead to imbalances in numerous processes involving B vitamin pathways.

Fallon is no more enthusiastic about the treatment of grains going into modern breakfast cereals. Dry breakfast cereals are produced by a process called extrusion. First the ground-up cereal grains are made into a slurry. At high temperatures and pressures, this slurry is then forced through a small hole whose shape creates whatever flake, shape or shred the manufacturer is looking for.

According to Fallon, the process destroys many of the nutrients in the grain, even the artificial vitamins the manufacturers have added. It also denatures amino acids, particularly lysine, sometimes rendering them toxic. She cites two unpublished experiments in which breakfast cereals were fed to rats that very quickly died.[18] All boxed breakfast cereals are made by the extrusion process, she says, including those sold in health food stores.

Britain and Ireland are the world's biggest consumers of processed breakfast cereals. Each year UK households spend over £1 billion on shaped, puffed, flaked, flavoured, sugared and salted cereals. And each year the manufacturers spend millions of pounds – £84 million in 2005 – trying to perpetuate the illusion that they're healthy.[19]

When bread and everyday wheat products have been so degraded it's hardly surprising wheat growers pay scant attention to the nutrient content of their crop. They no longer grow a food. Instead they are producing a raw material for an industrial manufacturing operation.

So long as they can meet the technical demands of the plant bakers and the breakfast cereals manufacturers, farmers have only one concern – the size of their harvest. Grain yield per acre becomes an obsession, a badge of achievement. Farmers are also subject to the baffling laws of agricultural economics which run counter to the usual forces of supply and demand. When the price drops in agriculture farmers produce more in a bid to maintain their incomes. This is why they must squeeze ever more production from their overworked soils.

The chief beneficiaries are the oil and chemical companies, global commodity traders, and the large-scale livestock farmers who take their animals off pasture where they belong and feed them the unhealthy grain. In this way commodity grain degrades the general food supply. Fortunately this way of farming is unlikely to survive for much longer, though the new subsidies on grains for biofuels has given it a major boost.

US agrarian writer Gene Logsdon expects large-scale industrial wheat-growing to collapse under its crippling burden of costs, those of the fertilizers, pesticides and machinery needed to keep the grain flowing.[20] Instead the western world will come to rely on 'pasture farming' for its food, with grazing animals providing meat, milk, eggs, dairy products, wool, and hundreds of other animal products at a fraction of the cost of producing them with current factory technology.

'Pasture farming is the first alternative to high-tech agriculture that has both short-term and long-term profit on its side,' says Logsdon. 'Industrial grain farming and animal factories may have had short-term profit advantage for a while. That's why they rose to prominence, but no longer. Over half the money to keep these operations afloat now comes from government subsidies.

'If there is any lesson of history that always remains true, it is that no economy can be falsely sustained when it can't compete with another economy. Neither all the king's horses nor all the king's men can make industrial farming survive with subsidies, just as fifty years of subsidies could not save the old family farm. Industrial farming is simply not profitable enough any more to compete with pasture farming.'

7

Look For The Pasture-Fed Label

Years ago I read and was moved by *The Farmer, the Plough and the Devil*.[1] In it Arthur Hollins tells of his struggle to bring health and fertility back to his farm after taking it over in 1929 at the age of just fourteen. At that time the farm had been brought close to bankruptcy by the overuse of chemical fertilizers which weakened and impoverished the soil.

Arthur was one of those remarkable people whose lives are imbued with an unquenchable spirit of discovery. Not for him the conventional view that farming's future lay with the new chemicals. He'd seen them fail and bring the land close to ruin. He was determined to find a new system of farming, one that would guarantee both healthy livestock and healthy foods.

He was extraordinarily successful. With his first wife May he built up a flourishing dairy business selling Fordhall products across the country. Chief among them was a high-quality yoghurt made from unpasteurized milk. At a time when few people in Britain had any idea what yoghurt was, May and Arthur were selling their classy version in Harrods.

It was a success based on a clear understanding of the natural world. Arthur studied carefully the natural processes at work in his soil, then developed a farming system that respected them. It was a case of the judicious 'tweaking' of a natural ecosystem rather than the full-scale attack practised by chemical agriculture. Because of this it produced healthy, nutrient-dense foods that tasted wonderful.

Arthur realized early on that fertile soils were far more than a collection of tiny, inert rock fragments. They were also 'a violent cauldron' of physical, chemical and biological activity, the site of a complex fight for survival between thousands of species, many of them microscopic in size. It was this ceaseless struggle between unimaginable numbers of organisms that produced the conditions for healthy plant growth and, ultimately, for healthy humans.

Knowing this, it made sense to apply organic materials such as farmyard manure to fuel the subterranean struggle. Better still were organic composts in which crop and vegetable wastes had been partially decomposed before they were applied to the soil. Composts, Arthur discovered, unleashed feverish activity in the soil, further improving the conditions for healthy plant growth.

Next he began questioning the use of the plough. What was the point in creating highly fertile conditions in the top few inches of soil, he reasoned, when you then buried it under several inches of poorer soil? So he stopped ploughing his land, choosing instead to use equipment that simply stirred and agitated those vital surface layers.

But he was not finished yet. In his search for the perfect conditions in which to grow healthy foods he began questioning the practice of leaving land crop-free over the winter in preparation for sowing in spring. He had noticed that land over-wintered beneath vegetation – even weeds – was softer, more crumbly and altogether a better growing medium when the seeds were planted in spring. It was this observation that led ultimately to his system of 'grass farming,' a system so simple and so productive it seems incredible that it has been ignored for so long.

Arthur decided to keep all his land as pasture. But unlike today's grassland farmers with their beloved monocultures, he encouraged as wide a range of species as possible. In his travels around Britain he would collect seed heads from some of the local fields, taking them home to spread on his pasture-land. He reasoned that if the soil and the climate suited them they would thrive; if not, they would fail. Either way he'd be left with pastures of such diversity they'd supply the full nutritional needs of his cows and enrich their milk with nutrients that would protect human health.

He made little hay or silage. Instead the cows stayed out all winter, grazing the driest pastures that had been 'shut up' since the summer for the purpose. He called this winter grass 'foggage'. It clearly suited the cattle. They stayed far healthier than if they'd been shut up together in sheds over the winter months.

I often wonder what Arthur's farming neighbours made of his rough and 'weedy' pastures as they glanced over the hedge. They must have shaken their heads in disbelief at his eccentric practices, no doubt convinced that he'd soon be bankrupt.

But Arthur and May were not bankrupted. Instead they made a lot of money. Their simple all-grass farm cost them nothing in chemical fertilizers or seeds, and next to nothing in vet bills because the cows stayed healthy. At the same time it produced dairy foods of quality.

So I decided to see what Fordhall Farm looked like today. I arrived feeling some trepidation. The farm, I knew, had become run down in recent years. The family had fought a protracted legal battle to prevent the land being sold by the landlord to developers. Most of the livestock had been sold to raise the cash to cover court costs. The historic farm was now safe thanks to the thousands of small shareholders who had been invited to invest in the land, each buying a tiny share of the farm. But would Charlotte and Ben, the new generation of farmers, be as determined as their father to produce healthy food?

I needn't have worried. As I walked the fields with Charlotte it quickly became clear that the fertile, herb-rich pastures, key to the production of nutrient-dense meat and dairy foods, were intact. We walked over pastures containing a clutch of different grasses, timothy, meadow fescue, rough-stalked meadow grass and the deep-rooting cocksfoot. Clovers, both red and white, enriched the soil with nitrogen without the aid of chemical fertilizers. And everywhere there were dozens of herbs and wild species, among them yarrow, chicory, vetch, plantain, even the humble dandelion.

Most farmers would view them as weeds, but to Charlotte they are part of the semi-natural ecosystem that ensures the health of the livestock and the healthiness of the foods they produce. She explained: 'This is the natural and sustainable way to produce food. Under the continuous cover of the turf soil microbes and other fauna steadily build fertility. And the diverse range of grasses and other plants provide the animals with all they need to stay healthy.

'Fertility-building in the soil is never disrupted by ploughing. The livestock are not stressed by being shut up in sheds for months every year. Best of all, this system produces foods that have all the nutrients to keep people healthy.'

The dairy cows have now gone from Fordhall Farm. Charlotte and Ben have replaced them with beef cattle, the traditional Hereford and Aberdeen Angus breeds, and sheep. There are also a few Gloucester Old Spot and Tamworth pigs. The species-rich grassland which once filled their father's dairy products with health-protecting nutrients now does the same for the meat his offspring sell at local farmers' markets and in the farm shop.

Most modern farmers, weaned on the chemical habit, would shake their heads in dismay at the sight of such traditional grazings, believing them to be hopelessly unproductive. The conventional view of a profitable grass field is one sown to perennial ryegrass and plastered with ammonium nitrate fertilizer. It's a notion that has done untold harm to livestock and robbed us all of the chance to eat healthy meat and dairy products. Almost daily the evidence mounts of the benefits of pasture-fed foods, particularly pastures containing a wide range of plant species.

Beef and lamb produced on almost any form of grass contain far more health-protecting fatty acids and antioxidants than meat from animals fed on sizeable amounts of cereal grain, as is much British livestock. Beef cattle, for example, incorporate up to ten times more beta-carotene and up to five times more vitamin E into their muscle tissues than grain-fed animals.[2] Beta-carotene – a precursor of vitamin A – and vitamin E are two of the fat-soluble vitamins the pioneering American dentist Weston A. Price considered most important to maintaining human health.

In addition, cattle fed chiefly on fresh grass produce meat with up to two-thirds more omega-3 fatty acids than animals fed grain-based diets. Omega-3s are vital for the prevention of heart attacks, depression and cancer, and their levels in proportion to the structurally-similar omega-6 fatty acids are a key measure of the healthiness of a diet. The proportions of the two fatty acids in grass-fed meat are far more beneficial than in grain-fed meat.[3]

Also found in beef and lamb is a group of compounds known collectively as conjugated linoleic acid or CLA. As well as being powerful cancer fighters, these are known to protect against heart disease, diabetes and obesity. In the meat from pasture-fed animals they are found at more than double the levels found in grain-fed animals.[4]

These are the general health benefits of raising cattle and sheep on grassland, including the chemically fertilized ryegrass monocultures which pass for grasslands in Britain. But new research from Bristol University shows that the benefits are even greater when the grassland in question is like the pastures at Fordhall Farm and filled with a variety of herbs and wild flowers as well as a range of grass species.[5]

The scientists compared the nutritional quality of lamb produced by grazing three classic types of grassland landscape – moorland, salt-marsh and heather moorland. As a control, they grazed lambs on what they called 'semi-improved' grassland, pastures dominated by perennial ryegrass and treated with chemical nitrogen fertilizers. All three natural grasslands produced meat with higher vitamin E levels than on the ryegrass monoculture. And all three produced meat with higher levels of omega-3 fatty acids, leading to a healthier ratio of omega-3 to omega-6 fats.

Saturated fat levels were lower in meat from the natural grasslands, and taste panel tests showed that the flavour was better. As if that weren't enough, levels of the powerful anti-cancer compound CLA were higher in the lambs grazed on the natural grassland. The reasons for this are clear from a remarkable piece of research done at Reading University.

The scientists investigated a range of common pasture plants species to find out how much of a substance called alpha-linoleic acid they contained in their leaves. In the rumen of ruminant animals such as cattle and sheep the compound is converted into CLA by the action of microbes. The scientists were surprised to find that the compound occurred in a large number of wild species including dandelions, knapweed, cat's-ear, ox-eye daisy, plantain, rough hawkbit, self-heal, bird's-foot trefoil, red and white clovers, sorrel and yarrow.

Most contained higher levels of the compound than the leaves of grasses. And in many of them – such as sorrel, knapweed and dandelion – the levels were higher in autumn than in spring. A century ago almost all Britain's grasslands contained this rich diversity of wild plants. It was these flower-rich meadows that inspired generations of poets and artists. Now it's clear they protected our health as well.

Tragically, most have now gone, victims of the modern farming obsession with 'clean' grassland and the chemical fertilizers and sprays that enable them to acquire it. No less than 97 per cent of Britain's flower-rich meadows have been destroyed, and our diets are less healthy for it. Today, most pasture-fed meat comes from chemically-fertilized ryegrass monocultures.

But there's real meat around if you look for it. From his farmhouse on a rocky outcrop in North Wales, sheep farmer Gwyn Davies looks down on the beautiful Dwyryd Estuary and, beyond it, the glittering waters of Tremadog Bay. Far away to the left stands Harlech Castle, while amid the tree-covered hillside to the right you can catch a glimpse of Portmeirion, the Italianate village dreamed up by Clough Williams-Ellis. But the sight that stirs Gwyn Davies's heart as he gazes from the dining room window are the 120 acres or so of *glas traeth*, or saltings, a patchwork of green turf on the shoreline.

This tidal grazing has a rich mix of saltwater adapted plants, including thrift, sorrel, yarrow, sea plantain, clover and samphire. Each year he runs his Welsh Mountain ewes and their new lambs on this nutrient-rich turf, turning them out on the shoreline when the lambs are about two weeks old. On this grass alone they quickly grow into sturdy, healthy animals, producing what Gwyn and his wife Rita consider to be the finest tasting meat around. From the make-up of the turf it's also likely to be among the healthiest of meats, well-endowed with minerals, antioxidants and protective fats.

Sadly the couple aren't able to sell it for a price that reflects its nutritional value. Gwyn has to sell his saltings lambs in the local livestock market, where they fetch the same price as lambs grown on chemically-fertilized ryegrass pastures. In up-market stores and supermarkets, salt marsh lamb sells for a sizeable premium, but like many other farmers who have resisted going down the chemical route he has found it impossible to tap into these outlets.

With the closure of a nearby abattoir the lambs would have to be trucked forty miles for slaughter and the meat brought forty miles back for packing. Marketing and Internet selling doesn't always come easy to farmers who have spent their entire lives rearing healthy stock, especially under the harsh conditions at Hafod-y-Wern, Penrhyndeudraeth, where the couple farm with son Rhodri. Apart from the saltings and a small area of low-lying water meadows, where Gwyn makes top-quality hay as winter feed for the ewes, the grasslands are on soils overlying rock.

Earning a living from such poor land is tough. He remembers how, back in the 1960s, the government's farming advisors were recommending that he put on heavy doses of nitrate fertilizer. As the thin turf began breaking away in clods from the rocky pastures he quickly realized that this was the way to ruin. Since then his management of the land has been strictly in line with organic principles.

For all its healthy qualities Gwyn Davies's lamb is lost in the torrent of second-rate foods flowing into the food chain. He once sent a sample of his lamb to the boss of a major abattoir. The meat-man cooked it, tasted it and pronounced it the best he'd ever tasted. But he still offered Gwyn the rock-bottom price for 'commodity lamb', the lamb that comes from chemically-grown monocultures.

Around the country there are dozens, perhaps hundreds, of farmers producing high-quality meat from traditional, mixed pastures. At the moment the mass market food chain ignores them. So do we when we shop exclusively at supermarkets. But the signs are there's going to be a great deal more of such quality meat around in the future if only we'll make the effort to find it.

Ironically, it's the very scarcity of traditional, flower-rich grasslands that has renewed interest in their products.

Many of the surviving meadows and pastures are now designated as nature reserves or are protected under wildlife management agreements. Conservationists have found that the best way to preserve them is to graze them in the traditional way using native breeds of cattle and sheep. As wildlife groups and conservation bodies set up these schemes, they look around for ways to fund them by marketing the meat as a premium product. The result is a lot more healthy meat and lamb on the market.

At Hilltop Farm, Malham, high in the Yorkshire Dales, there are cattle running on the flower-rich limestone grazings for the first time in 20 years. But they're not the fast-growing Charolais and Limousin animals so popular with today's commercial beef producers. The cattle chosen by farmer Neil Heseltine are of a native hill breed called the Belted Galloway. The animals are black in colour, with a white band that encircles the body just behind the shoulders.

The animals are hardy and slow-growing, thriving on the sort of rough moorland grazing that most farmers would consider poor. But the breed is also famed for the quality of its meat, and on the flower-rich pastures of Malham it's likely to produce some of the healthiest beef around.

The cattle have returned to Hilltop Farm because the unique grasslands of the 'limestone country' are scarce and under threat. The limestone areas of the Dales have, over centuries of grazing, developed their own characteristic pastures, dominated by blue moor grass and containing such species as bloody crane's bill, small scabious, rockrose and wild thyme.

Conservationists have decided that the best way to safeguard the species diversity of these pastures is to graze them with native breeds of cattle. Under a scheme known as the Limestone Country Project farmers in the area are given financial backing to establish new herds. Local marketing consultants have been taken on to help build new markets for the beef, particularly through direct sales to consumers.

Schemes like this are being set up by wildlife groups and nature conservation bodies across the country. The aim is to ensure the survival of species-rich grassland which is becoming increasingly rare in the age of chemical fertilizers. It means that healthy, nutrient-dense beef is slowly becoming more plentiful.

In a nation concerned with the health of its citizens all beef and lamb would be produced from species-rich grassland, as it was before the chemical age. Until the arrival of cheap nitrate fertilizer no self-respecting livestock farmer would have dreamt of sowing a new pasture, or ley, without including at least half a dozen different species in the seeds mixture. Diversity was seen as essential to the proper nutrition of the grazing animal. There would be, perhaps, two or three grass species along with at least one sort of clover to provide protein and minerals, and to boost soil fertility by fixing atmospheric nitrogen at the root nodules.

Some farmers went a great deal further. In Somerset, Newman Turner, author of the 1950s classic *Fertility Farming*, included more than twenty different species in the seeds mixture of every new grass ley he sowed.[6] Among them were nine varieties of agricultural grass and four types of clover, both red-flowering and white. The rest were herb species such as chicory, burnet, yarrow, sheep's parsley, kidney vetch, lucerne and plantain. Even seeds of the much reviled dandelion were included.

In the book telling the story of Goosegreen, his farm near Bridgwater, Turner wrote: 'A mixture containing deep-rooted herbs is essential to soil, crop and animal health, assisting in the aeration of the subsoil and the transfer from subsoil to topsoil of essential minerals and trace elements.

'Especially important are herbs like chicory, burnet, lucerne and dandelion, all of which penetrate to a depth of three or four feet or more in as many years.'

Turner shunned chemical fertilizers and pesticides. Having relied on them early in his farming career he had become convinced they were damaging to his livestock and ruinous of his land. Instead he came to depend on organic compost and herb-rich pastures for bumper crops and healthy cattle. And they proved to be remarkably successful at the job.

He claimed that by providing his cattle with organically grown, mineral-rich pasture he was able to prevent, and even cure, many of the most crippling animal diseases, including tuberculosis, infertility, mastitis and Johnes disease, a condition of the intestinal tract like Crohn's disease in humans, and thought to be caused by paratuberculosis bacteria in milk. Today these diseases remain rife in Britain's cattle population.

So confident was he of his methods that he was known to travel around local markets looking for sick animals, especially those that were clearly suffering from TB. He was confident he could cure them and return them to health and production, so making himself a pound or two.

More than thirty years after his book first appeared over five thousand British cattle herds are held under TB restrictions. Farmers blame badgers for the spread of the disease among their stock. They want government action to curb the rising badger population.

To Turner, the argument would have seemed pointless. What did it matter how any disease organism came to be in a particular place? It was the health of an animal's immune system that determined whether or not it contracted the condition. He was convinced it wasn't the TB bacillus that caused disease, but inadequate nutrition. While cattle remained well-nourished, disease organisms would do them no harm.

In *Fertility Farming* he tells the story of his favourite stock-bull, a prize-winning Jersey with the colourful name Longmoor Mogulla's Top Sergente. A routine TB test showed the animal to be 'a violent reactor'. The Ministry of Agriculture recommended that it be 'disposed of'.

Turner had different ideas. He isolated the bull on some off-lying land and put him on a carefully-managed diet of fresh, green foods grown on a fertile soil. Meanwhile, the Ministry vets continued to test the bull for TB. After a few months they declared he was free of infection. Five years later he was still winning awards and siring prize-winning daughters.

Turner concludes: 'All my work indicates that tuberculosis can be prevented and cured by food grown on a properly managed soil, provided an adequate ration of mineral-rich herbs is included.'

Half a century before Turner proved the health-giving properties of a species-rich Somerset pasture, a Scottish landowner (named by his neighbours as 'the daft laird') was carrying out similar experiments in the border country near Kelso.

Robert Elliot had made his fortune growing coffee in Mysore, in India. With his money he bought the Clifton Estate in Roxburghshire, and in 1887 began farming the land at Clifton-on-Beaumont. Until his death in 1914 his chief interest was in species-rich grassland and its capacity to produce fertile soils and healthy livestock.

Like Turner, he believed in using seed mixtures containing a variety of deep-rooting herbs. Burnet, chicory, alsike clover and yarrow were the key constituents. Elliot became convinced that not only were herb-rich pastures beneficial to cattle and sheep, but they greatly improved the health of the soil. Plants such as yarrow and vetch, burnet and chicory thrust their roots deep into the ground, breaking up any areas of compaction. As well as drawing minerals and moisture to the surface layers, they opened up the soil, or, in Elliot's terms, they 'disintegrated it', so allowing life-giving oxygen to penetrate the deeper levels.

Farmers had no need of chemical fertilizers, he later wrote. The cheapest soil conditioner was a turf made up chiefly of deep-rooting herbs. Plant roots were far and away the deepest and best tillers, drainers and warmers of the soil.

In his later years the old laird took to walking over his best pasture fields, 'mending' them with a garden rake and a little bag of seeds. During a wet summer the family coach would arrive early at Clifton Park to drive him and his equipment the four miles to the farm. These little excursions may have been the origin of the 'daft' epithet.

At the time Elliot was carrying out his experiments the country was awash, as now, with cheap food imports. A century ago the competition came from the virgin lands of the Empire, the prairie wheat lands of Canada and the wide, fertile grasslands of New Zealand and South Africa. Britain, the great industrial power, relied on her manufacturing industry to pay for food imports.

Elliot warned that the day would come when countries such as China, Japan and India would emerge as powerful industrial nations.[7] To survive in this new competitive world Britain would have to make use of her most valuable resource, her herb-rich grasslands and their ability to produce strong livestock and health-giving foods. The constant reliance on artificial fertilizers would cost farmers dear, he warned. In the end it would empty their bank accounts and exhaust the soil.

Raised naturally on fertile soil, beef could be one of the healthiest foods around. Red meat provides complete protein, including sulphur-containing amino acids such as cysteine. Beef is a rich source of taurine and carnitine, both needed for healthy eyes and a sound heart. It's also rich in co-enzyme Q10, which is important for the cardiovascular system.

Properly reared beef is also rich in essential minerals, including zinc, the prerequisite of clear thought and an active sex life. And it contains plenty of vitamin B12 – vital for healthy nervous and vascular systems – along with the fat-soluble vitamins A and D.

All these are well-known attributes of beef reared traditionally on fertile pasture. But modern science has uncovered a new benefit. Grass-fed beef is an important provider of essential fats, the polyunsaturated fatty acids. They include conjugated linoleic acid (CLA), together with the longer chain fatty acids EPA, eicosapentaenoic acid and docosahexaenoic acid (DHA). All are vital to human health.

CLA is highly protective against cancer.[8] It also promotes the build-up of muscle rather than fat tissue. When cattle are raised on fresh pasture alone, their meat and milk contains as much as five times more CLA than the products of animals fed modern, conventional diets.[9] EPA and DHA – which belong to the group known as omega-3 fatty acids – are needed for a number of vital body functions, among them efficient immune and nervous systems.

In ruminant animals these essential fatty acids are chiefly found, not in storage fats, but in muscle. That makes meat an important source of these nutrients. Along with oily fish, which is often contaminated with heavy metals, beef is a rich source of both EPA and DHA, so long as it is predominantly grass-fed.

Given the role of fertile grasslands in producing one of mankind's finest foods, it's hard to see why industrial societies have treated them so recklessly. Throughout the western world productive grasslands have been abused and squandered. Nowhere has the ruin been greater than on the American prairies.

Before the arrival of European settlers, species-rich grasslands stretched continuously across the North American heartland, from the forest edge in Canada to the Gulf Coast of south-east Texas; from the foothills of the Rockies to the plains of Illinois and western Indiana.

With up to four hundred different plant species in a single square metre of turf, these semi-natural grasslands were hugely productive. For thousands of years they supported vast numbers of bison, up to sixty million of them when the great, wandering herds were at their height.

Through drought and storm the grasslands fed them; through blistering hot summers and freezing winters –

and all without chemical fertilizers, pesticides, irrigation or any other of the technical aids without which modern farmers say production is impossible.

Like all grassland communities, the prairie plants gathered minerals from deep in the soil and concentrated them in the top few centimetres. Leaves and roots died and decayed, releasing nutrients to be taken up by other plants. Some leaves were grazed by bison or any one of a handful of other grazing animals such as the elk, deer and pronghorn antelope. The grazers built the plant nutrients into their bone and muscle. They left their wastes – and eventually their carcasses – to the unending cycle of decay and regrowth.

Nothing was lost to the system. Nutrients were constantly recycled through the great living powerhouse of the turf, in the rampant foliage above ground or in the myriad life processes below. It was a truly sustainable system.

The tribes of Native Americans, who hunted the bison, slipped easily into the cycle. From the bison they took meats that were rich in minerals and vitamins, the gift of a fertile soil. And in due time they returned those same elements to the soil and its permanent covering of grass.

For a brief period the Europeans respected this living producer of plenty. French traders bartered with Native Americans for buffalo meat and hides to ship back east to the towns and cities. Out west the cattlemen raised their hardy Texan Longhorns on the grass-draped plains. With federal help the railroads began to snake their way across the prairies. With them came the homesteaders and their steel ploughs. But their dreams turned literally to dust when the ruined soil blew away.

In Britain, there have been no dust bowls. On this side of the Atlantic the soils are deeper and more stable. But in a less spectacular way farmers have destroyed their own fertile grasslands as effectively as the American home-steaders. Many productive pastures were simply ploughed up and sown to the ubiquitous perennial rye-grass. Others were extinguished chemically by constant applications of nitrate fertilizer.

The outcome has been the same. British grasslands are now dominated by a single species grown on soils from which trace elements have either been eliminated or ren-dered unavailable to plants. Pastures robbed of their natural mineral balance now threaten the health of animals and human beings alike.

Industrial farming has mounted a second attack on the health-giving properties of British beef. As a farming student in the 1960s I was once given a glimpse of what was being hailed as a brave new world of food production.

Early one summer's morning a group of us 'agrics' piled into a couple of cars and set out on the long journey from North Wales to Lincolnshire. Our destination was a large shed on the edge of an arable field, the kind of build-ing that had begun to appear on industrial estates on the outskirts of towns. But this was no factory for manufac-turing screws or widgets. This was a factory for making red meat.

We filed inside to where a couple of hundred young cattle stood in the half light. Never in their short lives were these animals to experience the soft tread of a pasture. Instead they were destined to spend their days standing or lying on concrete slats and eating a diet made up mostly of barley grains.

The farmer thought it a wonderful development. He guided us round his beef factory with the pride of a developer opening up the show home. In the slanted light we watched the dismal beasts munching their rations.

'It's a fantastic system,' the farmer chortled. 'I can feed this little lot in no time at all. No more messing about with grazing and fencing and all that malarkey. Dead easy, this is. And the best thing of all, the buggers grow like hell. You take it from me – the way of the future, this is.'

Barley beef was the agribusiness answer to the threat of overproduction – a threat of its own making. The deluge of substandard grain that followed the widespread adoption of chemical fertilizers brought with it the risk of a market collapse. What better way to keep up the grain price than to convert it to meat and sell it on the hoof.

Unfortunately, putting cattle on a diet of cereal grains is dangerous to the animals and to the people who will one day eat the meat. Cattle are ruminants. They are adapted to eating large amounts of fibrous vegetable matter – in a word, grass. The rumen, the first stomach in a ruminant animal, is merely a large fermentation vessel in which microorganisms get to work on the cellulose in grass, breaking it down into compounds the animal can use in its own metabolism.

Small amounts of grain do little harm. In its natural grazing environment animals consume grass seed heads in summer. Cereals are simply highly-bred grasses. But large quantities of grain invariably make cattle ill. The rumen becomes inflamed and its delicate internal ecology is thrown into turmoil. The animal develops a kind of chronic acid indigestion. Toxins leak into the bloodstream, damaging the liver and causing a range of conditions from lameness to paralysis.

On too rich a diet the animal will die. But before that happens it's likely to put on flesh at a rapid rate, which is what appeals to farmers. The chances are the beast will be ready for the butcher at a young age, before too many of the health problems have become apparent.

Today, most American beef is fattened on grains. While United States citizens cherish myths of cowboys and the open range, their steaks are raised in feedlots, large-scale meat production yards that may hold tens of thousands of cattle. The animals are moved into the feedlot as well-grown calves or yearlings. They're held in open compounds and fed by highly-automated systems on a ration made up largely of maize and soya meal with added minerals.

It's the same prairie landscape, whose boundless grasslands once raised healthy meat, which now grows grains for the feedlots. With all the costly inputs of fertilizers, pesticides and irrigation, the prairie states, that supported sixty million bison, now produce the corn and soya to fatten an estimated forty-five million beef cattle.

To Richard Manning, American author of *Grassland*, it makes little sense. He says: 'Seventy per cent of the grain crop of American agriculture goes to the livestock that replaced the bison that ate no grains, and one wonders, what is agriculture for?'[10]

This change in the way beef is reared has had damaging effects on the health of Americans. When cattle are moved from pasture to a grain diet in the feedlot, their stores of omega-3 fatty acids – including the nutritionally important EPA and DHA – begins to fall. Each day the animal spends in the feedlot reduces the supply of omega-3 fats.[11] Only forty per cent of Americans are thought to consume enough of these essential nutrients. Twenty per cent have levels so low they cannot be detected.[12]

Feedlots on the American scale are rare in Britain, but the country once famed for its beef still manages to produce its own unhealthy, cereal-fed variety. I met a Somerset dairy farmer who fattened his bull calves like this. He kept them in a shed on a ration of wheat, with soya meal to boost the protein. These were calves whose mothers had been bred as milk factories, so there wasn't too much fat on them. And it's true that filling them with high-energy cereals quickly put the flesh on.

There was just one snag, the farmer told me in all innocence. If these young animals weren't fed precisely the right amount at exactly the right time, they had a tendency to keel over and die. I suggested that maybe it wasn't a great idea to feed a diet so unnatural the cattle were prone to sudden death. What might it be doing to the quality of the meat? The farmer didn't seem concerned. It was simply a matter of being careful, he assured me.

I asked him what happened to his finished bulls, the ones that survived, that is. He told me they ended up in the 'economy mince' of a major supermarket chain.

While few UK farmers rear their beef animals entirely in sheds, most beef animals spend a good part of their lives under cover, on rations rich in cereals or other high-energy foods. Traditionally, cattle housed for the winter would be fed on hay or silage, together with root crops and a small amount of cereal. Today's intensive beef 'finishers' feed, on average, more than a tonne of high-energy concentrate feed to each beast they fatten.[13]

The aim of feeding them is to keep the beast gaining weight fast and so speed the payback time to the producer.

High-energy feeds must be balanced by protein-rich foods that can be equally damaging to the animal. Among the most widely used is soya meal, the residue remaining from soya beans after the oil has been extracted, first by crushing, then by the use of an industrial solvent. High-protein soya meal is toxic to the animal's liver.

Taking beef cattle off pasture and feeding them on cereal-rich rations has had dire consequences for the nation's health. It has exacerbated a crisis which, according to Professor Michael Crawford of North London University, is more serious than obesity. It's the sickness caused by an imbalance of essential fats in the national diet.

To remain healthy, human beings need a variety of essential fats, including two types of polyunsaturated fats, the omega-3s and omega-6 fatty acids. It's the proportion of these two fats that's important for health. In a healthy diet the ratio of omega-6 to omega-3 fats should be no higher than four to one. In the diets of our Stone Age ancestors it was believed to have been in balance.[14] And in the traditional Greek diet – thought to be the healthiest in Europe – the proportion of omega-6 to omega-3 fats is less than two to one.

In most European and American diets the ratio can be as high as twenty to one. Because of the popularity of cereal foods and oils such as sunflower oil – all of which are rich in omega-6 fats – the level of dietary omega-3 fat has dropped dramatically.

In the body the two fats act as building blocks for the membranes surrounding neurones, the nerve cells. Omega-3 fatty acids enable the cells to function efficiently. They also help them to build links with other neurones, constructing the lattice of nerve connections which is the basis of intelligence.

The last three months of a pregnancy – and the early weeks in the life of the infant – are critical times for the laying down of this brain cell lattice. To ensure the child's healthy development the mother must be getting adequate levels of omega-3 fats in her diet. These essential fats are found in vegetables such as cabbage and broccoli. They are also plentiful in fish, and in the meat of cattle grazed on pasture. The rise of factory farming and the transfer of beef cattle from grass to cereal-based diets has steadily eroded an important source of omega-3 fats and contributed to a breakdown in mental and physical health.

Pregnant women on low omega-3 diets are at increased risk of depression,[15] and their children are more likely to suffer from behavioural and co-ordination difficulties. They are also likely to score badly in IQ tests. A number of studies have shown a link between aggressive behaviour in children and low dietary levels of omega-3 fats.[16]

The effects of this fat imbalance continue into adulthood. American researchers have shown that people with low blood levels of omega-3 fats are at a higher risk of heart attack than those with higher levels. Where the level of dietary omega-3s was considered ample, the risk of a serious heart attack was reduced by half.[17]

People whose diets are rich in omega-3s are also less likely to suffer from depression, schizophrenia, hyperactivity or Alzheimer's disease,[18] and they're likely to be at reduced risk from cancer.[19]

In the light of these findings food scientists are looking at ways of boosting omega-3 fat levels in meat by adding linseed oil to the rations of housed cattle. It's the classic industrial response to a threat caused in the first place by the industrialization of agriculture.

The traditional way to raise beef was to graze cattle on pasture. By restoring cattle to their natural environment farmers could again ensure that beef made a major contribution to the level of omega-3 fatty acids in the western diet. It would have the added advantage of raising dietary levels of CLA, the powerful protector against cancer.

The decline of beef as a healthy food is reflected in the breeds of cattle that now stock the fields and cattle-yards. In the nineteenth century British beef cattle were sought around the world. Famous native breeds such as the Hereford, the North Devon, the Aberdeen Angus, the Sussex and the Welsh Black were almost synonymous with tasty, succulent beef. For almost a century Britain was known as 'stockyard to the world'. Today, those once-great breeds are hard to find, even in their own native lands.

The great merit of the traditional breeds was their efficiency in converting grass to beef. This is the job they were bred to do. Most were early maturing, which meant they 'finished' quickly, with a good covering of fat. But it was a healthy kind of fat, rich in vitamins, minerals, and polyunsaturated fats with their essential fatty acids.

In the 1970s a number of events conspired to topple the native breeds from their elevated position as the main producers of the nation's beef. Animal fats were beginning to be stigmatized as the cause of heart disease. Suddenly the traditional breeds, whose very fats had given their meats such flavour, started to look suspect.

The fat theory of heart attacks is now largely discredited. Its proponents, writes James Le Fanu, glossed over the fact that the amount of fat in the diet predicted neither the cholesterol level nor the risk of heart disease in any single country.[20] The great cholesterol deception, as he calls it, was the result of the official endorsement of a false theory.

Nutritionist Sally Fallon believes that animal fats are not merely safe, but a vital part of a healthy diet.[21] In addition to vitamins A and D, beef fat contains important fatty acids, she argues, including palmitoleic acid, an antimicrobial that protects against pathogens in the gut. It's also a good source of CLA, the polyunsaturated fatty acid that protects against cancer and promotes weight loss, but only if the beef animal has been grazing fresh pasture.

Back in the 1970s, when the animal fat/heart disease theory seemed incontestable, beef production went in precisely the wrong direction. The growing use of chemical fertilizers and pesticides was flooding the market with cheap, industrial cereal grains. Beef farmers spotted an economic advantage in using a larger animal, one that would be fast-growing but slower to mature than the native breeds. They could safely take such an animal to higher live weights without the risk of it becoming too fat. And best of all, it could be kept in a yard and fed on the new, cheaper cereals.

Turning their backs on the British breeds, farmers looked to continental Europe for their stock. Today, modern intensive beef production is dominated by breeds such as the Limousin, the Charolais, the Belgian Blue and the Simmental. They were imported to produce a large, lean carcass. The farmer would make money by growing them quickly on energy-rich diets, and the butcher would make money because they could be processed efficiently.

But the bold new era of beef production has done little for the eating quality of the product, or the health of consumers. Far from enhancing the real health benefits of beef, industrial production based on global grains has done its best to obliterate them. It has been equally damaging to our environment. The route back to sanity lies in our long-neglected pastures.

In the Shenandoah Valley of Virginia is a small farm that is fast becoming one of the best known and most influential in the United States. It's called Polyface Farm, the 'farm of many faces'. It comprises just a hundred acres of pasture set in a patchwork within a large area of forest. But this small farm produces an enormous amount of good food, including beef, chicken, turkeys, eggs, rabbits and pork, together with sweetcorn and berry fruit.[22]

Underpinning all this production is grass; not just a single species but a grass 'community' made up of dozens of grass, clover, and herb species. Across these diverse grasslands the animals are 'pastured' in turn. The beef graze them, then, as they move on, the laying hens are introduced in their portable hen-houses, known as Eggmobiles. The hens peck grubs from the grass and cowpats, in the process spreading the dung and getting rid of parasites. The eggs they produce are tasty and rich in nutrients, while their own droppings fertilize the grass for the next batch of beef cattle that will move in once it has regrown.

This simple practice of rotational grazing, understood by generations of farmers before the industrial era, produces large amounts of food. Each year the hundred acres of pasture at Polyface Farm turns out around twenty tons of beef, fifteen tons of pork, ten thousand broiler chicken, twelve hundred turkeys, a thousand rabbits and thirty-five thousand dozen eggs. To produce yields like this industrial agriculture damages the health of both consumers and the environment. The extraordinary thing about grassland farming is that it enriches both.

For all their copious output, the pastures at Polyface Farm become more fertile and productive year by year. They require no pesticides or chemical fertilizers, and the food they produce is filled with health-promoting nutrients. It's a clear demonstration of how working with natural systems as opposed to waging war on them comes close to delivering the elusive 'free lunch', in the words of *New York Times* writer Michael Pollan:

> These days, Polyface Farm gets plenty of visits from the media and politicians. As the failings of industrial agriculture become ever more apparent, this earlier pastoral model of food production makes sense. Joel Salatin, who runs Polyface Farm, has described himself variously as a 'grass farmer' and as 'Christian-conservative-libertarian-environmentalist-lunatic farmer'. One thing he's clear about is that industrial agriculture has been a disaster. His solution is something he calls 'forgiveness farming'.
>
> He explains: 'Forgiveness farming encompasses everything we are and do. It includes how other people see our farms and how *we* want to see our farms. It's abundantly practical and it's totally opposite to the industrial food system. Forgiveness farmers can lie down at night knowing we have not violated creation, we have not raped the earth, we have not angered our neighbours, and we have nurtured our families. Let's go to it.'[23]

To find healthy beef today – or lamb, chicken, and eggs, for that matter – it's necessary to find animals that have been raised on fertile, species-rich grassland. Beef cattle must have been on pasture for a substantial part of their lives, not just for a period in the middle of the fattening process. The longer an animal has run on grass the higher will be the level of omega-3 fats in the meat. It's not hard to find beef like this today. It has even started to appear in supermarkets, though it's worth buying direct from the farm where you'll see the pastures and the animals, and where the money will go direct to the family producing this fine food. For those unable to make the journey there are a growing number of good sources on the Internet.

8

Good Soil = Real Food

Most farmers now function as dispensers of chemicals. When they want to grow a crop they turn first to chemical fertilizers. These supply the major plant nutrients, nitrogen, phosphorus and potassium, in a highly soluble form. Crop plants are able to take them up quickly and produce a vigorous burst of growth, but the weakened tissue has to be sprayed with an array of pesticides to stop it succumbing to pests and diseases.

The chemical approach to feeding plants dates back to the nineteenth century and to the work of a clever and charismatic German scientist called Justus von Liebig. Since the time of Aristotle philosophers had believed that plants were sustained by organic material gathered from the soil. Although this idea came under attack in the late eighteenth century it was Liebig who finally blew it out of the water.

In a paper to the British Association for the Advancement of Science he put forward the theory that plants obtained their carbon, oxygen, hydrogen and nitrogen from the atmosphere, and the other elements they needed from the soil. These essential elements included iron, sulphur and phosphorus in the form of phosphates.

But Liebig's theory was flawed. He was wrong about atmospheric hydrogen and, in the words of Colin Tudge, author of *So Shall We Reap*, 'spectacularly wrong' about nitrogen.[1] Liebig had proposed that ammonia produced by lightning in the upper atmosphere supplied all the nitrogen plants needed. After much argument he was forced to concede that this was not enough. Plants also needed some form of nitrogen at their roots.

Traditional agriculture depends on the recycling of nitrogen through the return of organic wastes to the soil. The other great providers of nitrogen are leguminous plants such as clover and beans, which form symbiotic relationships with soil bacteria of the genus rhizobium, capable of 'fixing' nitrogen from the atmosphere. By including legumes in their crop rotations, traditional farmers were able to boost the nitrogen fertility of their land. Otherwise the vast quantities of nitrogen present in the atmosphere were largely unavailable for crop production, except for a small amount converted to ammonia by lightning and carried into the soil with rainwater.

In spite of his error Liebig produced a radical shift in thinking as he travelled up and down Britain lecturing landowners and selling his own patent fertilizer (which didn't work). Through the power of his personality he demolished the idea that there was something special about living matter; that it contained some mysterious and indefinable 'life force'. Farming was simply a matter of calculating the amounts of essential elements removed in a crop at harvest time and replacing these in the soil with some form of soluble fertilizer.

Later in life Liebig recanted his early dogmas. In notes written in 1843 he comes across as almost wretched.

> I had sinned against the wisdom of our Creator, and received just punishment for it. I wanted to improve his handiwork, and in my blindness, I believed that in his wonderful chain of laws, which ties life to the surface of the earth and always keeps it rejuvenated, there might be a link missing that had to be replaced by me – this weak powerless nothing.

Whatever his own misgivings his philosophy became rooted in a Britain gripped by the possibilities of science and industrialism. Today's farming is built on the habit of applying the major plant nutrients – nitrogen, phosphorus and potassium – in the form of chemical salts. It has become known as the NPK philosophy, and the chemical industry (which benefits handsomely from it) has succeeded in spreading it around the world.

Around the world, traditional farming based on recycled animal and vegetable wastes has been swept aside before the relentless advance of chemical agriculture.

But chemical farming is leading the world to a precipice. In the end it is bound to fail because it has ignored the one element that can ensure human health – the life of the soil.

Liebig and his modern disciples were wrong in assuming that the flooding of crop roots with soluble salts would lead to healthy plant growth. Fertile soils produce healthy growth. And soils don't become fertile just because they contain high levels of organic matter and available minerals. To promote healthy growth they also need large populations of microbes and other soil organisms, an underground army which is constantly breaking down and rebuilding nutrients from plant and animal wastes; and in the process making minerals available to plants. About 5 per cent of soil is composed of organic matter, the wastes and decomposed residues of plants and animals, together with the billions of organisms that live in the air spaces between mineral particles.

It is the actions of this living community that enable plants to grow. They supply plants with the nutrients they need, provide them with water and protect them against toxins and disease. Without the activity of soil organisms, from microscopic bacteria to earthworms, life on the planet would quickly grind to a halt. Chemical farming subjects these living communities to a non-stop toxic barrage, wiping out whole species and disrupting the intricate, below-ground network that keeps plants healthy.

With their natural support systems severely weakened, crop plants become more dependent on pesticides to keep them growing – which is great news for the chemical industry. Many agricultural soils are now so damaged by chemical fertilizers and pesticides that they need ever greater amounts to produce any crop at all. They've been turned into agrochemical junkies, wholly dependent on the local chemical supplier for the next fix.

Sometimes when you kick over a clod of earth it's hard to grasp the complexity of it. We often call it dirt. Unlike 'land', with its real estate connections, we attach little value to dirt, but it keeps us fed and would, if only we looked after it better, take care of our health.

Just a teaspoonful of healthy soil contains over five billion living organisms representing ten thousand or so different species. Most are anonymous, like the crowds in a city street. The world a few inches beneath our feet is no better known than the life of deep oceans.

What is known is that soil bacteria are likely to be the most numerous group in the teaspoon of fertile soil. There will be two to three billion of them. In size and activity they'll range from the rhizobia, the family which 'fixes' atmospheric nitrogen in special nodules in plant roots, to the threadlike actinomycetes that appear more like fungi.

Bacteria get a bad press in our society mainly because there are dozens of companies trying to sell us products to wipe them out. But of the billions of bacteria in the soil the vast majority are beneficial. They are involved in almost all metabolic processes that go on below ground. Malign species only cause trouble when the soil has been so badly mismanaged that its normal life breaks down. That's their job: to clear up the mess.

Next in complexity come the protozoa. There are likely to be around fifty thousand of them in that teaspoon of healthy soil. These single-cell animals feed mostly on bacteria from which they differ in having at least one well-defined cell nucleus. They're classed according to the way they travel through water; amoebae get about by the flowing movement of their protoplasm, ciliates by the wave motions of their hair-like *cilia*, and flagellates by the rapid flexing of their whip-like *flagella*.

Another abundant group are the soil fungi which may be single-cell yeasts or the more complex multicellular moulds. These filamentous fungi are made up of long, branching chains of cells known as *hyphae* which may be interwoven to form *mycelia*, the thin, white strands some-times visible to the naked eye in leaf litter. Filamentous fungi break down most types of organic material, from tree bark to decaying animal remains. Some species form sym-biotic relationships with plant roots, supplying the plant with some of the essential elements it needs in exchange for energy-rich secretions from the root.

Nematodes also play a key role in the below-ground drama. This group is essentially made up of worms – roundworms, threadworms and eelworms. Originally water dwellers, some forms migrated to land and became adapted to living in the pores and films of water between soil particles.

Farmers see them as the enemy, mainly because they include crop pests such as the potato cyst eelworm. But in well-managed soils nematodes aid crop production by helping to recycle nutrients and by keeping root-eating species such as the potato eelworm in check.

Of the more visible players in the drama earthworms are the stars. Charles Darwin wrote his final book on the subject of earthworms.[2] He showed that the collapse and partial burial of many of the great monumental stones at Stonehenge had been the result of earthworm activity over many centuries.

Britain has twenty-five species of which ten are common. An earthworm can live for up to five years, ingesting many times its own weight of soil each day. In doing so it creates a network of pores which improve drainage and soil aeration. Along the walls it secretes calcium-rich mucus, and from time to time it expels casts containing a range of plant nutrients. Plants' roots snake their way through these underground channels, making good use of the nutrient-rich deposits so conveniently left for them.

If earthworms are the stars of the larger soil animals, there are many others playing supporting roles. Among them are soil arthropods, including mites, springtails and beetles. This group is important in breaking up organic wastes and starting off the process of nutrient recycling. A good example is the dung beetle, which stores balls of nutrient-rich animal dung in shallow, underground channels.

In Darwinian terms these myriad life forms are locked in an unending struggle for survival and genetic immortality. Yet the outcome is seldom, as in human economic systems, the emergence of a few dominant players. A sudden catastrophic change in conditions may lead to a collapse in some species, but the natural response of the soil community is to stabilize the situation and restore diversity.

For all its savage competition the soil acts almost as a single organism spread across the land surface of the planet. Within it the ceaseless building up and breaking down of living matter accumulates minerals and locks them in the system so they are not leached away in the groundwater. And it creates humus, the group of long-chain carbon compounds which links with clay particles to form a fine, crumb structure. In short, it maintains the perfect conditions for terrestrial life.

Down through the ages farmers, with no knowledge of science, have striven to build up the life of their soils. The more active the life of the soil, the greater the store of nutrients for crop growth. In a fertile pasture producing meat or milk there'll be at least twice the weight of 'stock' below ground than there is grazing on the surface vegetation.

Traditional farmers always knew this. The return of animal and plant wastes as manure and compost was aimed at stimulating the life of the soil. Bacteria and soil fungi need a constant flow of organic material to work on or their numbers will quickly fall. When this happens nutrients are lost from the system. In extreme cases the structure breaks down and the soil dies.

Most of the mechanisms through which soil organisms nurture crop plants remain shrouded in mystery, but at Oregon State University microbiologist Professor Elaine Ingham has started to provide answers.[3] Pared down to its essentials, fertility depends on the balance between decomposers – organisms such as bacteria, fungi and certain arthropods that break down soil organic matter – and their predators.

The decomposers are responsible for holding nutrients in the topsoil so they're not washed away in the ground-water. As they get to work on organic matter in the soil the nutrients they release are incorporated into their body tissue. Bacteria and fungi together account for a large pro-portion of the nitrogen, phosphorus, sulphur, and other minerals safely secured in the topsoil.

For these minerals to become available to plants once more they must first be freed back into the soil through the process of mineralization. This is where the predators come in. They include groups such as protozoa, nema-todes, small arthropods and earthworms which feed on the bacteria and fungi. In doing so they release much of the nitrogen and other minerals so they're available to plants.

Together, protozoa and nematodes regulate the process of mineralization. But their numbers in turn are controlled by a higher order of predators such as millipedes, centipedes, beetles, spiders and small mammals. It's this constant melee of life forms, from the simplest to the advanced, that is the foundation of fertility, the provider of plenty, the guarantor of health. Elaine Ingham calls it the soil foodweb. The greater its complexity – the more momentous the underground struggle between predator and prey – the more the earth will produce.

But the farming methods of industrial countries seem designed to wreck this ordered complexity. Chemical fertilizers, pesticides, soil fungicides, and fumigants (which sterilize the soil) – the whole arsenal used by industrial farmers in their battle with nature – all kill bacteria and fungi. Overwhelmingly it's the beneficial species that are hit hardest. That's when disease organisms seize the opportunity to strike at crops.

It's a similar story to the overuse of antibiotics. When antibiotics were first introduced they seemed to offer a miracle cure for some of the world's worst disease scourges. As they were used more widely, drug-resistant organisms began to appear. At the same time beneficial bugs were knocked out by the indiscriminate new products, leaving the field clear for more malign organisms.

In the same way, when chemical fertilizers or pesticides take out bacteria and fungi in the soil, a host of dependent organisms vanish along with them. Predators are knocked out with prey species. Soon the soil ecosystem starts to break down. The normal checks and balances no longer work and disease-causing species move into the vacant space.

The best way to take care of healthy soils is to heap on organic materials, straw and crop residues, manures, and composts. A soil that's fertile and productive doesn't need chemical fertilizers or pesticides.

A Cornell University study of America's longest-running investigation into organic farming showed that getting rid of pesticide sprays and chemical fertilizers leads to more biological activity in the soil, and ultimately to more food at lower cost.[4] Led by David Pimental, the study looked at a twenty-two-year-long trial at the Rodale Institute in Pennsylvania. In it chemical farming of corn and soya beans was compared with an organic rotation where no chemicals were used.

The research team compared the activity of soil fungi on the two systems as well as a number of other aspects, including crop yields, energy efficiency, costs, and the level of organic matter. The organic system produced yields that were as high as those of the chemical system, but they achieved it with 30 per cent less energy, less water, and no pesticides. Crop yields on the organic system were particularly high in drought years. This was because wind and water erosion degraded the soil on the chemical system. On the organic soil, by contrast, the level of organic matter steadily rose along with moisture levels and the activity of soil microorganisms.

Though they wouldn't have understood the science, farmers down the ages have been feeding soil organisms with organic material, in effect taking care of the soil ecosystem and allowing the soil to provide their crops.

Former farmer John Reeves learned the hard way that soil organisms are vital to the health of plants and animals. In the early 1980s he gave up his Devon farm and set off with his wife Kate and three children, Charlotte, William and Ben, to begin a new life sheep-farming in western Canada. The farm they bought on Vancouver Island had been cleared from forest over the previous thirty years.

The climate was benign, not unlike that of eastern England, and the native forest vegetation grew thick and lush. The family had every reason to expect a bright and rewarding future.

Instead the next few years turned into a nightmare. Their lambs were born stunted and sickly. They failed to thrive, and fattening them for the market proved almost impossible. Next there was a near epidemic of broken legs among the flock. That's when Reeves began to suspect a mineral imbalance.

There was a crop of other ailments. Some lambs developed white muscle disease, a form of dystrophy in which the legs become stiff and swollen. This can be corrected with an injection of selenium. Other lambs developed swayback, a type of paralysis caused by the poor development of myelin, the insulating material that surrounds the central nervous system. This is preventable so long as the ewe obtains adequate levels of copper in the diet.

Each year there would be several cases of thiamin (vitamin B1) deficiency. Animals would drop on their sides, their heads pressed back and their front legs pedalling the air. By now Reeves had become convinced that mineral imbalances lay at the heart of his problems. He started feeding his animals special supplements to restore the missing nutrients. At last the flock became healthy again, but the losses had cost the family most of their savings. They were forced to sell up and return to Britain.

Chastened by the experience Reeves spent the next twenty years carrying out his own research on soil minerals, and the way they're taken up by crops. He teamed up with a university chemist to get the necessary analysis done. He's now convinced of the vital role played by one particular group of soil organisms. Without them plants can't take up all the minerals they need so the animals, and people, eating them are more likely to become sick. But it's a group of organisms that industrial agriculture has done its best to obliterate.

These are a group of filamentous fungi known collectively as mycorrhiza. The threadlike fungi form intimate links with plant roots, actually penetrating the cells of the root cortex. It's a mutually beneficial arrangement known in biology as symbiosis. The plant supplies the fungus with carbohydrates and amino acids in its sap. In return the fungus supplies the plant with minerals, helps it to resist drought and protects it against soil-borne diseases and harmful nematodes.

In effect, mycorrhiza form an extension of the plant's root system. There are thought to be seven groups of the fungus, most of which are specialized for particular plant families. The largest group are the vesicular-arbuscular mycorrhizae (VAM), so called because they form little sac-like structures – or arbuscules – inside the root cells. These increase the surface area across which the plant can trade nutrients for minerals.

The VAM can increase the absorbing surface of the plant's root hairs by up to one hundred thousand times. And they can enhance the uptake of soil nutrients such as phosphorus, zinc, copper and magnesium by up to sixty times. That's why these little-known organisms are so essential to human health.

Mycorrhizae are thought to have evolved more than three hundred million years ago, in evolutionary terms not long after the appearance of land plants. They evolved to form symbiotic links with the roots of most plant species.

Biologists have known about them for a century. Because of the power of the chemical industry they've been largely ignored. But thanks to the conviction and dogged determination of a scientific amateur the human cost of that neglect is becoming clear.

I tracked down John Reeves in a tucked-away cottage on the edge of a small community in the Forest of Dean, in Gloucestershire. Since he returned from Canada he has carried out dozens of experiments on plant minerals. His aim was to find out how the presence or absence of mycorrhiza in the soil effects the mineral content of the crops it grows. He admitted to being sceptical at the start. The idea that a soil fungus could have a significant influence on the nutritional quality, as well as the yield, of a crop seemed fanciful.

He's sceptical no longer. Today, he's convinced we'll never again eat healthy foods until we return to a system of farming that protects these valuable organisms. And that means getting rid of most of our chemical fertilizers and sprays.

He carried out his experiments on a number of different soils, though many were done on his own land, a magnesium limestone soil to the south of the Forest of Dean. He enlisted the help of a university chemist to carry out the mineral analyses on his plant samples. A sympathetic scientist at Rothamsted experimental station in Hertfordshire supplied the innoculum of mycorrhiza.

Reeves devised his own mineral score sheet to represent the overall content of fourteen essential trace elements, including boron, cobalt, copper, iron, magnesium, zinc and selenium. He included in his trials a range of everyday vegetables: carrots, peas, onions, parsnips, potatoes and broad beans.

When the vegetables were grown on cultivated soils without chemical fertilizers their mineral scores were satisfactory, though not high. But when they were grown on soils that had been treated with chemical fertilizer, phosphate, they contained up to a quarter fewer minerals.

Innoculating soils with mycorrhiza had the opposite effect: the mineral scores soared. Comparing the two treatments, vegetables grown on soils with healthy populations of mycorrhiza contained up to two-thirds more minerals than those from soils fertilized by chemicals.

Reeves also looked at a number of farm crops, including wheat and pasture grass. As with vegetables, both the physical act of cultivating the soil and the application of chemical fertilizers destroyed mycorrhiza and depleted growing crops of minerals.

With wheat, he found that soil cultivation reduced the mineral content of grain by 25 per cent. Putting on chemical fertilizer reduced mineral levels still further, but when the cultivated soil was inoculated with mycorrhiza it again grew wheat containing the full complement of minerals.

Reeves made similar observations of pasture grasses. Grass leaves taken from long-established pasture contained high levels of essential trace elements, but when soils were sown back to grassland after five years of cultivation for crops, the resulting grass showed far lower levels of minerals. Selenium was reduced to almost half, boron and molybdenum by around 40 per cent, cobalt and copper by 30 per cent, and manganese and nickel by 20 per cent or more.[5]

Reeves believes his results show why there is so much ill health in western societies. They have relied on chemical fertilizers to grow most of their food. Yet those same chemicals, particularly phosphates, destroy the natural system for growing healthy, nutrient-filled crops.

And if that weren't enough, most farmers rely on fungicide sprays to deal with diseases on their crops. The irony is that these chemicals are also likely to be killing the very soil fungi that could prevent their crops becoming diseased in the first place.

Looking back, Reeves attributes the failure of his sheep farming venture to the absence of the *right species* of mycorrhiza on his land. It had been newly reclaimed from the forest, so the fungal species present would have been those adapted to forest trees. Even if they survived they'd have been unable to establish a symbiotic association with grass roots. This is why the pastures were depleted in minerals and the animals became sick.

All this was known by farmers a century and a half ago. In 1850, James Caird, a leading farming commentator, was commissioned by *The Times* to undertake a survey of English agriculture. In his report from Hertfordshire he describes a system for 'inoculating' new grassland so it would quickly become productive. Though the farmer would not have understood the science, the technique ensured that the new pasture contained the right types of mycorrhiza for healthy and nutritious grass.

> A small plough is passed along an old pasture, from which it throws out about three inches of turf and leaves a little more, returning again with another strip of turf, of the same breadth, until the requisite quantity is obtained. A corn drill is then passed over the ground to be inoculated, the coulters of which mark it off in rows at eight inches apart. The sod is

then cut into little pieces and laid down in the rows, each piece about four inches apart, by men who then tread it into the ground. This must be done in damp weather in September or October. In spring the ground is rolled and a little Dutch clover is sown, after which the whole is allowed to seed itself, and stock is put on in autumn. By this process a fine pasture is rapidly formed.[6]

Today, the essential role of mycorrhiza in maintaining the nutrient content of crops has been forgotten. According to Reeves, modern farming methods are fast destroying soil organisms that have supported plant life for millions of years. He explains: 'There's no need for pesticides or chemical fertilizers. By inoculating soils with mycorrhiza we could easily restore the natural systems that keep plants healthy and adequately supplied with minerals. Our crops would be protected against disease, and the foods they produced would be rich in nutrients. It's not credible that plants, animals and humans could have evolved with the requirement for higher levels of minerals than were provided by nature, but until we restore these natural systems we can't rely on the food supply to deliver them.'

Reeves wants to see food producers introduce quality controls for their products that take account of nutrient content as well as cosmetic appearance. In the meantime, he believes, consumers will have to rely on mineral supplements to make up the shortfall in everyday foods.

The chemist who analysed the mineral content of plants in Reeves's investigation was Neil Ward, of Surrey University's School of Biomedical Molecular Science.

Ward, too, thinks the reintroduction of mycorrhiza in agriculture would do much to enhance the nutrient status of foods.

A New Zealander, he grew up in a farming community where many of his relatives still farm. As a result of the UK trial results he suggested that an uncle farming in an arid region of New Zealand try using mycorrhiza to improve the pastures.

The advice proved very sound. Inoculation of the soil with the beneficial fungi resulted in an immediate improvement, Ward reports, with the turf growing thicker and more lush.

He'd like to see mycorrhizae sold in garden centres throughout Britain, though he has no great hopes that mainstream agriculture will embrace the technique. The chemical industry has too much to lose. With colleague John Reeves he has made the findings available to the Department for the Environment, Food and Rural Affairs (Defra). So far there has been no government commitment to research funding.

Ward is currently involved in research on the use of mycorrhizae to establish grasslands in arid regions of several South American countries. While there's plenty of backing for the development of genetically modified crops in such areas, there's less interest in mycorrhiza, the natural way of protecting plants in unfavourable climatic conditions.

In Scotland, I called to see another amateur farming sleuth who's convinced chemical farming damages our food. Former farmer Tom Stockdale once worked for the fertilizer company ICI. Now he thinks the high-nitrogen fertilizers sold by chemical companies have harmed many

UK soils. As a result they've been the cause of ill-health among both human and animal populations.

He has good grounds for his claim. During his time as a farmer he became very ill as a result of a mineral imbalance. The crisis spurred him to carry out a detailed study of soils and the way they're managed. Today, he's more than ever convinced that the wide-scale use of high-nitrogen fertilizers is neither safe nor sustainable. And he fears the world's much-vaunted 'green revolution', with its dependence on fertilizer nitrogen, is doomed to fail.

Stockdale is now retired, though his interest in soils and their effects on health remain undimmed. I met him in his solid, stone-built house on the outskirts of Dumfries. The day I called the dining-table was covered with technical books and papers, so we chatted in the sun-filled conservatory.

The son of a Cambridge chemistry don, he has had a lifelong passion for farming. With his Cambridge agriculture diploma, he joined ICI in the late fifties. He recalls with a wry smile that the day he started with the company was April Fools' Day.

'I was interested in the science of farming,' he says. 'But ICI was mainly interested in selling fertilizer. So it was pretty obvious we weren't going to be together for long.

'Up until that time most fertilizers were impure, which was an advantage in that it meant they contained trace elements. For example, most farmers used basic slag, a by-product of the steel industry, containing a lot of minerals. But ICI was just introducing its new, high-nitrogen fertilizers, so pure they contained no trace elements.

'The company was pushing them hard. Selling fertilizers wasn't a job I relished, so we decided – as a family – to go farming.'

Tom and his wife Margaret took the tenancy of a small hill farm in Scotland. There he started applying all 'the wonderful new methods' he'd learned at ICI, especially the use of high-nitrogen fertilizer. It soon became apparent something was going badly wrong.

His barley crops germinated well, then quickly began losing ground. The plants were stunted and the leaves turned purple. The plant roots were short and jagged – 'fanged' is how he described them. Eventually the plants became so frail and light that they seemed about to blow away.

At the same time the black coats of his Aberdeen Angus cattle started turning a dirty brown colour. Many of them 'scoured' – the cattle equivalent of getting diarrhoea. Slowly their grazing fields were taken over by moss.

A farm advisor he'd called in to help criticized him for failing to control the weeds in his crops, although he'd already sprayed them many times. After each dose of herbicide the weeds seemed to come back stronger than ever, even though the crops had failed. In desperation he resorted to even stronger, and more expensive, weed-killers, all to no avail.

It wasn't just the livestock that were ailing. Soon Stockdale himself became ill. On two occasions he was poisoned by the element molybdenum after it had found its way into the farm's private water supply.

When soils become anaerobic, lacking in oxygen, and lose their structure, the living processes that normally regulate the release of minerals break down. So potentially toxic elements such as molybdenum appear in ionic form in the soil water to act as rogue poisons.

Stockdale's condition worsened. He lacked energy and hardly dared look in a mirror, so awful had his appearance become. In his search for answers he began talking to specialists in trace elements. One of them commented that his symptoms sounded like selenium deficiency. So he and his family started taking selenium tablets. Very soon the symptoms disappeared.

Since his health crisis Stockdale has spent many years studying the role of selenium in the metabolism of plants and animals, and in the way chemical fertilizers disrupt natural processes. The findings have confirmed his belief that today's heavy use of high-nitrogen fertilizers is leading Britain, and other countries, to a health disaster.

When these products were introduced back in the 1960s they were tested mainly on the alkaline soils of southern and eastern England. On the basis of these findings the fertilizer companies introduced recommendations for their use across the country. However, most of UK soils are not alkaline but acid. They're on the igneous and metamorphic rocks that make up the bulk of the country. In these areas high-nitrogen fertilizers damage soil structure and produce crops that are depleted of minerals.

It's the deficiency of selenium that worries Tom Stockdale most. Since his own illness he has become an expert on the physiological effects. With insufficient selenium the body is unable to activate the thyroid hormone thyroxine, he says. The body is starved of energy, and any of a number of vital functions are likely to break down.

A marginal deficiency of selenium over many years can lead to coronary heart disease, he says, while those severely affected can suffer conditions such as obesity, depression and late-onset diabetes.[7] Some of these conditions can induce stress, leading to panic attacks or outbreaks of irrational anger.

Chemical farming is portrayed as a great triumph of western technology because it produces mountains of grain and tanker-loads of milk. But it's hardly a triumph to ruin the nation's health. And who can take pride in a system that destroys the earth's most precious asset – its soil?

9

Butter, Cholesterol And Omega-3

Today, milk and dairy products are demonized by diet propagandists. This is because a large proportion of their fats are in the form of saturates, and these are believed to be unhealthy. The idea originates from the theory, developed in the fifties and sixties, that animal fats and cholesterol in foods raise blood cholesterol, which then builds up in the arteries to cause heart disease. The theory has now been largely debunked.[1] Experimental evidence finally refuting the diet/heart disease theory emerged in the early 1980s.[2]

Far from being harmful, saturated fats play an important role in human nutrition. They enhance the immune system, protect against pathogens, provide energy to the heart and are essential to the function of the kidneys and lungs.[3] Despite this, many now believe saturated fats to be wholly bad.

As if this weren't enough, a growing number of people now appear to be intolerant of milk. Medical journals have run a string of articles on milk allergies in babies and young children. What the authors seldom reveal is that almost all these allergies are to pasteurized milk. The process of pasteurization, heating it to a high temperature for a short period, can denature the milk proteins.

A century ago a diet of unpasteurized, whole milk was widely recommended as the cure to a range of conditions including diabetes, gastric ulcers, obesity and kidney disease. In the United States a doctor called Charles Sanford Porter published *Milk Diet as a Remedy for Chronic Disease*, a book which ran to eleven editions. In it he wrote: 'A good food is a good remedy, and, as disease is only a disturbance of the mechanism of nutrition, it is only natural that the use of milk in ill health should be almost as old as its use as a food in health.'[4]

Porter insisted that the milk must be unpasteurized. 'What is required is good, clean milk as it comes from the cow, without the removal or addition of any substance whatsoever. Boiled, sterilized or pasteurized milk – or milk artificially preserved in any way – cannot be used for this treatment. Pasteurizing milk renders it unsuitable for human use.'

There's a sound basis for Porter's argument. Pasteurization destroys milk enzymes, which would other-wise help the body assimilate nutrients, including calcium.[5] It also destroys the lactic-acid-producing bacteria which protect against pathogens. It destroys vitamins and makes many of milk's most valuable trace elements less available.

In 1929, Dr J. R. Crewe of the Mayo Foundation, in Rochester, Minnesota, published an article on the benefits of milk in the *Certified Milk Magazine*.[6] In it he claimed to have used unpasteurized milk to improve a variety of health conditions, including obesity, heart disease, diabetes, prostrate enlargement, tuberculosis and high blood pressure.

Modern science has confirmed the health benefits of milk and dairy foods produced in the traditional way from the milk of cows grazing on fertile, fast-growing pastures. Cows are adapted to eating grass. It is their natural food. Evolution has equipped them with a large fermentation chamber, the rumen, in which fibrous materials, low in energy, are broken down by resident microorganisms. This is, after all, why human beings domesticated them in the first place. Ruminants have the capacity to convert inedible roughages into food.

In Europe, cows were traditionally calved in spring. So the peak demand for milk came at the time when the growth of fresh green grass was at its most vigorous. Many rural peoples, like those of the Loetschental Valley, placed a special value on the deep yellow butter made from the milk of cows feeding on this early spring grass. They knew intuitively that its life-enhancing qualities were especially beneficial to children and expectant mothers.

Milk from cows feeding on young fresh grass contains high levels of the fat-soluble vitamins A, D, K and E. So butter made from this milk is a rich source. Vitamin A is more easily absorbed from butter than from other foods.

Vitamins A and E are powerful antioxidants. They protect the body against damaging pollutants and free radicals, so acting as anti-cancer agents.

Vitamin D, like vitamin A, is needed for calcium and phosphorus absorption. It is essential for strong bones and teeth, and for normal growth. Vitamin K is a key factor in blood clotting. Like the other fat-soluble vitamins, it also plays a role in bone formation.

Milk from grass-fed cows contains high levels of essential fatty acids, particularly omega-3 linoleic acid together with CLA, with its strong anti-cancer properties. Even small amounts of milk and cheese from pasture-fed cows have been linked to a significant fall in the cancer risk. One researcher estimated that eating one serving daily of grass-fed meat, plus one ounce of cheese and one glass of whole milk from a grass-fed cow, could significantly reduce the risk of cancer.[7]

CLA is produced in large amounts by cows eating fresh, green pasture.[8] But when cows are fed on small amounts of grain, or even on grass that has been cut and conserved in the form of silage, its level in milk falls away dramatically.[9] And as with beef there's evidence that traditional pastures containing plants like plantain, self-heal, rough hawkbit, red clover, and bird's-foot trefoil produce milk with higher CLA levels than all-grass pastures.[10]

When milk is turned into cheese, the way the cheese is made has a big influence on the level of CLA it contains. In general, the longer a cheese is aged, the lower the CLA. So hard cheeses such as Parmesan will contain less of this health-promoting compound than softer cheeses like cream cheese, cottage cheese, Feta and Brie.[11] A serving of high-fat cheese will usually contain more CLA than a similar serving of low-fat cheese. There's also evidence that artisan cheeses aged by 'bacterial surface ripening' contain more CLA than cheeses not matured this way.

Organically produced milk is known to be richer in many nutrients than conventional milk because, under European law, organic dairy farmers are required to feed a high proportion of home-grown forage feeds to their cattle. In practice, this means cows spend a lot of time grazing on grass and clover pastures. As a result, organic milk has been found to be 50 per cent higher in vitamin E, 75 per cent higher in beta-carotene (converted in the body to vitamin A), and two to three times higher in the anti-oxidants lutein and zeaxanthine.[12]

Research at the University of Aberdeen showed that levels of omega-3 fats were, on average, 30 per cent higher in organic milk than in non-organic milk.[13] But the differences were far higher in the summer months when the organically farmed cows had greater access to fresh grass and clover-rich pastures.

Without the benefit of modern scientific knowledge the traditional dairy farmers of Europe knew their summer pastures delivered the healthiest and most nutritious dairy foods. It's a belief that persisted well into the twentieth century. A Dairy Council advert of the time showed three young boys sharing a glass of milk. The caption read: 'You'll feel a lot better if you drink more milk.' Today's dairy advertising still targets young people.

On its stand at the 2004 Dairy Event, the national show for UK dairy farmers, the Milk Development Council displayed life-sized cut-outs of two smiling teenage girls. Surveys had shown they were the group most likely to be short of calcium in their diet. In response the industry's 'Three a Day' campaign warned that low-calcium diets could lead to osteoporosis in later life. Three portions of milk, yoghurt, or cheese every day were a simple way to meet calcium requirements, said the advert. Among other benefits, milk and dairy products were claimed to give protection against colon and breast cancer, a benefit thought to be linked to their calcium and vitamin D content.[14]

What the adverts don't tell you is that damaging changes in the way milk is produced has depleted it of the vitamins the body needs to make use of calcium in the diet. And that far from enhancing its natural, cancer-fighting properties, the changes have blunted them.

In a little over a generation, dairy farming has been transformed from a natural process into an industrial operation. In that time the health benefits of milk have been systematically eroded, and the role of the dairy cow has changed from one of generous companion to abused and over-exploited slave.

In the 1960s, the average yield of a British dairy cow was a little over three thousand five hundred litres a year. Today, the average is almost double this, with some high-production herds notching up ten thousand litres or more. The cow is able to transfer only a fixed amount of vitamins to her milk. The greater her milk volume, the more dilute its vitamin content, particularly for vitamin E and beta-carotene, a precursor of vitamin A. The unimproved cows may have put less milk in the tank at the end of every day, but while they were grazing fresh pasture it was milk packed with nutrients.

The modern Holstein super-cow is little more than a walking milk generator. To achieve these levels of output the cattle breeders have selected from animals with over-active pituitary glands. The pituitary not only secretes hormones that stimulate the production of milk, it also produces growth hormones. These inevitably turn up in the milk. High levels of pituitary hormones have been linked to the formation of tumours.[15]

The development of what nutritionist Sally Fallon calls the 'freak pituitary cow' has led to dramatic changes in the way herds are fed. Grass, the natural food of ruminants, is unable to provide the energy-rich and protein-dense rations these high-performance animals need in their genetically programmed drive to produce vast quantities of milk. Unless they are fed nutrients in concentrated form they will break down their own body tissue to the point of collapse.

No longer can they be left to graze pasture alone for a large part of the year. Grass must now be supplemented with a range of industrial feeds, many of which spoil the nutritional value of the milk.

Cereals such as wheat, maize and barley are among the starchy foods chosen to boost energy levels in the diet of high-yielding cows. These industrial grains are cheap and plentiful. But there are other, equally damaging foods on offer: potato waste; bread discarded by the factory bakers; breakfast cereals that for one reason or another have been rejected for the human food chain.

These energy-rich foods have to be 'balanced' with feeds supplying concentrated forms of protein. This is why dairy farmers embarked on the disastrous practice of feeding meat-and-bone meal to their cows, a move that may have caused the spread of mad cow disease and its human equivalent. Had dairy farmers not chosen to base their production on 'abnormal' cows they wouldn't have needed to resort to abnormal diets to sustain their excessive output.

Today, farmers rely heavily on soya bean meal to supply protein in concentrated form. Unfortunately most soya, like cereals, is grown with heavy inputs of pesticide and chemical fertilizer. Other widely used protein feeds include groundnut meal, rapeseed meal and cottonseed meal.

On today's factory farms, grazed grass produces less than one-sixth of the milk that goes into the food chain.

The rest is produced from other feed materials. That's why our dairy foods no longer have the health-giving properties of those from traditional farming systems based on flower-rich pastures.

The healthy omega-3 fats of grass-fed milk are largely eliminated on these industrial rations. Instead, the milk fat is almost entirely made up of saturated fats together with omega-6 polyunsaturated fats which occur too widely in western diets. These high-octane dairy rations also depress the levels of CLA in milk, so reducing its protective effects against cancer. Fat-soluble vitamins are reduced; so are the antioxidants lutein and zeaxanthine.

The findings explain why milk produced by traditional methods was so widely regarded as a healthy food. Under the rules of organic production cows eat large amounts of fresh grass and clover, just as they did on the Swiss mountainside visited by Weston Price.

Taking ruminants off grass is as damaging for dairy cows as it is for beef cattle. Too much starchy food in the diet increases the acidity of the cow's rumen, particularly when it's fed in large amounts. The rumen microbes respond by producing excess lactic acid, some of which is absorbed into the bloodstream where it disrupts the animal's normal metabolism.

Toxins, too, are released into the bloodstream. These are produced by the decay of microorganisms killed in the over-acid conditions. Other pathogenic microbes seize the opportunity and multiply rapidly. This is why high-yielding cows are beset by ill-health.

There are dangers for consumers, too. In the highly-acid intestinal conditions of cows fed mainly on grain, the bacteria that thrive include the acid-resistant pathogens most harmful to human beings. Among the most dangerous is the *E. coli* strain O157. It takes as few as ten organisms to cause illness, even death in humans. Their numbers in cattle fed inside on grain and silage are far higher than in cattle fed mainly on grass and hay.

Disease is endemic in modern intensive dairy units. As many as 40 per cent of the national herd suffers from some form of mastitis, or udder infection. A Bristol University survey put the average incidence of clinical mastitis in Britain's dairy cows at almost 70 per cent.[16] This means they are secreting pus cells into the milk which ends up in our 'healthy' yoghurt or milkshake.

In a bid to limit the epidemic, farmers routinely squirt antibiotics up the teats of their cows during the 'dry' period, the short period between lactation cycles. But antibiotics deal with the symptoms, not with the cause of disease. Cows are ill because of the way they're managed.

Faulty feeding lies behind another modern affliction of dairy cows, lameness. Around a quarter of the national dairy herd suffers from lameness, commonly caused by a restriction in the blood supply to the feet. Toxins and histamines in the blood, the result of over-acidic conditions in the rumen, permanently damage the blood vessels supplying the tissues of the foot. As a result the feet of many modern dairy cows are susceptible to damage and infection.

As if this weren't enough, the stresses on these high-performing cows have led to a rising tide of infertility. Conception rates have fallen dramatically, chiefly because the overworked animals cannot meet the huge physical demands made on them.

In the early weeks of each lactation they are expected to produce up to fifty litres of milk every day. In an instinctive drive to meet their genetically programmed targets they 'milk off their backs,' in the old farming expression, metabolizing their own body tissues and diverting the products into milk. At the same time they are expected to get into calf again. Not surprisingly, many fail to achieve this.

The excessive breakdown of body tissue clogs up the liver with fat. Hormone secretion is disrupted and conception rates fall away. More often than not the stressed-out animal is labelled as infertile and sent off to market.

In the face of such abuse it's not surprising that the average dairy cow is worn out by the time she has completed her third lactation cycle. Traditional breeds grazing naturally on herb-rich pastures for much of the year will remain productive for ten years or more.

Today, half of all UK dairy cows are sent for slaughter after just two years of milking. The chief reason given by farmers is that they failed to get in calf quickly enough. The sensible solution would be to return dairy cows to the habitat evolution prepared them for, open grassland, but the economics of modern milk production don't allow this. So an army of scientists are kept busy searching for technical fixes to add to the growing list of disasters resulting from industrial agriculture.

The current method of feeding cows is by a system called TMR (total mixed rations). All the ingredients that go to make up a cow's diet are blended together in a large, mobile mixing tub. The TMR is carefully formulated to keep the animal on her production target.

First there are fibrous foods or forages, mostly grass and maize silage, to keep the cow's digestive system in some sort of order. The mix will also contain energy-rich cereals and high-protein feeds to push up milk yields. Because these are mainly grown by intensive methods and are dependent on chemical fertilizers they're likely to be deficient in essential minerals. So an artificial mineral supplement is added to the mix, though it can be no substitute for nutrient-rich feeds.

TMR is the dairy technologists' answer to the problems of feeding the yield-freak cows they themselves have produced. The aim is to churn out the milk to a minimal quality standard at the lowest possible price.

A great deal of science goes into ration formulation. There's much discussion between farmers and feed company specialists about such things as energy density, starch-to-sugar ratio and the level of utilizable protein. The animals must be goaded into producing their fifty litres a day.

But what TMR doesn't deliver is milk rich in health-giving CLAs, omega-3 fatty acids, vitamins and minerals. This is the product of cows on their natural food, especially the fast-growing green grass of spring and autumn. Grass preserved for winter in the form of silage cannot produce the CLAs of fresh pasture.

In May 2005, the dairy company Dairy Crest launched St Ivel Advance, an omega-3-enriched milk.[17] It was endorsed by Professor Robert Winston of Imperial College's Institute of Reproductive and Developmental Biology. On the Dairy Crest website he warned parents that today's children were not getting enough omega-3 in their diets, and he welcomed its availability in a user-friendly format. It was sound advice. The supplementation of children's diets with essential fatty acids has been found to improve reading, spelling and behaviour of schoolchildren.[18]

There are benefits for the rest of the population, too. Omega-3 fats protect against heart disease and strokes, reduce joint pain and inflammatory conditions, and improve foetal development in pregnant women. The Dairy Crest marketing experts clearly believed the benefits of omega-3 fats were well enough known to stimulate a keen demand for their product.

Of course, you might wonder why milk needs to be enriched in this important nutrient. It's plentiful in the milk of cows that spend much of the year grazing pasture in the traditional way. If cows were put back on the grass the levels of omega-3 in their diet would rise along with vitamins, CLA, and possibly many other valuable nutrients that the scientists have yet to evaluate. But livestock nutritionists have discovered that they can raise the omega-3 content of milk by boosting the levels of oils such as flaxseed oil in the rations of housed cattle. So the cows stay in their sheds instead of treading the fresh green sward.

On average, British dairy cows spend only half their lives on pastures. The average includes a number of smaller herds still managed by traditional methods. At the other end of the scale are large herds whose cows hardly set foot on grass at all.

An increasing number of large herds are today kept in sheds for months on end. Inside, their rations can be more carefully controlled. Why go to all the trouble of turning them out to grass when cheap, chemically-grown grains and industrial by-products will keep milk flowing into the tank?

The big dairy processing companies are adding to the pressures on natural production methods. On traditional farms cows calved in the spring. The flush of grass in early summer coincided with the peak in the cow's lactation curve, and it was this seasonal surplus of milk that was turned into butter. This was the deep yellow butter, rich in antioxidants and protective fats.

In today's dairy industry the efficient running of processing plants has become more important than the nutritional quality of the product. The dairy companies understandably want to see their plants running at optimum capacity throughout the year, so they offer farmers substantial bonuses on the milk they produce in autumn and winter, when grass is hardly growing. This forces them to use even larger amounts of grain and industrial by-products in the ration.

Early in 2004 the weekly farming paper *Farmers Guardian* featured the 'revolutionary' new milking parlour of a West Country dairy farmer. The paper reported that he had travelled to California to look at large-scale dairy farms. He had come back determined to set up something similar in the UK.

According to the report he now had a building big enough to accommodate up to six hundred cows. The roof area totalled more than an acre and a half. Though it was made up partly of translucent panels, ensuring that the interior was very light, the building was equipped with 170 electric lights to provide round-the-clock daylight if needed. This was the result of American research showing that extended daylight could increase milk production.

For high-yielding cows this vast new building was to be their entire world. While lower yielders were turned out to grass for a few weeks in summer, said the report, the top yielders were housed all year round. At milking time they simply walked from their cubicles to the central milking parlour and gathering yard. 'The new system has been designed around maximizing production and minimizing labour input while maintaining high welfare standards,' stated *Farmers Guardian*.

While the scientific basis of healthy milk and dairy products is becoming ever clearer, the ruthless economics of modern milk production are driving farmers in precisely the wrong direction. Modern dairy farming has increasingly confined animals to sheds and to steel-and-concrete cubicles. Though all-year-round housing is still uncommon in the UK, many cows spend the greater part of the year shut away in buildings. When they are out on grass in summer, it's a pasture very different from that grown on the traditional mixed farm.

The temporary grass 'leys' on which the cows grazed were part of the arable rotation. After two or three years under grass the field would be ploughed up for wheat. Even though a pasture was only due to stay down for two or three years, the farmer would sow a mixture of grasses and herb species. It was considered important to provide grazing animals with a variety of nutritious vegetation.

Through the 1950s and 1960s government farm advisors worked closely with fertilizer companies to cajole farmers into abandoning their species-rich pastures and relying instead on grass monocultures.

Modern ryegrass varieties, like wheat varieties, are bred to respond to high levels of chemical fertilizer. In 1950, British farmers spread just five kilograms of nitrate fertilizer to every acre of grassland. Today, they are using twenty-five times as much, with some using almost one hundred times more.

As chemical nitrogen rates went up, so the ryegrass monocultures put on more growth, allowing the farmer to keep more cows on fewer acres. No one worried too much about the nutrient content of the extra grass. Nor were they concerned with the effect on milk quality.

Next came a campaign to convert dairy farmers to silage-making. Until the sixties most farmers made hay as their chief winter fodder crop. The chemical companies weren't happy with this. Hay meadows were cut just once a year and were rich in fertility-building clovers and wild plant species. They didn't need much fertilizer to produce a good crop.

Working with the government's farm advisors, fertilizer representatives mounted a vigorous campaign to persuade farmers that they should rely on silage instead of hay. Silage, grown as a ryegrass monoculture, is cut two or three times in a season, and requires large amounts of chemical fertilizer,

Today, Britain's flower-rich hay meadows have largely vanished, killed off by chemical nitrogen. Instead of hay, cows munch grass silage in their TMR diets. Like chemical wheat from the arable fields, this 'forced' grass is depleted of minerals and vitamins and therefore the milk that goes into the farm tanker is too. Milk produced by cows eating hay contains far more healthy omega-3 fats than the milk of cows on silage.[19]

Though it was British politicians who first began the process of ruining the nation's milk supply, it was the EU that completed the job. Under the common agricultural policy farm ministers worked unstintingly to 'modernize' Europe's more 'backward' farms. This meant promoting large-scale industrial farming. Through the 1970s and

1980s they offered dairy farmers huge grants and loans to enlarge their herds and put up vast sheds to house them.

Alongside the grants they operated market support arrangements that consistently favoured large-scale producers and discriminated against small farmers. Long after the butter mountains and the milk lakes had become a political scandal, Britain's dairy farmers were being exhorted to increase production by feeding ever more starchy cereals to their overworked cows.

By the early 1980s the politicians knew that milk quotas were inevitable if Europe's growing surpluses were to be reined in. Milk quotas, when they came, heaped rewards on intensive farmers, those who had pushed their animals to the limit in the race for higher output. Those who had refused to farm that way – and who had maintained the health of their cattle by keeping them on forage diets instead of starchy foods – were penalized with lower quotas. Many never recovered and were forced out of business.

The industrialization of milk production has brought few benefits for dairy farmers. Today, they're getting out at an unprecedented rate. In the early seventies there were a hundred thousand dairy farmers in Britain. Four out of five of them have now gone and the drop-out rate is increasing. By the autumn of 2007 there were just fourteen thousand dairy farmers left in Britain, and the drop-out rate was still running at three a day. Among the casualties were some of the best farmers in the country.

Those that remain are turning themselves into factory-scale operations. Many modern dairy units are little more than a collection of industrial sheds, surrounded by acres of concrete and lit by security lights.

These are no longer farms. They are rural factories driven by the ethics of industry. The overriding aim is to drive down costs, to produce every litre of milk at the lowest possible price. 'Get bigger or get out' is the background refrain of bankers, accountants, management consultants, and the vast army of advisors who have their own reasons for seeing farming behave like any other business.

To be fair, many dairy farmers feel they no longer have any choice in the matter. They feel they're being pressed like some gigantic Cheddar cheese, and turning the screw are the supermarkets and the big milk processors.

A study by the Milk Development Council shows just who is making money out of today's commodity milk.[20] Over the decade to April 2004, prices received by farmers fell by a quarter. Prices to processors, the big dairy companies and co-operatives that buy milk from farmers and sell it on to supermarkets, remained fairly stable. The big winners were the supermarkets, dominated by a handful of giant multiples, Tesco, Asda, Morrisons and Sainsbury's. Their margins almost doubled over the ten-year period.

In 2003, the retail price for liquid milk averaged 47 pence a litre. Of this, farmers received just 18 pence. The processors took 16 pence, and the big retailers 13 pence. In the autumn of 2007 the milk price at last began to rise, the result of a surge in demand for milk products in China and the Far East, but the improvement came too late to save many dairy farmers.

To stay in the game dairy farmers pack more cows into their sheds, and constantly search for cheaper materials to feed them on. It's a game that has few winners. Farmers come under increasing strain while making little profit. Their long-suffering animals are goaded into producing even more milk, despite the toll in ill-health, and consumers are supplied with products that are, at best, depleted in nutrients, and may at time be downright hazardous. The supermarkets, by contrast, make bigger margins than ever.

Predictably the same social and economic forces that have downgraded British milk are at work in the United States. There, too, herds have grown larger, cows are increasingly kept in 'confinement' rather than outside on pasture and small family farms are being driven to the wall. Food campaigners have had enough. They're intent on turning the tide, and the method they've chosen is modelled on a small revolution that took place in the UK.

In 1999, the Weston A. Price Foundation of Washington, a non-profit-making organization set up to disseminate the discoveries of the nutrition pioneer, launched 'A Campaign for Real Milk'. It was inspired by a group of English men who sat in a pub back in the 1970s and bemoaned the rise of the corporate brewers and the threat to British ale. Out of that meeting sprang the Campaign for Real Ale (CAMRA), the movement which saved traditional beer.

According to the Real Milk Campaign website, 'Back in the 1920s, Americans could buy fresh raw whole milk, real clabber and buttermilk, luscious naturally-yellow butter, fresh farm cheeses and cream in various colours and thicknesses. Today's milk is accused of causing everything from allergies to heart disease and cancer, but when Americans could buy Real Milk, these diseases were rare. In fact, a supply of high quality dairy products was considered vital to American security and the economic well-being of the nation.

'What's needed today is a return to humane, non-toxic, pasture-based dairying and small-scale traditional processing.'[21]

Ron Schmid, naturopathic physician and author of *The Untold Story of Milk*, writes of buying 23 acres of land at Watertown, Connecticut, land that had once been a small dairy farm.[22] With partner Elly the plan was to stock the farm with a few hens, plus six to eight Jersey cows, and begin supplying grass-fed raw milk, meat and eggs to the local community. It's a step he'd like to see duplicated thousands of times across the length and breadth of America.

'What the dairy industry has striven mightily to eradicate – wholesome milk and independent dairy farmers – is growing up like new grass on a spring morning,' he writes. 'Every week hundreds of consumers discover that raw, whole milk products from grass-fed cows represent the answer they are seeking to their health problems; and every week dozens of farmers wake up to the fact that the direct sale of raw milk, raw cheese, raw butter and raw cream is the answer they were looking for, the way to save the family farm.

'Raw milk is the key to the health crisis, the farm crisis, the economic crisis, the small town crisis, even the environmental crisis.'

Eighty years earlier an English farmer beset by the same difficulties came to a similar conclusion. Threatened by low prices and cheap imports, Arthur Hosier took the radical step of keeping his dairy cows outdoors on his rolling chalk downland for 365 days a year, even milking them outside in mobile milking units.

The measure dramatically cut his costs, enabling him to make good profits while other dairy farmers were struggling to break even. What's more, the milk he produced was purer and healthier than most other milk around. In a speech to the Farmers' Club in London he said: 'Milk produced from cows living in the open air is better in every respect... The milking outfit being moved frequently prevents the land becoming foul, and there is no need for expensive and palatial buildings.

'There is not the slightest doubt that milk produced under such conditions is of much higher food value than milk produced in stalls (inside). It keeps longer, and is higher in butterfat. Infectious diseases of the udder are almost unknown.'[23]

Hosier delivered his speech in 1927, when the world economy was in recession and farmers were struggling to make a living. He showed that by producing healthy milk from pasture, and selling direct to the public, there were good profits to be made. Today, a handful of dairy farmers have made the same discovery.

10

Reinventing Farming

Since the Second World War food growing has been transformed by two, relatively new technologies – farm chemicals and large-scale mechanization. But just because technologies exist isn't in itself a reason for using them.

Modern, industrial farming with its sophisticated machines appeals to our taste for everything new. We take it for granted that the new will be an improvement on the old. In the wake of wartime food shortages it may well have been.

But the world is different now. We face a new set of challenges – climate change, the loss of natural resources, water shortages, flooding, food insecurity and the need for sustainability in food production. In this new environment high-input intensive agriculture doesn't look so great any more. There's a need for new approaches to food growing, ones that address the challenges to the modern world.

Since alternatives to chemical farming have been largely ignored by mainstream science, it's necessary to look at anecdotal accounts for pointers to the way ahead. Fortunately there's no shortage of them, and while they don't necessarily involve organic methods, they're all rooted strongly in traditional farming.

In Japanese farmer Masanobu Fukuoka's book *The One-Straw Revolution*, there's a picture of the author standing in a field of ripening barley.[1] The crop looks thick and strong. Fukuoka expects it to yield as well as any in the district, perhaps in all Japan. This crop was grown without sprays or chemical fertilizers. And it's growing on land that hasn't been ploughed for twenty-five years.

To grow his crops Fukuoka simply scatters the seed on the ground in autumn. The seeds are sown in a standing crop of rice that's still a few weeks from harvest. A winter grain such as barley or rye, clover seed, and the seed for next year's rice crop all go on the unprepared seedbed in autumn.

In early November the rice is harvested. Fukuoka thrashes out the grain, then spreads the straw back on the field to cover the newly sown seeds and seedlings. After that there's no more work to be done until the early summer next year.

Through the autumn and winter the barley and clover seeds germinate and grow up through the straw mulch. In spring, the rice seeds germinate and start to grow. In late May, the barley is ready for harvest, a little earlier than if it were growing alone. Once more Fukuoka thrashes out the grain and returns the barley straw as a mulch on the growing rice and clover plants.

In autumn, when the rice is ripening, it's time to sow next year's seeds by scattering them in the standing crop. And so the cycle begins again. Year after year the land produces two crops, a winter grain and rice. There's no ploughing or cultivating to do. No costly and damaging sprays or fertilizers are needed. Yet the yields are comparable with any chemical farm in the land.

To western eyes it seems almost too good to be true. In our experience food crops must be worked for, sweated over, protected with costly sprays, but here it's as if the land were providing something for nothing. That, according to Fukuoka, is exactly what the land will do if we allow it.

He calls his method 'do-nothing farming'. He also calls it 'natural farming'. Fukuoka, who trained originally as a microbiologist, believes it is appropriate since his system works by 'co-operating' with nature rather than trying to improve on it through conquest.

The Fukuoka system relies on soil microorganisms to prepare the soil, nourish the crop, and supply all the trace elements it needs. Clover is there to provide nitrogen by fixing it from the atmosphere. The all important straw mulch gives the soil microbes the organic material they need to stay active.

The results, achieved over more than thirty years, contradict the agribusiness claim that traditional forms of farming are unproductive. When the Soil Association, which represents Britain's organic farmers, launched a campaign to highlight the danger of pesticides in everyday foods, they provoked a storm of protest from farming leaders.

One irate member of the National Farmers' Union wrote a letter to the weekly *Farmers Guardian* denouncing the Association's 'scare-mongering'. He accused the organic movement of wanting to 'go back to the Dark Ages and see a starving population'.

This is the common jibe of modern agribusiness, that traditional forms of farming lead inevitably to food shortages. It's a myth. Across the world millions of people are fed well by methods that don't rely on the fertilizers, agrochemicals or the GM seeds of a few multinational companies.

Up until the Second World War, Japanese farmers practised highly productive forms of agriculture, though for Fukuoka there was rather too much work involved. By careful timing they were able to take two crops a year from their fields, rice and a winter grain, and by rotating crops, applying compost and manure, and growing cover crops, they succeeded in maintaining soil fertility.

After the war the Americans introduced chemical agriculture to the country. Although farmers produced no more food than before, they achieved it using far less labour. This seemed like a great advance, and soon all farmers had switched to the chemical system.

Fukuoka was horrified by these developments. He believed it should be possible to grow crops without chemicals, and with a lot less work than traditional methods demanded. He hit on the idea of how to achieve it when he saw healthy rice seedlings growing up through a tangle of weeds in a field that had been neglected for years.

He realized there was no need to flood the land to grow good rice crops. Seed could be scattered directly on the land, as happened naturally in the wild. And why bother to plough in order to get rid of weeds when they could be controlled with a permanent covering of straw?

'This method completely contradicts modern agricultural techniques,' Fukuoka tells visitors to his farm on the southern island of Shikoku. 'It throws scientific knowledge and traditional farming know-how right out of the window.

'With this kind of farming, which uses no machines, no prepared fertilizer, and no chemicals, it is possible to attain a harvest equal to, or greater than, that of the average farm. The proof is ripening right before your eyes.'

According to Fukuoka, the reason modern chemical methods appear necessary for food production is that the natural balance has been so badly upset by those methods, the land has become dependent on them. Nature, left alone, is in perfect balance, he says. Harmful insects and plant diseases are always present, but do not occur in nature to an extent requiring poisonous chemicals. The sensible approach to disease and pest control is to grow sturdy crops in a healthy environment.

His philosophy differs greatly from western ideas about agriculture, but it clearly works. He expects a yield of twenty-two bushels of rice and twenty-two bushels of winter grain, barley or rye, from each quarter acre of land. In a good year the harvest for each grain can be as high as twenty-nine bushels per quarter acre. This converts to more than six tonnes per hectare in western agricultural terms. In 2004, the UK barley crop averaged just under six tonnes a hectare for both the winter-sown and spring-sown crops.[2] The UK yield was achieved with the whole arsenal of chemical fertilizers, sprays and hybrid seeds, and, of course, there was no second crop of rice from the same land.

Fukuoka applies four cardinal principles in his farming system. First, there must be no cultivation, no ploughing or turning of the soil. The earth cultivates itself naturally, he says, by means of the penetration of plant roots and the activity of microorganisms, earthworms and small animals. Secondly, no chemical fertilizer or compost must be used. If left to itself, the soil maintains its fertility naturally, in accordance with the orderly cycle of plant and animal life.

The third rule is there must be no weeding, either physically or by the application of chemical weedkillers. Weeds play their part in building up soil fertility and in balancing the biological community. They need to be controlled, not eliminated. Finally, there must be no dependence on chemicals, he insists.

The same four principles are applied to the growing of vegetables. The traditional Japanese way of growing vegetables for the kitchen blended well with the natural pattern of life. In his book Fukuoka explains:

> Children play under fruit trees in the back-yard. Pigs eat scraps from the kitchen and root around in the soil. Dogs bark and play, and the farmer sows seeds in the rich earth. Worms and insects grow up with the vegetables. Chickens peck at the worms and lay eggs for the children to eat.
>
> The typical rural family in Japan grew vegetables in this way until not more than twenty years ago.
>
> Plant disease was prevented by growing the traditional crops at the right time, keeping the soil healthy by returning all organic residues to the soil, and rotating crops. Harmful insects were picked off by hand, and also pecked by chickens. In southern Shikoku there was a kind of chicken that would eat worms and insects on the vegetables without scratching the roots or damaging the plants.
>
> Some people may be sceptical at first about using animal manure and human waste, thinking it primitive or dirty. Today people want 'clean' vegetables, so farmers grow them in hothouses without using soil at all. Gravel culture, sand culture and

hydroponics are getting more popular all the time. The vegetables are grown with chemical nutrients and by light which is filtered through a vinyl covering. It is strange that people have come to think of these vegetables grown chemically as 'clean' and safe to eat. Foods grown in soil balanced by the action of worms, micro-organisms and decomposing animal manure are the cleanest and most wholesome of all.[3]

Fukuoka had rediscovered a secret known to many primitive peoples, that the land can be bountiful when natural laws are respected. It's a discovery that farmer Newman Turner made in the years following the Second World War.

When he took over as manager of Goosegreen Farm, during the war, he unashamedly used every pound of chemical fertilizer he could lay his hands on.[4] But he struggled with diseased animals and crops, and the farm made a massive trading loss even though wartime prices to farmers were high.

So he gave up using chemicals or the plough. Instead he decided he would work *with* nature. He sowed his cereal crops into soils that had been merely cultivated with disc harrows. If there was too much weed or stubble 'trash' on the surface for the seed drill to work properly, he scattered the seed on the surface, or broadcast them, just as Fukuoka had done.

He soon started to harvest bumper crops. Following an unusually dry summer in 1948, for example, his wheat crop yielded almost five tonnes per hectare. Modern wheat growers would expect to harvest eight tonnes a hectare in a 'normal' season, but only after applying a battery of fertilizers, pesticides, and growth regulators. More than half a century ago Turner was achieving two-thirds as much with scarcely any inputs. There were no expensive sprays and fertilizers to pay for. Neither he nor his staff were spending long hours on the tractor, ploughing, cultivating, and working the land to get a fine seedbed. The UK average wheat yield in the early fifties was just three tonnes a hectare.[5]

For his pasture fields he included clover and deep-rooting herbs in his grass seeds mixture. The clover supplied nitrogen, while the herbs brought up minerals from deep down in the subsoil. On these mineral-rich pastures, the herd of pedigree Jersey cows stayed healthy and productive and Turner's milk sales rose steadily. During the war, when he had used chemical fertilizers, half the cows were infected with TB, calf abortions were running out of control, and the herd was losing nearly £300 a year. By 1950, it was making a profit of more than £2,000 pounds (worth £120,000 pounds today).

The cows had recovered their health and many lived for twenty years or more. They grazed the herb-rich pastures most of the year, so it's likely the milk would have been of the highest nutritional quality, high in vitamins, minerals and protective fats. This quality of milk is difficult, if not impossible, to buy today. Most farmers would deny that such achievements were possible without chemicals.

As an agricultural student in the sixties I was inspired by a book that was by then more than twenty years old. George Henderson's *The Farming Ladder* had been published during the Second World War.[6] It told the story of a small farm on the edge of the Cotswolds, and of the two city-born brothers who ran it through the tough years of the Depression between the two wars.

When the book appeared in 1944 it became an immediate bestseller, selling in the tens of thousands and running to more than six editions. Many of those who bought it were young servicemen and women dreaming of a better life after the war, for *The Farming Ladder* showed how any hard-working youngster could make a good living from farming.

It didn't take a vast acreage; nor did it take a huge amount of capital. When George Henderson and his brother Frank moved into Oathill Farm in the early 1920s they had only one aim, to raise the fertility of their poor, stony-brash soils. This they achieved by steadily increasing the number of livestock, and by returning all waste, from both animals and crops, to the land.

On their little farm they introduced almost every form of livestock, including cattle, sheep, pigs, hens, geese and working horses. And despite the number of animals, they also sowed a large area with arable crops each year, chiefly wheat, barley and oats. It was the ordinary British mixed farm, the sort you see illustrated in children's picture-books. But there was nothing ordinary about its results.

As the copious amounts of animal manure built up the levels of humus and organic matter in the soil, so crop yields rose year by year. Within ten years the Henderson brothers had made enough money from their small rented farm to buy the freehold outright, though land prices were relatively cheap in the years before World War Two. Even so it was a remarkable achievement at the end of the deepest farming depression of the twentieth century.

By the onset of World War Two, Oathill Farm had become so productive it was held up as an example to other farmers of how they could feed the nation during the U-boat blockade. A report by the local 'War Ag (War

Agricultural Committee),' the official committee which took over the wartime administration of food production, showed that, on a per-acre basis, the little Oxfordshire farm carried three times the cattle, four times the breeding sheep, ten times the pigs and twenty-five times the sheep of the average farm for the county. At the same time, it had a higher percentage of its land in arable crops.

Henderson, whose farm and book made him something of a celebrity, advocated his style of small-scale mixed farming as the way ahead for British agriculture after the war. Applied across the country, it would, he claimed, make Britain self-sufficient in all but a few tropical foods, such as tea and bananas. And it would give opportunity to talented youngsters who wanted to farm the land them-selves. He might have added that the rich, fertile soils it produced would lay the foundations of good health in the population at large.

The politicians had other ideas. Following intense lob-bying by fertilizer manufacturers, the post-war Labour government introduced a farm subsidy system that rewarded large-scale chemical farming. Britain, along with other industrial countries, had been set on the route to rural decline. And the book that might have prevented it today gathers dust in second-hand bookshops.

George Henderson was one of those farming fanatics that urban societies seem to produce from time to time. Though he grew up in London there was nothing else in life he wanted to do. From his earliest youth, he once wrote, he had believed 'there was only one thing worth doing on earth – farm it!'

Having taken a correspondence course in agriculture, and worked on a number of farms to gain experience, he went to the bank with an offer they could very easily refuse. It seemed a ridiculous idea. He wanted a loan to go farming; this at a time when farm prices were tumbling and established farmers were going bust. Here was a nineteen-year-old with no capital, proposing to start from scratch. The manager practically laughed him out of the door.

But the Henderson brothers weren't easily put off. They managed to borrow enough cash from their mother to cover the cost of the 'in-goings.' With a little over £200 in working capital they took over eighty-five acres of stony Cotswold brash in the spring of 1924, just as the farming recession was starting to bite.

The brothers had a master plan. They would adopt a system that had stood the test of time, mixed farming. What had been good enough for British farmers over a century and a half was good enough for them, but they would push the system to its limits. They would discover whether a farm based on natural biological cycles could also be an intensive farm.

With their small amount of capital they started building up the livestock numbers. They reared chickens in outdoor arks, watching them grow strong and healthy on fresh grass and the insects they found in it. They also reared geese on fresh green crops of grass, mustard and trefoil clover planted in the corn stubble.

As poultry numbers grew, they took to rearing young pullets in fold units, portable arks with wire runs attached. These were moved daily to a fresh patch of grass or stubble. The rich manure left behind by the chickens helped to build up the soil fertility, laying the foundation of bumper crops when the time came to plough up the grass and sow cereals.

Next the brothers began building up a herd of pedigree Jersey cows, rearing up to twenty-five heifer calves a year for sale to milk producers. The cattle remained remarkably healthy. In twenty years of farming the brothers didn't suffer a single case of bovine TB in their herd, even though the disease was rife among dairy cows. Mastitis was another disease that never appeared at Oathill Farm.

As they accumulated more cash they expanded their flock of pedigree Border Leicester ewes until they numbered forty. The lambs were sold for meat or as breeding stock. Though the enterprise seldom made big profits the Hendersons were glad of it. After all the sheep flock had been known as 'the golden hoof' throughout Britain's farming history because of the invaluable part it played in improving soil fertility.

There was another reason George liked having the sheep around. There was nothing to match 'the pleasure of seeing lambs playing in the spring sunlight,' he wrote, 'running races up and down the banks of our clear-flowing stream, leaping over it, and getting such fun out of life as only lambs can'.

As if there weren't enough livestock, the brothers ran a herd of twelve pedigree Large White sows on their little farm, selling many of the offspring as breeding stock and fattening the rest for bacon.

The pigs, like the other animals, remained largely free of disease. The piglets got off to a good start by being fed Jersey milk at weaning time. As older animals they were allowed plenty of 'green' feeds, such as kale, rape, vetches and root vegetables with tops attached. Breeding sows enjoyed a run of fresh grass growing on an increasingly fertile soil.

To modern farming eyes this little holding in the foothills of the Cotswolds must have looked like a scene from Beatrix Potter, with its cows, sheep, poultry and pigs all sharing the same green turf. George Henderson would have cared not one jot. He knew the fertility they brought to the soil was helping to grow cereal crops of up to two-and-a-half tons to the acre, an outstanding yield for the time. Today's cereal growers might expect a ton an acre more. But they'd make precious little profit. Much of the return would be swallowed up in the cost of chemical fertilizers and sprays, without which there'd be no crop at all on their impoverished soils.

Any lingering doubts about the credibility of this little farm are quickly dispelled by a glance through the penultimate chapter of *The Farming Ladder*. In it George Henderson sets out the full farm accounts for three sample years. The figures for 1942, the last full year before the book was published, show an extraordinary profit of nearly £4,500. At today's values that's equal to up to half a million pounds.[7]

Admittedly, it was midway through the war, a period of high prices following lean inter-war years. But even in 1932, the low point in the farming depression, Oathill Farm notched up a profit of nearly £600 (£95,000 pounds in today's money).[8] Suggest to any modern farmer that there was money like this to be made from just eighty-five acres of less than ideal land and they'd laugh in your face. It's more than a farm ten times the size would be likely to make today – and that's with the taxpayer putting in thousands of pounds in subsidies.

It's no surprise that the Hendersons' farming system should have been so productive. Biologically, it was far more diverse than today's specialist industrial farms with their monocultures and paucity of crops. Farms, like natural ecosystems, are likely to be more productive the more complex they are, as science writer Colin Tudge observes in *So Shall We Reap*.

> The mixed farm is the key to the future of all humanity. For when crops and livestock are judiciously mixed, agriculture mirrors nature, and nature works... Animals, plants, fungi and all myriad variety of other organisms complement each other, and feed off each other. Plants create organic material by photosynthesis. Animals eat plants, and return the materials to the soil in their manure, in forms that the plants in turn can feed upon. Fungi, bacteria, and other 'detritivores' mediate the interactions. This simple cycle is elaborated in myriad ways but this is the essence of it. The key issue is that of ratio: the right proportion of animals to plants.[9]

The Henderson brothers understood this essential relationship between plants and animals and adopted a farming system that made use of it. They weren't alone. At the time tens of thousands of other farmers were doing something similar up and down the country. It was an ancient wisdom they had inherited. Not all of them did it as efficiently, or as profitably, as the Hendersons. But all were hard-working, resourceful, and independent. And all were producing nutritious, uncontaminated food.

Today, we'd probably think of them as 'food heroes'. That was the view of one contemporary commentator, the author H. J. Massingham, an astute observer of rural matters in the thirties and forties. In his book *The Wisdom of the Fields* he describes some of the small peasant farmers he met in the part of England where I live, the 'hillock and dingle country' between the Quantocks and the Brendons in west Somerset.[10]

There was the couple who grew enough food on their tiny smallholding, just four-and-a-half acres on the side of a steep hill, to feed a small village. Their wartime crops included strawberries, early and maincrop potatoes, orchard fruits, plus a greater diversity of vegetables than many a grower 'with four hundred acres of fat and level land'. In addition, there were enough pasture, fodder crops and flowers to support a pony, over a hundred chickens, goats, ewes, a breeding sow and her litter of eight, and thirty hives of bees.

Not far away lived another couple with a farm of seventy-five acres. With the help of one woman worker, a girl from the wartime Land Army, they grew wheat, barley, oats, kale and root crops. They milked a herd of eleven cows, carting all the manure out to the fields. They also fattened sixty yearling sheep on root crops, corn stubble and pastures. In six years they had doubled the output of the farm, writes Massingham, as well as the fertility of their soil.

Before the advent of chemical farming, small, traditional farms like this were the mainstay of British agriculture. Then, as now, they were often portrayed as backward and inefficient. Yet they cost taxpayers nothing in subsidy and supplied natural, healthy foods to local shops and markets.

A 1955 report by the independent policy group, the Rural Reconstruction Association, was in no doubt of the value of small, traditional farms. They were, according to the association, 'as efficient as large farms in the production of corn crops, rather more efficient in the production of potatoes and root crops, and markedly superior in the growth and utilization of grass and *forage* crops'.[11]

George Henderson would have agreed. He compared the output of his small, traditionally run farm with that of what he called well-managed, large-scale farms. He quoted wartime figures published in the *Daily Telegraph* for three well-known estates, ranging in size from eleven thousand acres to thirty thousand acres. Their outputs were one-third or less than that achieved by the Henderson brothers on their little Oxfordshire farm.[12]

Modern farmers become defensive at any suggestion that the food they produce is less than the best. At a farmers' conference I was once almost lynched for suggesting the food I ate as a youngster in the forties and fifties was healthier and more nutritious than the foods on offer today. But the facts are inescapable.

Before chemical fertilizers and sprays were freely available, farmers had no option but to care for their soils. Their business survival depended on it. The land had to be kept in good heart if there were to be crops to sell next year and the year after.

In the same way there was a real incentive to keep cattle healthy by giving them natural feeds and avoiding the overcrowding that might encourage disease. Before the advent of cheap antibiotics there was no other way to keep stock fit and productive. Almost by definition, foods produced by traditional methods were healthy and nutritious.

Small, mixed farms, numerous at the end of the Second World War, had mostly emerged from the pre-war depression in good shape. The collapse of the international wheat price had taken a heavy toll of specialist arable farms, but the markets for beef, mutton, bacon, chicken, eggs, milk, cream and vegetables had all remained strong.

Back in the twenties, farmers growing commodity grains for a global market had struggled to survive but those growing nutritious foods for the people of their own country thrived. When I grew up in the forties and fifties, the daily doorstep milk delivered to our council estate came from a dairy set up by a local dairy farmer in the twenties.

Traditional mixed farming gave family farms a survival strategy through the bad years. And when food prices bounced back after the outbreak of war, they were able to enjoy better times. In *The Farming Ladder*, George Henderson urges farmers to use their new, wartime prosperity to 'put their farms in order', to stock up with healthy, disease-free cattle and sheep. To depend on corn alone was to 'live in a fool's paradise', he warned.

Henderson believed the future for British farming lay with small-scale mixed farms. On a per-acre basis, he argued, they would always produce more and better food than large mechanized farms. Only the small farm could achieve the necessary intensity of production by building up livestock numbers and returning all manure to the land.

He wanted to see the big landed estates broken up and split into small farms run by youngsters who, as farmworkers, had proved themselves capable. He didn't expect state handouts to finance them. They would work on profit-sharing farms while they built up the capital to take on farms of their own. As he himself had shown, there were plenty of profits to be made from well-farmed fertile soils, even in lean times.

He pointed to Ireland and Denmark as examples of the kind of farming he wanted to see. In 1923, the Irish Free State – later to become the Irish Republic – had begun buying up land from the big landlord-owned estates and selling it off to the tenants. The change had increased production per acre three-fold, said Henderson. In Denmark, a country similar to Britain, the farm output per acre had doubled during a period when the average farm size had been halved.

But if Henderson expected to see good farming and a prosperous countryside emerge in peacetime Britain, he had counted without the muddled minds of politicians. The government had taken a large measure of control over farming with the outbreak of war. The 'War Ags' were given tough powers to tell farmers what crops they ought to grow, even to throw them off the land if their standards didn't come up to the required level.

The 'War Ags' were generally unpopular, and most farmers expected them to be scrapped with the ending of hostilities. But the post-war Labour government of Clement Atlee had plans for the countryside. Under the watershed Agriculture Act the 'War Ags' were to continue. The government also declared its intention to work for 'a stable and efficient agriculture' by means of 'guaranteed prices and assured markets'.

It was a piece of legislation that would sound the death knell for traditional mixed farming and undermine the whole basis of healthy food production. With the government guaranteeing prices for all the main farm products, there was no longer any need for balanced production. The more of a commodity you produced, the more money you picked up in state subsidy.

It was simply a question of deciding which product to specialize in, then going flat out to produce as much of it as possible.

In place of mixed farming, large-scale specialist agriculture became the norm. Many farmers, especially those in the drier east of the country, got rid of their cattle and sheep, devoting themselves instead to growing monocultures of wheat or barley.

Soon the supply of manure began to dry up. As a result soil fertility started falling. But the new grain barons weren't worried, for help was at hand. The fertilizer companies had seen an opportunity denied to them in the pre-war days of mixed farming when farmers had been largely self-reliant. Soon the grain barons were relying on chemicals to maintain crop yields. This was more costly, of course. But public subsidies made it worthwhile. By 1960, just one thousand large farms in eastern England were collecting more from the taxpayer than all seven thousand farms in the county of Carmarthenshire.

Livestock farmers, too, began reinventing themselves as large-scale factory producers. This meant putting ever higher doses of chemical fertilizer on their pastures so they would carry two or three times the number of livestock. Along with the nitrate overdose came big sheds for housing the super-herds. There the healthy forage diet was diluted with cheap, chemically grown cereals. In this way the taxpayers of Britain were duped into funding the degradation of their own food supply.

To George Henderson it was profoundly depressing to watch his fellow farmers and their leaders looking more and more to the state for help. For him the Agriculture Act had been 'a crowning folly' in which farmers acquiesced to control by officialdom, bartering their right to farm as they pleased for an ephemeral guarantee of prices and markets.

He added: 'To invoke government assistance is like tying a brick to a cow's tail when she has flicked you in the face. The next time she swings it you'll be hit on the head with the brick.'

The destruction set in train by the national government was brought to completion by the European Union. Through its common agricultural policy the union has waged ceaseless war on good farming and wholesome, natural foods. The rules of the European subsidy system virtually obliged farmers to become large-scale specialist producers. Small farmers were offered bribes to get out, and large farmers were offered inducements to get even bigger.

There were generous capital grants for livestock farmers prepared to double the size of their herds. In the process many of them doubled the size of their debts and were forced to pile on more chemical fertilizers, and stuff more chemical grain into their long-suffering cattle.

On croplands, there were handsome rewards for those who sprayed their wheat a dozen times through the season, then drilled the next crop almost as soon as the first had been harvested. The principle of balanced agriculture, with animals and crops mirroring the natural world, was consigned to history. So, too, was the idea of fertile soils based on organic matter and natural cycles. Farming was made an industrial process, a factory operation carried out in the open countryside.

The first farming revolution – the revolution of rotations and mixed farming – doubled crop yields and fed the nation during its emergence as an industrial power. The farming revolution of the twentieth century took away farmers' independence, ruined their soils and made the nation dependent on imported chemicals and oil for its food supply. And the foods themselves were degraded.

George Henderson warned that this kind of farming posed dangers for the nation. When Britain went to war it was the fertile mixed farms that were able to meet the demand for more food. The large, specialist farms had been unable to cope. For the future he wanted to see a nation of independent, family-run mixed farms. They would deliver large amounts of healthy, wholesome food, he argued, while maintaining the biodiversity of the countryside.

Had Britain chosen to go down this route we would all now be eating the kind of food that a few now pay a fortune for in fancy West End restaurants and Hampstead butchers' shops. One of the consequences of our global industrial food system with its array of hidden subsidies is that real food, natural food, is made to seem expensive.

Organic food often sells at a hefty premium and has come to be seen as a niche product for the well-off. Farmers' markets with their restrictive rule requiring the farmer to stand behind the stall all day add unnecessary costs. What matters is that the foods are local and that the sales staff know about them. Making the producer stand there taking the money is as daft as making the shoemaker serve in shoe shops or recording artists take a turn on the till in record shops. Running farmers' markets this way is costly and elitist.

TV chefs add to the idea of good food as something precious and scarce. They make heroes of farmers and growers who choose to produce food by natural methods, often, it must be said, in return for fancy prices. In a sense, what these people are doing is very ordinary. It is, after all, no more than traditional farmers have done for centuries.

This is not to denigrate the work of today's natural food producers. Most are highly principled, and they've been courageous enough to swim against the industrial tide. But their scarcity should not be taken as a sign that good food is only for the few.

The kinds of food grown by George Henderson and his contemporaries were not expensive or elitist. They sold everywhere at prices ordinary, working people could afford. They are made to seem expensive by modern production and marketing patterns. Industrial farmers are dependent on expensive fossil fuels, chemicals, buildings, and machinery that are not required to anything like the same extent by traditional farmers.

Also, we as consumers choose to buy our food in supermarkets, and supermarkets choose to source their foods centrally. This means unnecessary costs are built into food prices, not least transport costs and the retailer's margin. If we all bought locally, and direct from the producer, there's no doubt that the cost of real food would be within reach of almost everyone, even allowing a decent margin for the farmer.

Japanese farmer Masanobu Fukuoka believes natural food should be cheaper than industrially grown food. No costly agrochemicals or fertilizers are used in its production and, in his version of natural food, far less effort is required from the farmer so it should be the cheapest food around. Unfortunately we have come to expect natural foods such as organic foods to be expensive. If they're not we worry they may be fakes.

'If a high price is charged for natural food, it means that the merchant is taking excessive profits,' says Fukuoka.

'What's more, if natural foods are expensive they become luxury foods and only rich people are able to afford them.

'If natural food is to become widely popular, it must be available locally at a reasonable price. If the consumer will only adjust to the idea that low prices don't mean the food is not natural, then everyone will begin thinking in the right direction.'[13]

Buying local and buying direct are, for most of us, the best means of obtaining healthy food at a reasonable cost. They're also the only way we're going to save real farms from extinction. Can there be a bigger challenge?

11

Time For Change

Investors have begun talking of soft commodities – the great global farm products such as corn, wheat and soya – as the hot new stock. Thanks to such pressures as a growing demand for wheat created by the biofuel industry in America, changes in Chinese diet and the Australian drought, the price of wheat – which had been moribund for years – climbed by almost 100 per cent within twelve months. As dealers scrambled to convert their bonuses into real estate, the price of farmland soared.

But despite the hype the commodity boom will do nothing to improve the nation's health. Commodities are not the same as foods. Nutritionally they are often inferior, and their highly-mechanized production damages the environment and impoverishes rural communities. It has been the singular achievement of the EU's Common Agricultural Policy to transform farmers into commodity producers. In their droves they reinvented themselves as specialist cereal growers, relying entirely on fossil-energy-dependent chemicals for their crops. In the words of

Indian writer Vandana Shiva, author of *Earth Democracy*, we stopped eating food and took to eating oil.

Under EU diktats UK farmers have doubled their acreage of cereals and doubled the yields from those acres. But it is a spurious productivity gain. The nitrate fertilizer they use has destroyed soil organic matter, releasing megatonnes of carbon into the atmosphere.

Through commodity agriculture we commit the same environmental vandalism that we condemn in poor countries. In the absence of decent levels of organic matter crops grown in these impoverished soils are, as we have seen, unable to take up trace elements efficiently. This means the grain that pours from today's combine harvesters is frequently deficient in essential elements. Yet EU and American subsidies have ensured that this sub-standard product is maintained in structural surplus around the world, putting poor farmers out of business and undermining the market for nourishing, healthy food in the west.

Just as western politicians have at last begun to recognize the folly of subsidizing food commodities, the corporations have come up with a new wheeze for getting their hands on taxpayers' cash – biofuels.

If you're looking for the very worst way to counter climate change it would be to divert food grains such as wheat and maize to biofuels. Yet the US is now spending $10 billion a year bribing Mid-West farmers to do just that. Not to be outdone, the EU wants 10 per cent of its transport fuels to come from biofuels by the year 2010.

Simply diverting crops from food use to industrial processing takes no extra carbon from the atmosphere. Making one litre of ethanol from corn uses one litre of oil in fertilizers, pesticides, transport and processing.

The Brazilian practice of making ethanol from sugar cane waste and using it to power buses makes a lot more sense. The process cuts the amount of carbon released per mile travelled by 90 per cent. For developing countries it gives a boost to rural incomes while raising the local technology base.

But for northern industrial countries to turn their temperate food crops into biofuel benefits no one but agribusiness companies. Like factory farming, it wouldn't have happened but for hefty government subsidies. The reward for citizens who hand over their taxes to fund the process is higher food prices in the shops.

With the world facing cataclysmic climate changes there's never been a greater need for the traditional approach of the peasant farmer. Communities who depend on the soil for their lives as well as their livelihoods have no option but to farm sustainably. They must produce foods that will keep people healthy, while at the same time keeping the land fertile so it will go on feeding them year after year.

By happy coincidence fertile soils can make a valuable contribution to countering climate change. Sustainable farming which relies on the recycling of organic wastes to keep soils fertile has the great advantage of taking carbon from the atmosphere and depositing it in the 'carbon sink' of soil organic matter. Farming in an age of climate change will mean returning to traditional methods.

It's easy to be pessimistic about the future for real food. It's still there if you look for it. For a small, well-off section of the population with time to spare, there's good food on offer at farmers' markets and farm shops around the country. But the supermarkets grow stronger by the day. Having established the habit of a weekly 'big shop' in the local superstore, they're now busy driving out corner shops by moving in with their pared-down city centre outlets. They've even managed to 'dumb down' organic foods by restricting their buying to a small number of large-scale producers.

There's a growing counter-culture trying to shift things in the opposite direction. Organic sales are booming. In newspaper and magazine articles food writers decry the falling standards of everyday foods. Celebrity chefs and 'foodies' are becoming as concerned with the way food is produced as they are about preparing and cooking it. Following a seemingly endless series of food scares from BSE to Sudan Orange, there's clearly a rising groundswell in favour of real food.

Could such a movement topple the edifice of industrial food production, shored up as it is by so many powerful interest groups? It's starting to look possible, even likely. There are signs that Britain could be on the verge of a social revolution.

The government, if they chose, could make the neces- sary changes with ease. With sensible legislation they could bring real food within reach of the whole popula- tion and, at the same time, provide a brighter future for family farms. Some would claim the politicians were under an obligation to act. After all, it has been sixty years of ill-judged farm policies that have robbed people of their food heritage, in effect, selling out agriculture to the chemical industry. But to take strong action now, govern- ment ministers would first have to acknowledge the mis- takes of the past.

Politicians don't quite 'get' farming. If they think about it at all they see it as an activity much like the IT industry, an enterprise that must be forever reinventing itself, constantly grasping at new technologies to be successful.

This would seem to be the view of the previous Prime Minister. In a speech to the Royal Society Tony Blair warned that without advanced technology, and in particular genetic engineering, the growing world population could not be fed. By implication anyone opposing genetically modified crops was a romantic Luddite prepared to see half the world starve.

But this view is flawed. In his critique of industrial farming, *So Shall We Reap*, science writer Colin Tudge argues: 'Genetic engineering has so far contributed nothing of significant use in feeding the world. Its contributions have purely to do with ease of husbandry, and hence the reduction of costs. There is no good reason to assume that genetic engineering will contribute anything that the world actually needs within the next half century, in which time the world population will have stabilized, and the heat will be off.'[1]

Industrial agriculture is the offspring of outdated 'reductionist' science. It works by looking at the effect of a single measure or action taken in isolation. This might be the application of a new pesticide or the introduction of a novel crop variety. Whatever the innovation, when it leads to an increase in yield, commercial farmers quickly grab it in their frenzy to produce more at lower cost.

In the biological world things are never that simple. In complex living systems like the soil, there will be a range of, sometimes subtle, effects. For example, a new chemical fertilizer may reduce the activities of soil microorganisms that would otherwise make essential trace elements available to plant roots.

Such subtleties are ignored in industrial farming, until, that is, they begin to have damaging consequences. Then the 'agri-technologists' embark on a frantic search for some new technical 'fix'. In this way, the business of growing food is turned into one unending battle with nature.

In mainstream biology the reductionist approach has been largely discredited. Modern genetic research shows it to be a poor explanation of the way living organisms work. For years, genetic scientists searched for genes that might be responsible for conditions such as heart disease, schizophrenia and autism. But they've proven to be remarkably elusive. Rather than being 'caused' by particular genes, these diseases are more often the result of small actions by a large number of genes.

The idea of the gene at the centre of living processes – a concept given credibility by the 'selfish gene' theory – has now given way to the view of the 'multi-tasking gene' operating as part of an integrated network. In response to this new way of thinking, courses in 'systems biology' are springing up on campuses around the world. In most of them physicists, mathematicians and engineers work alongside biologists in a network that mimics the natural systems they're studying.

In farming, the outdated reductionist view still holds sway. Agronomists still throw chemicals at crops and look for yield advantages. It's the chief reason for our spoiled food and polluted environment and because it fails to account adequately for living processes, it seems destined to collapse.

The irony is that the traditional farming systems adopted the same integrated approach as modern biology. Traditional farmers knew they were managing complex living processes. When they returned plant and animal wastes to the soil, they were simply creating the conditions that would allow soil organisms to flourish and so nourish their crops.

The post-industrial view of biology has, until now, failed to register with the policy makers. Organic farming, which embodies the new 'systems' approach, was left to fight it out in the market place, where the die were loaded in favour of large-scale commodity production. Organic food was downgraded into a simple lifestyle choice. All food was nutritious and wholesome, the politicians argued. If a well-off minority wished to pay over the odds for biologically grown produce, that was their business.

It's a policy that suited both chemical farmers and the supermarkets. It effectively defused any concerted campaign for real foods. Consumers had the choice, therefore governments need take no serious action to confront the agribusiness lobby and raise food standards. Now, at last, there's a mood of change in the air.

High-input agriculture has flourished in an environment of generous public support. For decades, western industrial countries have channelled tax revenues into farm subsidies. Now most governments have begun to realize that it's not such a good idea.

In the European Union, the subsidies have already been 'de-coupled' from production. This means that farmers are no longer paid by the state for the crops they grow. They're paid instead for the 'public goods' they deliver – a cleaner environment, greater biodiversity, a more beautiful landscape. So long as they keep the land in good condition, they don't have to grow crops at all to receive the cash.

Some European countries are pressing for far deeper cuts in public payments to farmers. On the other side of the Atlantic there are moves for reciprocal cuts in the Unites States. State subsidies have supplied the 'oxygen' that allowed chemical agriculture to grow and prosper. With the ending of state support there's every chance it will collapse as dramatically as the old Soviet state in the closing years of the twentieth century.

There's far more the politicians could do to hasten change and repair the damage done over decades by their disastrous farm policies. To qualify for the new 'de-coupled' support payments, today's farmers have to show they are maintaining their land in good agricultural order. The present rules on 'cross-compliance' set out measures they must take to protect wildlife and avoid physical damage to the soil. What's missing is any requirement to keep soils fertile with a healthy balance of minerals.

It's a simple procedure to analyse soils for important trace elements such as zinc, boron, calcium and selenium, and then make good any deficiencies. A small number of farmers already do it, often because some health disaster has befallen their crops or their animals. If the government were to make this simple step a condition for collecting support payments, they'd see a dramatic and immediate improvement in the quality of everyday foods.

After decades of neglect, organic farming is now the recipient of new support measures. It's clear the government sees an expansion in organic farming as a way of improving the nation's diet. But it will take years, perhaps decades, to convert Britain to a mainly-organic form of agriculture. Nor is there any guarantee that the foods produced this way will contain the necessary complement of essential minerals.

By introducing the requirement that all farmers balance the mineral levels of their soils, the politicians could, at a stroke, improve the health prospects of millions. Under the present rules of 'cross-compliance', food quality ranks below wildlife when it comes to qualifying for the 'single farm payment' scheme.

There are other measures the politicians could quickly take to restore sound husbandry and healthy food. The substitution of green waste compost for chemical fertilizers would produce a near-instant improvement in the health of soils, and with it the health of crops and animals raised on them. Since local authorities were prevented from putting organic wastes into landfill sites, small mountains of compost are building up in municipal sites across Britain. It's this that should be fertilizing the fields, replacing the chemical cocktails produced by the oil industry.

Intensive livestock farms and nitrate fertilizers – the two are usually linked – cause widespread pollution of watercourses and river estuaries. Under EU legislation farmers in many areas are restricted in the total amount of nitrogen they are allowed to apply per acre. But following intense chemical industry lobbying, the politicians have so far shied away from putting an outright tax on chemical fertilizers.

Yet such a tax would be perfectly justifiable under the 'polluter pays' principle. For a start, it could include the £16 million it costs the water companies each year to remove nitrates from drinking water.[2] A nitrate tax would put the cost back where it belongs, with the user.

There's an equally strong case for a tax on pesticides, though the government shows every sign of bowing to industry pressure for a voluntary code of practice instead.

The water companies spend £120 million a year removing pesticides from drinking water.[3] They don't remove them all, just enough to comply with legal limits. The cost is included in water charges to consumers. This represents a hidden subsidy to those who pollute watercourses and degrade our food.

The Danish government introduced a pesticide tax in 1996.[4] Weedkillers and fungicides are now taxed at the rate of 34 per cent of the wholesale price, while the rate for the more environmentally damaging insecticides is more than half. Most of the money raised by the tax is returned to farmers in the form of support for more sustainable methods. Along with other measures to curb pesticide use, the Danish tax has succeeded in cutting the amount of agrochemicals used on farm crops by more than half.

British governments have been far less willing to take on agribusiness interests. It also has to be admitted that in the modern world the freedom of politicians to take decisive action is strictly limited. In all directions they are confronted by powerful political and economic groups, including multinational trading companies, the EU and international regulators such as the World Trade Organization.

There are signs that many in government now recognize the need for radical changes in the way we produce our food. But faced with intense lobbying from special interests, it seems unlikely that they'll act.

The agricultural lobby, dominated over the years by large-scale producers, is likely to oppose the restoration of traditional farming and real food, though most family farms have been severely damaged by the shift to commodity production.

Since agriculture came under state control during the Second World War, the economic climate has grown ever more hostile to small family farms, and ever more favourable to large landowners. For decades, the subsidy system has heaped rewards on the large commodity producers and disadvantaged small farmers. The planning system has been equally biased against family farms.

Despite it all, Britain still has more than two hundred thousand small family farms. Disadvantaged by the subsidy system and ignored or opposed by the planners, they have somehow survived. Though their markets have been undermined by commodity producers, they remain more or less intact, awaiting better times. And the better times may yet arrive.

Large-scale industrial farmers cannot easily convert to good husbandry. Their dependence on agrochemicals and giant machines renders them largely incapable of producing healthy, nutrient-rich foods. By contrast the small family farm can easily adapt to traditional, biological methods. After all, they're the methods most small farms have been using for centuries.

Opponents may argue that a return to traditional farming will put up the cost of food. There's no disputing that sound farming carries costs that chemical producers manage to avoid: labour costs, for example, are inevitably higher on farms that rely on human skills in place of chemicals and machinery. But industrial agriculture imposes hidden costs on the community, the cost of healthcare to combat nutrition-related disease; the cost of cleaning up polluted watercourses and drinking water supplies. The nation as a whole would benefit from a farming system that protected human health and the environment.

The amount we spend on food has dropped from 25% of the average family's household bill, to just 9% in the last two decades. No one's suggesting that food should become substantially more expensive than it is today, but the constant pressure on farmers to produce more cheaply is incompatible with the provision of a stable supply of nutritious, healthy food. We ought to be able to pay the true cost of fertile soils and a skilled farming community.

There's one group powerful enough to improve food quality almost at will: the supermarkets. With 80 per cent of the grocery trade,[5] supermarkets control what we eat, and, to a large extent, how healthy we are. They don't need to wait for government action. If they chose they could make real food available at a price all their customers could afford.

It's doubtful they'll do so without prodding by consumers. Not long ago I stood on a motorway bridge with the idea of counting the food lorries that passed by in an hour. I was on the M5, just north of Weston-super-Mare, at a little after eleven o'clock on a Wednesday morning. After twenty minutes, I'd had enough and went home. By then, the total stood at thirty-six, most of them in the livery of the major supermarkets. And I hadn't even counted the unmarked refrigerated trucks that seemed very likely to be carrying food. Every hour of every day thousands of food products are hauled across the road system of Britain. Food transport now accounts for a quarter of all the miles driven in the UK by heavy goods vehicles,[6] and it's responsible for almost ten million tonnes of carbon dioxide emissions a year.

Environmentalists worry about the pollution caused by the air-freighting of green beans from Kenya or tomatoes from California, but the environmental damage is trivial compared with the trucking of food within Britain. If we were all able to buy food produced within twenty kilometres of where we live, environmental and congestion costs would fall by 90 per cent, or more than two billion pounds.[7]

For all their efficiencies, supermarkets, as they're now structured, are incapable of delivering truly healthy food, because their centralized buying arrangements mean that even fresh foods must spend hours in warehouses and refrigerated trucks before they even get near the shelves. The supermarkets' cool-chain transport system may well represent a triumph of logistics, but it's no substitute for truly fresh food. The supermarkets need to address the problem of sourcing and stocking locally produced food. By and large, local food produced by small producers *is* real food.

Local food aside, there is much more the major retailers could do to make sure all their customers enjoyed the benefits of real food. They could, for example, insist that their suppliers grew food crops on fertile, well-mineralized soils. It would cost them little. An annual soil audit would quickly highlight fields in which mineral levels were unbalanced, and whose biological activity was in decline. To sell their produce farmers and growers would have to remedy soil deficiencies. In doing so they might start to question the practices that led to the imbalance in the first place.

From this simple step the retailers would earn much kudos, while suffering no great blow to their margins. They could, if they chose, print on the package a symbol or statement verifying that the product, or its ingredients, had been grown on fertile, well-mineralized soils.

Nor is it beyond the capabilities of fresh produce managers to certify that fruit and vegetable items contain minimal levels of key trace elements. In any food, the level of any particular mineral will vary widely according to the variety, growing conditions, climate and so on. Yet in his experiments in the Forest of Dean, amateur investigator John Reeves devised his own 'mineral score' sheet to represent the overall content of a range of essential trace elements. What's to stop the supermarkets guaranteeing that their products contain minimal levels of important trace elements?

They could go very much further to improve the quality of everyday foods. For example, they could insist that at least two-thirds of the milk going into their dairy foods, such as yoghurt and cream, is produced by cows grazing fresh, green grass. This would ensure that the products contained decent levels of fat-soluble vitamins, healthy fats (including the protective CLAs) and other important antioxidants. For that matter, what's to stop the retailers setting minimum levels for vitamin and omega-3 fatty acid content?

They could equally insist that their beef was produced largely from grazed grass in summer, and clover-rich hay or silage in winter. So long as the grass is grown on fertile soils, this would result in meats that were truly healthy, at the same time answering many of the criticisms of vegetarians.

Sadly, none of these things is likely to happen without consumer pressure. The reasons are embedded deep within the culture of modern retailing. Like everything else on the high street, food is principally marketed on price.

'Two for the price of one,' shouts the point-of-sale poster. 'Buy one, get one free', or 'Fifty per cent extra free'.

Price is the only measure of worth. Foods are seen as no more than material goods, intrinsically no different from cars, freezers and digital cameras.

But food is different. Every fresh item, from an apple to a steak, is infinitely variable in its nutrient content. To begin with, there are the macronutrients, the proteins, carbohydrates, fats and fibres the food contains. It's not simply the total amounts that matter, it's the quality, too. Nutritional value is determined by the form of the proteins, fats, and fibre as well as the amount present.

At the micro-nutrient level things get even more complicated. The range and proportions of minerals and vitamins have a major bearing on the health-giving quality of foods. Then there are the secondary nutrients, or phytonutrients, a bewildering array of up to ten thousand compounds believed to play a part in human health. They include the cancer-preventing glucosinolates found in cabbage, broccoli and Brussels sprouts; the flavenoids that occur widely in brightly coloured fruits and vegetables; carotenoids, the antioxidants found in red or green leafy vegetables; and the sulphur-containing compounds in onions and garlic that protect against heart disease.

Since the role of most of these micronutrients still has to be established by science, the safest policy would be to ensure their presence by growing foods organically on fertile, well-mineralized soils. Yet supermarkets have little to say on this. They merely ensure that their products are uniform in size and free of blemishes, then sell them as cheaply as possible, always provided there's a good margin in it, of course. It's a policy which is almost bound to depress the nutritional quality of food, and ultimately lead to widespread malnutrition.

The current epidemic of chronic diseases marks the failure of the entire food system, not just of the policymakers. In that failed system the multiple retailers are major players. By simply offering their customers a choice between chemically grown 'commodity' foods and organic produce, the big retailers shirk their responsibility to customers. Fruits and vegetables that are poorly mineralized – meats that are deficient in omega-3 fatty acids – are not fit for consumption by anyone at any price.

In the end it must be consumers themselves who bring about change. By the way we vote we can make good farming and healthy food a real political issue. And through our dialogue with shops and supermarkets we can begin to make the nutritional value of foods a retail priority.

Given the supermarkets' sensitivity to consumer trends, the transformation could come about very quickly. One of the chief drivers in modern retailing is the fear of losing market share. So obsessed are the major players to stay ahead in the race, they watch tirelessly for new and changing customer attitudes. Complaints and suggestions are usually monitored at board level. Anything that looks like a genuine shift in consumer tastes – a growing interest in 'real food', for example – is quickly picked up and acted upon. In the world of multiple retailing, a demand for better food from even a small percentage of a supermarket's customers could spark a small revolution at store level.

That's why a few simple buying rules could become a powerful force for change. For example, when buying beef it's worth asking the butcher or fresh produce manager if the cut on offer is from a mainly grass-fed animal. Get the manager to outline the full history of the animal, or at least point you to a website where it's all set out. Failing that, get a phone number for the supplier. What you need to find out is: how much of its life did the animal spend grazing grass, and for those periods it was inside, what was it fed on? Small amounts of grain are acceptable so long as the diet was made up principally of fibrous feeds such as hay and grass silage.

As an extra safeguard it's well worthwhile seeking out beef from the traditional British breeds like the Hereford, Devon, Welsh Black and Aberdeen Angus. These animals were bred to thrive on pasture. It's unlikely that any farmer stocking them would be interested in feeding them on grain.

There's just one caveat: some supermarket schemes claiming to support traditional beef breeds only require that the farmer uses a bull of that breed. The beef may well come from a cross-bred animal in which the benefits will be considerably diluted.

What you're looking for are full details of the way the animal is produced. Good butchers, in supermarkets or in the high street, should be able to supply the information. If they can't, go to the producer. Without a full knowledge of the production process it's impossible to make a judgement about which foods are healthy and which are best left alone. It's like buying a used car without a full service history.

For milk and dairy products, too, it's well worth asking the supermarket how big a proportion is from cows grazing fresh grass. The question is likely to bring a blank stare, but the point will have been made. Since New Zealand butter is produced from grazed grass, it might be worth asking whether there's a British brand that can make the same claim. There probably won't be, but again the point will have been made.

For butter, cheese and milk from exclusively grass and forage-fed cows, the best places to look are farmers' markets and the Internet. But when the multiples start getting asked for the real stuff, it won't be long before they talk to their suppliers about sourcing it. Until that day the best policy is to choose organic. This will at least ensure that a large part of the animals' diet is in the form of grass and forage crops.

When it comes to bread, biscuits and cakes made from properly mineralized wheat, there's a battle ahead. Today's wheat growers are in the business not of producing food, but turning out a raw material for the manufacturing industry. When they speak of quality it's not the nutrient content of the grain they're talking about, but how closely their physical characteristics meet the requirements of industrial millers and plant bakers.

Since the milling process itself removes a sizeable proportion of the nutrients, why worry about the levels in the grain? Nutrient content can be left to the bakers. They will 'fortify' the flour with whatever vitamins and minerals the law tells them to, or with those they think will give them a marketing edge. In practice that means just a handful of nutrients to replace the dozens that are lost or depleted during milling and baking.

Ultimately, it's we as consumers who will bring about the food revolution. By insisting on 'real food' we could transform the health of the nation. Even the notorious fast-foods we have become so attached to, the pizzas and the burgers on sale in every high street, could be made to deliver more of the nutrients that protect health rather than undermine it.

12

Break The Supermarket Habit

It's as familiar a part of the weekly routine as the journey to the office or the school run – the big supermarket shop. Tens of thousands of everyday products together in a single space, with plenty of parking outside.

What other pattern of shopping for basics could be more time-efficient? We take it as writ that the weekly shop supplies our everyday needs at the lowest possible cost and for the least effort and inconvenience.

But what if supermarkets – through their particular supply and selling practices – were almost guaranteed to deny us and our families the healthiest foods? Would that seem like such a great bargain?

In her powerful critique, *Shopped – The Shocking Power of British Supermarkets*, Joanna Blythman sets out the case against the chilled sandwich.[1] Pioneered by Marks & Spencer, this product has been copied by all the major supermarkets along with practically every highway service station. As one food industry observer commented: 'The M & S sandwich is now an icon, representing freshness, quality and flavour.'

But according to Blythman, the modern chilled sandwich – pre-packed in its plastic carton – encapsulates much that is bad about British food. The basic concept is flawed because, as every baker knows, bread should never be refrigerated. Refrigeration with its associated coldness and dampness removes any possibility of a proper contrast between crust and crumb.

In reality the best sandwich is the sort that any small shop can put together: fresh bread and rolls straight from the local baker, filled on the spot and sold within hours. It is, says Blythman, a simple, straightforward and sustainable process capable of delivering an end product worth eating.

In its place the supermarkets have developed a sandwich which can be mass-produced on a factory scale. From the factory, sandwiches are trucked to regional distribution centres, and then on to stores. To satisfy the hygiene requirements of such an extended food chain, the products have to be chilled to glacial temperatures. This means that special 'technobreads' have to be developed, breads that won't fall apart under the cold, damp conditions.

Fillings are made in the supermarkets' own food factories. They include such tempting items as soggy chopped salad leaves, tikka chicken, industrial block cheese, salty tuna and egg mayonnaise that doesn't actually taste of eggs. Not surprisingly such industrial sandwiches make unrewarding eating. What they do instead is attack sensitive teeth with their extreme coldness. 'We buy them, even though they aren't cheap, because we have got used to them since that's the sort of sandwich supermarkets want to sell us,' says Blythman.

The big food retailers claim to offer 'food democracy'. They provide an unprecedented range of safe food, all the year round and at prices people can afford wherever they live in the country. Supermarket chiefs claim to have been successful by giving consumers what they want.

But according to Blythman, it's more a case of the supermarkets giving us what they want us to have – then convincing us it's what we really wanted anyway. Like the chilled sandwich, the foods they offer are not principally chosen for their taste or their nutrient content, but because they fit with the large-scale production processes and centralized distribution patterns that suit their interests. They also want to stock foods that – like the chilled sandwich – have a lengthy shelf life. 'In the guise of giving us choice, they simply sell us what suits them,' concludes Blythman.

In one local Tesco store no fewer than thirty-eight different kinds of milk are on offer. They include skimmed and semi-skimmed, omega-3-enhanced, soya milks, locally-produced milks, flavoured milks, goats' milks, whole milks and filtered milk. None of them represent a truly healthy, nutrient-dense milk.

A healthy milk isn't difficult to define. It's the whole milk of cows fed principally on grazed grass. It'll be fresh (less than twenty-four hours old when it reaches the customer) and it'll almost certainly be unhomogenized.

No supermarket in the country supplies milk like this. Instead they provide the illusion of real choice by putting dozens of different types of milk on their shelves. But it doesn't suit their production or distribution practices to provide really healthy milk, so they don't bother.

By contrast, local farmers with on-farm pasteurizers and their own doorstep delivery rounds could supply this kind of milk easily and cheaply. The reason most of them don't is that we've all allowed the supermarkets to decide the foods we should eat. Far from creating a food democracy, we have voted with our feet for a kind of food dictatorship.

Perhaps this wouldn't matter so much if the supermarket chiefs were all in competition with each other to supply us with the healthiest foods possible. Unfortunately, like most dictators, they're more often in the business of deception. They want us to believe we're getting the best when mostly they give us the second-rate and the dumbed-down.

The bewildering array of products on offer in a major superstore – often more than thirty thousand items – can confuse or even depress customers. The sheer effort of choosing between so many items can leave people feeling powerless. Having to consider every aspect – including food miles, animal welfare, taste, ingredients and carbon footprint – can make it seem impossible to ever make a decision.

In *Straight Choices*, co-author psychologist David Shanks examines the complexity of decision-making in the modern world.[2] Faced with a perplexing array of options, almost any choice leaves shoppers feeling bad. They feel they have missed opportunities and so are dissatisfied.

Because they can't cook gourmet meals like Jamie Oliver – and don't know what to do with the new foods and ingredients that are constantly appearing in supermarkets – they feel inadequate. As a result they opt out, often buying and eating the same foods over and over again.

The solution, according to psychologists, is to simplify the decision-making process. This may mean making use of smaller shops where the range of goods on offer is more limited. It can also mean deciding on priorities; for example, choosing foods that are rich in health-giving nutrients. When healthy eating is the main criterion, large superstores are probably the worst places to shop.

In Sevenoaks, Kent, Matt and Harriet Rudd tried a month boycotting supermarkets. Would shopping for local foods at independent retail outlets prove easy, they wondered? Or would the inconvenience and extra expense of supermarket-free living prove unbearable?

Though Kent is widely known as 'the garden of England', the rise of supermarkets in Sevenoaks has been – as everywhere – relentless. The town has two Tescos, a Sainsbury's, an M&S and a Waitrose. But the independent fishmongers, bakers and grocers have all gone.

When they started their experiment the Rudds set themselves a few ground rules. For a month there would be no supermarkets, no chain food shops and, wherever possible, they would buy locally-produced food. It didn't prove easy, as Matt Rudd later wrote in *The Sunday Times*.[3] But the family adapted and survived.

'We did things people complain they can't do any more,' he said. 'We met local people. We escaped our car. We enjoyed a meal that was an event rather than a means to refuel. If this hadn't been a proper challenge we would never have bothered because supermarkets are, on the face of it, just so easy.'

The Rudds' first step in their non-supermarket month was to sign up to a vegetable box scheme. They loved the freshness of the vegetables that arrived each week, and they also valued the sense of staying in touch with the seasons. They also shopped at the local butcher's, buying Angus fillet steak, home-made burgers and a locally-raised organic chicken.

At the end of the first week they had spent less than a week's shopping at Tesco, though their diet had included a lot less meat. In the second week they found a farmers' market about ten miles from town. With much excitement they bought Kentish eggs, Kentish goats' cheese and wild sea bass caught near Rye. But the real triumph was finding free-range chicken which had been raised within ten miles of their house.

'All the food tasted good,' says Matt. 'Our house smelt nicer and our fridge looked less like an advert for obesity. We had less rubbish to throw away each week. While the trip to the farmers' market cost £47 and took three hours longer than the trip to Sainsbury's one month earlier, it was a great deal more fun.'

Londoner Katie Austin also tried living without supermarkets. Instead of giving up chocolate or alcohol for Lent, she decided to give up supermarket shopping.

'I would spend forty days ignoring the easy option of nipping out twenty-four hours a day to pick up whatever I wanted at the cheapest price,' she wrote in her *Evening Standard* diary of the experience.[4] 'Instead I would discover a new way of shopping and eating. I'd search out the best butchers, bakers and candlestick makers.'

Before the forty-day experiment, Katie and her boyfriend carried out a test-run while on holiday in Phuket in Thailand. They were horrified to discover a local Tesco in Phuket, but were determined to use markets and independent shops. The food they found was locally-sourced, fresh and delicious. But would it be possible to live that way back in London, they wondered?

Looking back on the Lent experience, Katie concludes that living without supermarkets was time consuming and more expensive. But she has no intention of going back to her old way of shopping. For the most of her needs she will go on using independent shops.

Katie's new shopping pattern included the local butcher and deli. She also shopped at Borough Market – though it's quite a trek from where she lives – and at Portobello Market, which she found a lot cheaper. Pimlico Farmers' Market turned out to be a great place to buy sausages from a farm in Suffolk, vegetables and artisan cheeses.

In the course of the no-supermarket Lent, Katie discovered that she was eating better quality food than before, and that she and her boyfriend felt healthier. She noticed that there was a lot less packaging material going into her recycling bin every week, and because she was using cash instead of chip and PIN, she was more aware of what she was spending her money on.

'The shopping experience is now far more interesting,' says Katie, 'and I'm talking to people and learning about food. I'm thinking more about our meals so they're more inventive. One other plus for independents – fruit and veg are far cheaper than at supermarkets."

Like the Rudds in Sevenoaks, Katie found that non-supermarket shopping usually cost more money and took up a lot more time. But the benefits of better and healthier food – plus a more rewarding shopping experience – left her determined not to rely on supermarkets any longer. From now on they'll be strictly for emergency buys.

Not surprisingly the supermarkets are responsive to the growing demand for healthier foods from farms and market gardens close to home. All the major retailers now stock 'local foods'. Their quality ranges often feature named farmers standing among their livestock or leaning on the farm gate. Food labels carry short narratives about welfare-friendly production methods and fields alive with butterflies, bees and wild flowers.

Leading the field is the up-market store Waitrose which has, arguably, the most affluent customer base of any major supermarket. Waitrose has won many plaudits for its policies on animal welfare, local sourcing and environmental sustainability. Their current large expansion programme reveals the increasing store set on these principles by today's consumers.

The opening of the US-owned Whole Foods Market in Kensington, in 2007, gave a new boost to the market for fresh, seasonal produce. It's a market in which most of the major multiples now want an increased share.

However, it's doubtful whether any big supermarket will offer the healthiest foods. By their very nature they must deal in large volumes and be competitive on price. Though they may raise the standard of supermarket food in general they will never be able to offer the best.

The healthiest, most nutrient-dense foods come from farmers and growers who follow what used to be known as 'good husbandry' without compromise. They're the vegetable and fruit growers who use plenty of well-made compost on their soils; the producers of beef and dairy products who shun chemical fertilizers and whose pastures are filled with wild herbs and flowers.

These are not the kind of farmers who will ever be 'volume producers'. Nor are they farmers who would thrive in the price-driven market of modern supermarkets. This is not to say that their foods are unaffordable. In terms of nutrients delivered they're likely to represent superb value for money. But you're far more likely to find them in a farm shop or local market than in the neighbourhood superstore.

That's the true price of convenience and low-cost eating – we and our families are deprived of the foods that will do most for our health and well-being. The obvious question is: wouldn't it be worth going to a little more expense and trouble if it means we'll find the foods most likely to promote good health?

The supermarkets have made food shopping seem quick and easy. They've also made it both mind-numbingly boring at and the same time fraught with fears about making the wrong choices. We accept this because we feel that as part of the bargain we've been given extra time for the fun things that we'd rather be doing.

But by choosing to make more effort to find truly healthy foods wouldn't we begin making the whole process more interesting, even enjoyable? We'd be returning to 'man, the hunter-gatherer' in a contemporary setting.

Unlike supermarket foods, 'real foods' become desirable objects as they must have been for the hunters of the primeval forest. There's real satisfaction in tracking down a healthy, wholesome food, then cooking it for supper – just ask the average angler or rough shooter.

In modern, urban Britain there are few of us who would go to these lengths, but the satisfaction of searching the local markets, independent shops and farm-gate suppliers for that special food can be just as great. Far from making food shopping more burdensome, the quest for real food can become an enjoyable, informative and enriching activity.

Some people find it easiest to view supermarket shopping as a bad habit like smoking, one to be given up outright in a test of resolve and will-power. But it's not essential to adopt the all-or-nothing approach. For many of us it's easier to start by using markets and farm shops to source a special meal – a Saturday-night supper for friends or a special Sunday lunch for the family.

Once you've done this a few times you'll have built up a useful bank of knowledge about the best local producers and food suppliers. You'll then be more confident about using these trusted sources as part of your regular shopping pattern. Before you know it, the supermarket will no longer seem so central to your life and well-being.

It'll become like clothes shops and shoe shops, just another specialist retailer to be used when you feel the need. The umbilical cord will have been broken. You'll no longer view the supermarket as an essential life-support system. Who knows, you might even discover that you don't need it at all.

So here are 39 steps to breaking the supermarket habit and getting the best out of buying locally:

---

1. SPLIT YOUR SHOPPING INTO BASICS VS. FOOD

Divide your shopping between household basics which you buy in the supermarket and food which you buy from specialists. Food is for pleasure and good health.

---

2. BUY BASICS ONLINE

Buy the household basics online from the supermarkets and source your good food locally. In the **Local Food Directory** on page 263 of this book, you'll find information on locating good suppliers in your area.

3. DON'T FILL UP THE FRIDGE

If you do go to the supermarket take the smallest trolley available: you'll spend less. Try to get your supermarket shopping down from the largest trolley to the smallest trolley; use a basket if you can.

4. SUPPORT THE SMALL SHOPS

The small, family-run suppliers need you to shop with them; the supermarkets don't. Try to spread what you spend.

5. CONVENIENCE ISN'T EVERYTHING

We shop in supermarkets because it's convenient. But convenience isn't the whole point of living. Work out what you can source locally that is more interesting, more fun and better tasting and work out how you can work it into your routine.

6. BUY LOCAL

Buy locally and buy direct from the farmer or grower if you want the freshest, healthiest food at the price of supermarket food. But there are pitfalls, so do your research (turn to page 263 for an excellent place to start).

7. SHOP IN MARKETS

Local markets and farmers' markets are showcases for local suppliers. Try them out on a sunny day and try to shop there once a month or more often if you can. Farmers' markets are good places to find healthy, local food and they're also places to meet farmers and talk about production methods. Don't expect the lowest prices here, but expect to buy better-tasting, better quality food than you would be able to find in a supermarket. Farmer's markets are listed county-by-county in the **Local Food Directory** or can be found on the internet at www.wewantrealfood.co.uk.

8. VEGETABLE BOXES

Organize a vegetable box delivery online (see page 357). Some schemes are better than others and some times of year are better than others. It isn't all or nothing: you can stop and start, but do start!

9. DO WHAT YOU CAN

Don't be a puritan: do a bit if you can't do a lot. Not everyone can reduce their shopping in supermarkets, but some people can and if we all do a bit it'll add up to a lot.

10. ASK, ASK, ASK …

Don't be afraid to ask about food. All good food retailers will welcome polite questions about how their food is produced.

11. SHOP ONLINE FOR REAL FOOD PRODUCERS

Whether you're in a town, city or the countryside the Internet is your best bet. The net is a lifeline for embattled producers of healthy food. Start your search using the information listed in the **Local Food Directory**, which starts on page 263. Look into national box schemes (a selection of websites is listed on page 357). If the producers' websites look promising, get in touch. Tell them what you're looking for and if their production methods make the grade, strike a deal. Then celebrate. Whether they supply by mail order, box scheme or direct delivery you're likely to be getting better food than you've ever tasted before.

12. KEEP IN TOUCH

Once you've found your preferred suppliers, start communicating. Send e-mails. Phone them up. If you get the chance, visit them and look at what they do. Ask questions. If there's something about their production methods you're unhappy with, say so. With luck this will be a long-term and productive relationship.

13. MIXED FARMING

Try to buy foods that come from traditional mixed farms – that is, farms with both animals and crops. It's this balance of animals and plants that – as in nature – retains nutrients in the top few centimetres of soil. Avoid farms that use a lot of chemical fertilizers. Nitrate fertilizers are especially damaging. They break down the natural soil processes and weaken plants and animals.

14. PASTURE-FED MEAT AND POULTRY ARE BEST

If you eat meat choose beef, lamb and offal such as liver from pasture-fed animals. Try to buy farm-fresh poultry direct from the producer. But make sure the farm allows the birds to range freely over herb-rich pastures. Look out for fakes where the so-called free-range birds rarely venture out, or where they go out to a muddy, worn-out patch of ground instead of being moved frequently to fresh grass.

15. AVOID SKIMMED MILK

Unless you have to be on a low-fat diet, choose whole milk. Avoid homogenized milk too if you can. It's a process in which the natural fat globules are smashed into smaller ones. Dairies do it for purely commercial reasons, among them extended shelf life. The jury's still out on the health implications.

The fat in the milk of pasture-fed cows is of the healthy sort. It'll supply fat-soluble vitamins, minerals, protective fats including omega-3s, and CLA, a powerful anti-cancer agent. If you know it's from a healthy herd, buy 'raw' or unpasteurized milk. Other healthy dairy foods include yoghurt, cream and unpasteurized cheeses.

16. CHANNEL ISLAND MILK

If you have to buy milk in the supermarket, choose organic milk or go for one of the Channel Island brands; that's the milk of Jersey or Guernsey cows. CI milk is likely to be from cows fed mostly on grass and forage. The downside is that the pastures may well be heavily fertilized grass monocultures, so it's worth asking questions. If you don't get answers, organic is the safe solution.

17. DOORSTEP PINT

Find a local dairy farmer who delivers to your area and sign up. The chances are you'll get a fresher pint than you've ever had before. Don't worry too much if the production process isn't exactly as you'd like it. With a bit of customer feedback the farmer may improve things.

18. BUTTER FROM PASTURE-FED HERDS

Don't worry about eating butter if you can get the deep yellow butter that comes from grass-fed cows. It's not easy to find, so you'll need to check out farmers' markets and the local smallholders' groups. Alternatively, New Zealand butter is made from the milk of grass-fed cows and is widely available in the UK.

19. UNHEALTHY SPREADS

Avoid vegetable oil spreads and margarines. They claim to be healthy, and many contain added nutrients such as vitamins, omega-3s and plant extracts. Despite this they're over processed, not healthy and best avoided.

20. RAW MILK CHEESE

If unpasteurized milk isn't for you, try eating cheeses made from raw milk. Since they will retain their full complement of enzymes they are more easily digested than pasteurized-milk cheeses. To maximize your CLA intake go for quick-ripened hard cheese or cheese with a bacterially ripened rind.

21. REAL CHEESE

Stick strictly to natural cheeses and avoid factory-made processed cheeses. These are liable to contain emulsifiers, extenders, phosphates, hydrogenated oils and other nasties.

22 GO WILD

Whenever you get the chance supplement your diet with wild foods. Edible salad leaves, wild mushrooms and blackberries will supply more protective nutrients than their cultivated equivalents. So will venison, pigeon or wild duck.

23. MINERAL ACTION

In Farmer's markets or at farm shops, ask about the farm's mineral policy. Many farmers feed mineral supplements to their animals because they know their feeds are deficient. But minerals work best and are most beneficial when they're present in the grass, so try to find a farm where they monitor soil mineral status. Check on the grazing pastures. Do they contain clovers and deep-rooting plants, as well as a variety of grasses? Species-rich grasslands supply the most minerals. Visit the farm if you can. You can learn a lot about the nutritional quality of the meat by checking out the cattle and the grassland. On the best farms the animals are quiet, alert and curious. Pastures should have plenty of clovers, flower and herb species, as well as grasses.

24. FIND A GOOD LOCAL BUTCHER

If you can't buy beef and lamb direct, find a good family butcher who really knows his animals and how they're produced. You need to be sure they've been raised principally on grass.

25. STICK TO TRADITIONAL BREEDS

Choose meat from one of the traditional beef breeds – the traditional Hereford, the Devon or Red Ruby, the Welsh Black, the Lincoln Red, the Beef Shorthorn, the Galloway, the Aberdeen Angus and the Sussex. They will almost certainly have been grass-fed. When it comes to lamb it's also worth going for traditional breeds if it's taste and nutritional quality you care about. Try the Shropshire, Southdown, Portland, Llanwenog, Cheviot or Hampshire. If your butcher can't supply them try the local farmers' markets.

26. SEARCH OUT A RARE BREEDS BUTCHER ONLINE

For rare breeds that thrive on grass — such as the Dexter and the White Park — log on to the website of the Rare Breeds Survival Trust (www.rbst.org.uk). You'll find details of your nearest accredited rare breeds butcher. For an extra-special taste experience try rare-breed lamb. Look for primitive breeds such as the Soay, the Hebridean, the Manx Shetland, the Castlemilk Moorit, the North Ronaldsay and the Herdwick.

27. LAMB RAISED ON WILD GRASSLANDS

If you're buying lamb, look out for meat that has been raised on salt-marshes, heathland pastures and moorland. But beware of fakes — the traditional grasslands that have been 'improved' with chemical fertilizers.

28. CONSERVATION GRASSLAND

Contact your local wildlife trust (www.wildlifetrusts.org). They should be able to help you find sources of beef and lamb from animals used for grazing conservation grasslands such as species-rich chalk grassland or heather moorland. This is likely to be superb meat.

29. BEST EGGS

The most nutritious eggs come from hens that scratch about in fresh grassland every day. They're not easy to find. The best bet are local 'good-lifers' or friends who keep laying-hens. For smallholders, try the Wholesome Food Association (www.wholesome-food.org).

30. REAL BREAD

Say 'No' to factory-made bread. The high-speed production process will have destroyed many nutrients. Find an artisan baker who selects good ingredients and takes care over the production. Avoid white bread. Nearly all nutrients will have been discarded or damaged in the milling process. Any minerals and vitamins listed on the wrapper are later additives. They're no substitute for what's been lost. Choose naturally fermented or slow-rise breads such as sourdough. Cereal grains contain an organic acid called phytic acid. In whole-grain breads made by fast, factory processes this blocks the absorption of trace elements in the gut. Fermentation neutralizes the acid and aids digestion.

Better still, buy some organic flour and make your own bread using traditional, slow-rise methods. This allows time for the phytic acid to break down.

31. REAL SALT

Replace table salt with sea salt produced by traditional methods. Commercial table salt is an adulterated product in which valuable trace elements have been removed and potentially toxic additives introduced.

The best salt is produced by the action of sun on seawater in clay-lined lagoons. This natural salt is light grey in colour and contains about 82 per cent sodium chloride. It has around 14 per cent macrominerals – particularly magnesium – plus nearly eighty trace elements. Sun-dried sea salt contains traces of marine life which provide organic forms of iodine, an element often missing from damaged soils and the crops they grow. There's evidence that this form of the element is better utilized by the human body than the potassium iodide added to table salt. Some of the purest commercial supplies of unrefined sea salt come from Brittany and are available at some UK farmers' markets.

---

32. GIVE UP BREAKFAST CEREALS

No matter how many times the manufacturers use the word 'healthy' on the box, don't believe them. They're not. The high-pressure extrusion process that forms the flakes and shapes destroys nutrients and may render some proteins toxic.

---

33. REAL PORRIDGE

Try traditional porridge instead. Use pinhead oatmeal and be sure to soak it overnight in water made acidic with a few drops of lemon juice. This will neutralize the phytic acid. Serve with cream or a knob of real, yellow butter. The fat-soluble vitamins will help mineral uptake.

34. REAL MUESLI

A good organic muesli makes a nutritious alternative to porridge. Choose one with seeds, nuts and dried fruit in addition to oat flakes. And soak it overnight to break down the phytic acid.

35. SEALED PACKET

When buying oat flakes for porridge or for making your own muesli, choose those in a sealed packet. Don't buy them loose from bins, as they have a tendency to become rancid.

36. MILL YOUR OWN

Wholegrain flour quickly deteriorates after milling. If you're serious about healthy bread buy a small grain mill. Using organic or biodynamically-grown cereals, you will then have a source of freshly-milled flour whenever you want it.

37. STEER CLEAR OF FOOD SOURCED FROM DAMAGED SOILS

Assume all non-branded, commodity foods are from damaged soils and are therefore depleted of nutrients. Branded foods such as milk from Jersey cows or beef from Hereford cattle are more likely to be from better managed soils, but there's no cast-iron guarantee, so don't be afraid to ask questions.

38. TRUST ORGANIC

If you can't avoid buying fresh food from a supermarket, make sure it's organic. That way you'll know the soils that produced it haven't been ruined by nitrate fertilizers.

39. NATIONAL POLICY

Ask your MP to press the government for a national strategy to reduce the level of nitrate fertilizer used in food production. Nothing would improve the quality of British food faster than a sizeable cutback in nitrate use. There would be great benefits for the environment too.

13

Where To Buy Real Food

Imagine a company whose new products are inferior to what has gone before, a computer firm whose latest model is slower than the old one, a car company whose new model has a top speed of thirty miles an hour and needs a starting handle to get it going. The odds are that sales would be slow.

Yet in the world of everyday foods this is the norm. Many of the familiar staple foods that fill the shelves of modern supermarkets are nutritionally inferior to those our parents and grandparents ate. Unlike car and computer manufacturers, food producers can get away with this dumbing down of their products simply because science has yet to find a way of analysing the total nutrient content.

The big retailers stock their stores with foods that look fresh and unblemished, but in terms of their power to promote health and fitness they are mostly second rate. There are still good, healthy foods out there, mostly in small quantities that are easily lost in the jungle that is the modern food system. They're known only by those intrepid 'foodies' who take the trouble to seek them out.

For most of us who visit supermarkets and want fast, hassle-free shopping, it's the second rate we get. In modern food retailing this is the default position. Finding nutrient-rich foods that will promote the health of our families takes time, and until now few of us have been prepared to go to the trouble.

Yet is it really such a commitment? It needn't take any more effort than arranging the annual family holiday, and the pay-off in good health will be a lot longer lasting. There's also the satisfaction of knowing that the more of us who go to the trouble of seeking out real food, the faster it will become available in the mainstream food outlets.

In the search for real food, there's one vital step that will help to ensure success. Wherever possible choose food with an 'identity'. For fresh foods this means those that come from identified farms, with the full farm details supplied by the retailer or printed on the accompanying packaging.

Knowing the origins of a food changes the relationship between producer and consumer. If you know where a food comes from you can act on your experience of it. If you've been disappointed you can complain; if you're worried about some aspect of the production process, you can call the farmer and discuss it; if you're still unhappy you can walk away and buy elsewhere.

Of course, you may be perfectly happy with a food and feel no need to contact the producer. The mere fact that you have the farm details will ensure the farmer works hard to bring you a good product that you'll want to go on buying in the future.

One of the most damaging consequences of the political management of agriculture is that it placed bureaucracy between farmers and their customers. Farmers quickly lost interest in what happened to their products once they'd disappeared through the farm gate. All they had to do was ensure their products met the minimum standards of the Ministry grader or the official EU intervention store. After that they could forget them. Their products would be lost in the great sea of commodity foods everyone was obliged to eat.

For the consumer there was no one to complain to, no one to listen to concerns about aspects of the production process. There were officials to take care of all that. As far as food was concerned this was very much a 'Big Brother state', where the interests of consumers were looked after by Whitehall and by Brussels.

It was an arrangement that managed to swamp farmers beneath a torrent of form-filling and bureaucracy while giving them little incentive to improve the nutritional quality of their products. Britain was still subjected to regular food scares, from BSE and its human equivalent, new-variant CJD, to bovine tuberculosis, yet ordinary citizens were denied any say in the way their basic foods were produced.

Today, the gateway to farming and food production is guarded, not by the ministry bureaucrat, but by the supermarkets and the big food companies. With the politicians now largely discredited as protectors of the food supply, the retailers and the food industry are trying hard to win the nation's trust. They, too, have an interest in keeping their suppliers anonymous.

In order to minimize procurement costs, they want the freedom to switch easily from one supplier to another. In this way, producers can be played off against each other, so driving down prices. By identifying the producer of a particular food they risk turning it into a brand with its own loyal following, a development that would severely limit their control and, ultimately, their profitability.

I know an organic dairy farmer who has for years packaged his milk in his own distinctive cartons and supplied one of the major supermarket chains. Recently the company decided it wanted to 'rationalize' the supply of organic milk, selling the output of fewer producers under its own label. My friend was told his milk was no longer required and his cartons were removed from the chill cabinet.

Within days the volume of customer complaints had swelled to an avalanche. They demanded that the familiar cartons be returned to the shelves. They had grown to love the delicious, creamy milk produced from clover-filled pastures, and they were determined to get it back. In the face of such clear customer demand, the supermarket was forced to reinstate the product.

Knowing the origins of foods puts power back in the hands of consumers and keeps producers on their mettle. Increasingly the best fresh foods carry the name of the producer. Under the weight of public pressure, even the supermarkets are adorning their stores, and their packaging, with photos of smiling farmers standing in front of grazing cows or a bunch of outdoor pigs. At the moment they're largely restricted to the 'premium' end of the market, particularly organic foods, but in other retail outlets such as farm shops and farmers' markets the farmer ID has become standard.

The Supermarket

If you're a regular supermarket shopper it's worth starting the search there. Real food isn't unheard of in the giant superstores; it's simply that the cut-price culture of modern grocery retailing is more likely to drive down food quality than force it up, even for premium foods such as organic.

While the organic label will certainly steer you away from foods that are laden with pesticide residues, it won't be a foolproof guide to foods that are nutrient-rich. For example, organic apples are not guaranteed to be well endowed with trace minerals. You'll need a Brix refractometer or a set of well-educated taste buds to find that out.

An organic label on a milk carton will guarantee that at least 60 per cent of the cows' diet was in the form of fibrous fodder, fresh or dried. What it won't tell you is how much of the diet was in the form of fresh, grazed pasture, the food that secures the highest content of health-giving vitamins and omega-3 fats in the milk. While supermarket organic milk may meet the minimum standards, it won't compare in its health-giving properties with the milk of spring-calving cows grazed on fresh pastures until December.

The chances are the close scrutiny of most supermarket foods will point up serious deficiencies for those in search of truly healthy foods. That's when it's time to start looking elsewhere.

Farmers' markets

Farmers' markets have produced something of a food retailing revolution over the past few years. The first opened in Bath in 1997, and there are now around five hundred operating across the UK. They are now used by almost one third of the population.[9]

The basic principles of farmers' markets are that the food on sale must have been produced locally, often within fifty miles, and that the person selling the produce must have been involved in its production. These rules make farmers' markets an ideal place to meet farmers and quiz them about aspects of the production process. There's a chance to ask beef producers how long their animals spend grazing and how many plant species there are in the pastures. On stalls selling vegetables there's the opportunity to find out from growers how they ensure the soil is fertile and rich in available minerals.

Farmers' markets vary widely in the range of produce they offer and their general dynamism as retail operations. The odd rules that govern them make them more expensive than they ought to be, though not necessarily more than the supermarkets. A survey of farmers' markets in the south-west region showed that shoppers could expect to pay one-third or more less at farmers' markets than for items of a similar quality bought at supermarkets.[10]

Source
http://www.farmersmarkets.net

Farm shops

A farm shop is another good place to meet farmers and find out more about their production methods. As the name implies, farm shops are generally attached to farms with at least some of the produce being grown and raised on the home fields. Many shops stock meat, eggs, fruit and vegetables, plus a range of local and regional products such as jams and chutneys.

There are now more than three thousand farm shops in the UK, excluding farms that simply sell the odd item at the farm gate. Since most of the foods are produced 'at home' or on an identified local farm, there's a chance to make contact with the producer and discover more about how the foods are grown.

It's not easy getting to Lizzie and Rob Walrond's farm shop near Langport, in Somerset. Though the sign's prominent enough on the B-road from Langport to Somerton, you have to plunge into deep, hedge-bordered lanes and pass mellow, ham-stone cottages to reach the little shop in the yard of Glebe Farm, Pitney. But each week dozens of people make the trip. They know this is a place where they can buy the natural foods of the Somerset countryside at their freshest and best.

In the shop, Lizzie and Rob sell their own, organically grown vegetables, meat and eggs. The meat cabinet is stocked with cuts of beef, pork and lamb produced from native breed beef cattle, Saddleback pigs and the small sheep flocks that graze the farm's flower-rich pastures. Also on offer are packs of dry-cured bacon and Italian-style cured meats and burgers, all prepared on the farm. The sausage range includes a spicy Tuscan, together with the Pitney Porker made from pork, gammon and Dijon mustard.

The shop sells farm-grown vegetables, local cheeses and preserves produced in the area. The free-range eggs are laid by the hens that scratch about in the adjoining field. This is a truly local enterprise where even the ice cream is made on the neighbouring farm. In summer, the shelves are often stocked with produce such as rhubarb and plums from local gardens.

Through the farm shop the Walronds have found a way to keep the natural wealth of the land within the community, not allowing it to leach into the balance sheets of global corporations. They've also found a way of securing the future for their small farm.

'In these days of commodity farming, there's a limit to what you can do on a hundred acres,' Rob told me as we sat drinking tea in the homely farmhouse kitchen. 'The soil isn't particularly good here. It's limestone brash, thin and stony, overlying blue Lias clay. It used to be a mixed farm. When I came back from university I tried running the place more intensively with sheep and barley beef, but it wasn't really the way we wanted to go.

'Then after the BSE crisis, when the market suddenly disappeared, we tried selling beef direct. We had a couple of carcasses back and boxed them up in freezer packs. After that we started selling at village markets. In 2001, we went fully organic and the following year opened the farm shop.

'Our aim is to sell only local foods, what we produce on the farm, and what we can source from other farmers and food producers in the area. About the only things we import are lemons. As I see it, this is the best future for the small family farm. Building strong local food networks benefits everyone, farmers and their customers who enjoy fresh, quality food.'

In addition to the traditional farm shop there's now a new breed of town centre store, a sort of hybrid between farm shops and farmers' markets. The Goods Shed in Canterbury describes itself as Britain's first daily farmers' market and food hall. It was set up by a group of Kent farmers, growers, fishermen and cider producers who wanted a permanent outlet for their products. They operate it along co-operative lines, employing paid staff to run the stalls.

Though farmers aren't actually on site at this type of shop, staff are well informed about the produce they sell. For detailed explanations of the production process they may need to refer back to producers.

Sources
http://www.farmshops.org.uk;
http://www.farma.org.uk

Box schemes

Box schemes represent one of the fastest growing forms of direct marketing in the UK. Originally developed by organic vegetable growers who wanted to short circuit the lengthy food supply chain, they have now been taken up by producers of fruit, dairy produce, meat and wine. They have become a principal means of getting food direct from farmers to consumers.

There are now around four hundred box schemes operating in Britain, three-quarters of them supplying organic produce. They provide a means for entering into a long-term relationship with food producers. Box scheme customers are encouraged to provide feedback to the producer about what they've enjoyed and what they don't like. There's no reason why the dialogue shouldn't be expanded to include the production methods used and how they could be improved.

When a vegetable supplied in a box scheme lacks flavour, for example, there's a mechanism for alerting the producer and pressing for improvements. If you have a

Brix refractometer, back up your complaint with the readings. Suggest that the farmer has the soil analysed, and where it is deficient takes steps to remedy it.

Box schemes have many benefits for farmers and growers. They offer a secure market, stable prices and a regular income. That's why few producers running them will want to lose customers. There's every incentive to keep consumers happy by growing better foods.

Sources
http://www.alotoforganics.co.uk;
http://www.livingethically.co.uk

The Internet

A UK web search for grass-fed beef produced around ten thousand pages. Many were on the science of pasture feeding and its effects on omega-3 levels in the meat. There were also a fair number of sites offering grass-fed beef for home delivery. One of the best sites, a resource called Seeds of Health, featured a number of articles on the health benefits of pasture-fed beef and milk, together with a list of suppliers.[11]

The Internet has become an important route for sourcing real food. Farm websites generally give a brief outline of their production process. In the case of beef they'll normally identify the breeds used and whether they're mainly grass-fed. When in doubt there's always a phone number and an e-mail address for further contact.

Run a search for 'organic, food, direct' in the UK and you'll come up with more than a million pages. Type in 'natural, food, direct' and you'll come up with nearly five million pages. Direct sales of food are booming. In 2006, direct organic food sales grew by 53 per cent to £146 million, double the growth of sales through supermarkets.[12]

The Internet is proving a powerful force in the struggle for healthier foods. It is enabling health-conscious consumers to make direct contact with producers without having to go through the tangle of processors, distributors and large retailers that make up the modern food system. It gives consumers a fast, direct means of making their requirements clear to farmers, and it gives farmers a clear incentive to respond. The Internet looks capable of making real food available to everyone.

The Wholesome Food Association

A network of growers, processors, suppliers and distributors of locally grown wholesome food, this is a campaigning organization that promotes smaller-scale, sustainable food production. All their producer 'affiliates' use traditional and 'natural' methods of food growing, such as crop rotations, composting and mulching, and all shun the use of harmful chemicals.

One of the association's key objectives is to help rebuild and renew local communities by encouraging people everywhere to produce and buy food locally. Their aim is to see wholesome food traded and consumed within a short distance of where it was grown.

'We believe that everyone should have access to land and the opportunity to grow at least some of their own food. Most of what they cannot grow, they should be able to obtain locally from people they know and trust,' it says.

Sources
http://www.wholesome-food.org.uk

Community-supported agriculture

Close to the Moray Firth, in north-east Scotland, there's a small herd of dairy cows. They're not the familiar black and white Holsteins that currently produce most of Britain's milk. These are red and white Ayrshires, the native Scottish cows once famed the world over for the quality of their milk.

Unlike the overworked beasts that stock today's intensive herds, these cows live to a great age. Most of their placid, measured days are spent on the fertile pasture that covers this little farm. It contains plenty of clover to harness the fertility-building microbes that enrich soils with nitrogen. There are also deep-rooting grasses and herbs such as cocksfoot and chicory to pull up trace elements from deep in the earth, and raise the mineral content of the vegetation.

The milk produced on these fertile grasslands is turned into traditional cheese. Here at Wester Lawrenceton Farm they make a traditional Scottish cheese of the type known as 'dunlop', a product long associated with the Ayrshire breed. This particular one is called 'Sweetmilk'. It's based on the cheese made by Barbara Gilmour, a seventeenth-century Scottish exile who returned from Ireland with the recipe.

The other cheese made on this small, east coast farm is a full-fat version of the traditional crofter's cheese, usually made from skimmed milk because in this moist coastal climate it was found to keep better. The new full-fat version is called 'Carola'. It's made by a sort of hybrid method that blends the practices of Scottish crofters with those of the makers of French *tomme* cheese.

The most remarkable feature of these Scottish cheeses is that they combine both the taste and the health-giving properties of traditional 'peasant' cheeses like those produced by the robust people of the Loetschental Valley, in Switzerland. Like Alpine cheeses, they're made from the milk of cows grazing species-rich pastures, so they're high in minerals and fat-soluble vitamins. And because the milk used is unpasteurized, their power to promote good health and vitality is undiminished.

In an age when most cows are managed in ever larger herds – and cheese-making has become a factory operation – Pam and Nick Rodway have found a way of producing cheese of the highest quality. They've done it with the help of a group of friends and relatives who have become 'cow-sharers' in their project to produce healthy, life-enhancing food.

When Pam and Nick started farming at Wester Lawrenceton, their aim was to produce organic eggs and goat's milk cheese. Though friends wanted them to keep dairy cows, they didn't have the capital to establish a new herd. So their friends offered to finance the project by making them long-term loans. Each contributed £500, roughly the price of an Ayrshire cow. In return, the cow-sharers receive annual interest of 8 per cent, paid out in the form of cheese.

Through this novel partnership the sharers get health-giving cheeses at a price far less than they'd pay in a specialist cheese shop. The arrangement also gives them an added extra, a commodity impossible to put a value on. It gives them an involvement in real farming, a stake in the cultivation of land and the care of livestock.

The Rodways do all they can to encourage cow-sharers and their families on to the farm. Many come and lend a hand at busy times. Children are invited to share in the naming of animals. That's why there are cows called Rhubarb, Crumble, Custard, and Syllabub at Wester Lawrenceton.

At Christmas, sharers join in the custom of singing carols to the animals in their byres. Then on February 1st, the feast day of St Bride, patron saint of dairy women, everyone joins in the special celebration for the healthy, natural foods of the countryside.

The feast day falls exactly forty days after Christmas, the day before Candlemas. Everyone gathers to walk the boundaries of the farm in a re-enactment of the Celtic custom of 'encompassing', or blessing the land. A fire is lit to burn the Christmas greenery, the flame being later brought into the house. Celtic songs and blessings are sung, most being taken from the ancient collection known as *Carmina Gadelica*.

Afterwards there's a feast to celebrate healthy local foods. The farm's cheese-makers bring in small, celebratory cheeses and decorative butter. To accompany them there's a traditional bannock, a round, unleavened loaf made from oatmeal, wheatmeal, a primitive form of barley and buttermilk.

It's a custom with echoes of the spring celebration in the Loetschental Valley, in Switzerland. There candles are made from the season's first butter, and the whole community gathers in the village church to thank God for this nutritious and life-preserving food.

The cheese-making venture at Wester Lawrenceton Farm is an example of the most demanding, and perhaps the most rewarding, way of securing healthy food for the family. It's known as community supported agriculture (CSA).

Basically a group of consumers get together and contract a local farm to produce the kind of foods they want using the methods they're happy with. Sometimes it's simply a matter of guaranteeing farmers an agreed annual income in return for producing the right kinds of food. In a few cases, community groups have taken on farms themselves, simply engaging local farmers to manage the holdings on a paid basis.

In all its forms, CSA demands a big commitment from consumers. To a greater or lesser extent they are taking on responsibility for the production and delivery of healthy food. In Stroud, Gloucestershire, one hundred families make a fixed monthly payment to Stroud Community Agriculture. The money pays for the services of three part-time farmers, the rent on twenty-three acres of land, and everything else needed to produce vegetables, beef and pork from healthy, fertile soils.

The scheme aims to share the risks and rewards of good farming between farmers and consumers. Consumers make a commitment to support the farm and provide a fair income for the farmers. This means the farmers then have the security to develop the health and fertility of the land. The produce is shared among the supporting members. When there's a surplus it's sold locally, though with a waiting list of families keen to join, there are few surpluses these days.

Sources
http://www.cuco.org.uk

The Local Food Directory

The following two sections of the book are designed to provide detailed and useful information about how and where to find real food. The **Local Food Directory** (page 263) is organized by county and lists as varied a selection as possible of farm gate suppliers, farm shops and farmers' markets in each area. Details of national box schemes are listed on page 357. Obviously there are more, and do hunt around, but these popular schemes should help you on your way. **Which Foods To Buy** (page 359) takes a detailed look at readily available foods, which can contribute to a nutritious, balanced and pleasurable diet. It offers advice on what to buy, what to avoid and why it is important to track down these real foods.

We have done our best to list a fair and comprehensive representation of sources of real food. We are aware that we do not have the space to include everyone, and there are new suppliers being established all the time. If you'd like to make a recommendation or comment on the places we have listed, please visit www.wewantrealfood.co.uk where you'll find details of how to get in touch, and how to find out more about various subjects covered in this book.

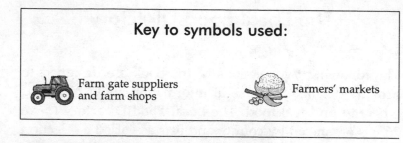

Key to symbols used:

Farm gate suppliers and farm shops

Farmers' markets

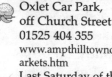

BEDFORDSHIRE

Ampthill

Oxlet Car Park,
off Church Street
01525 404 355
www.ampthilltowncouncil.org.uk/markets.htm
Last Saturday of the month, 09.00 to 13.00
Wide range of produce including fresh fruit and vegetables; fresh meat, poultry and game; and buffalo cheese and milk.

Bedford

Buy-Local.Net
PO Box 1279 MK41
01234 302 325
Online local farmers market. Buy quality local goods online ranging from organic veg, free-range meat to organic dairy produce.

St Paul's Square
MK40 1SQ
01234 221 672
Second Thursday of the month, 08.30 to 14.30

Studham

T Harper and Son,
Bell Farm,
Near Dunstable LU6 2QG
01582 872001
www.tasteandtry.co.uk
Wide range of deli products including salt beef.

BERKSHIRE

Eton

Eton Court,
off Eton High Street
01628 670272
www.tvfm.org.uk
Third Friday of the month, 08.30 to 13.30

Hungerford

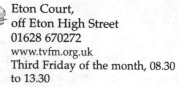
Highclose Farm Shop,
Bath Road RG17 0SP
01488 686211/686770
www.thefarmshop.co.uk
Farm shop sells own soft fruits and vegetables. Also locally sourced meat, free-range eggs and dairy produce.

Lambourn

 Sheepdrove Organic Farm
RG17 7UU
01488 674747
www.sheepdrove.com
Organic beef, lamb, mutton, pork
and poultry reared on one farm.

Pangbourne

 Garlands Organic,
6 Reading Road RG8 7LY
0118 984 4770
www.garlandsorganic.makessense.co
.uk
Organic shop selling seasonal
fruit and vegetables plus local
honey, bread, cheese, fish, chilled
and frozen foods.

 Tolhurst Organic Produce,
West Lodge,
Hardwick Estate,
Whitchurch-on-Thames
RG8 7RA
01189 843428
Box scheme offers a wide variety
of organic vegetables. An
impressive 90 per cent of annual
production is grown on the
owner's farm.

Reading

 The Cattle Market,
Great Knollys Street
0870 241 4762
www.tvfm.org.uk
First and third Saturday of the
month, 08.30 to 12.00

Slough

 Southlea Farm
SL3 9BZ
01753 542892
Milk from Friesian cows, grass-
fed in summer and GM-free
dairy cake in winter.

White Waltham

Waltham Place Organic Farm,
Waltham Place Estate,
Church Hill SL6 3JH
01628 825517
www.walthamplace.com
Sells organic fruit and vegetables
from the farm. Also home-made
butter and chutney.

Windsor

Windsor Farm Shop,
Datchet Road SL4 2RQ
01753 623800
www.windsorfarmshop.co.uk
Farm shop selling produce of the
Royal Farms. Includes beef,
lamb, free-range pork and
poultry, milk from its own dairy
and fruit from Sandringham.
Also local fruit and vegetables.

Woodley

Oakwood Centre,
Headley Rd, RG5 4SZ
0118 921 6920
Third Wednesday of the month,
09.00 to 14.00

BRISTOL

Corn Street
BS1 1HQ
0117 922 4016
Every Wednesday, 09.30 to 14.30,
and slow food market on the first
Sunday of the month, 10.00 to
15.00

Farrington's Farm Shop,
Main Street,
Farrington Gurney BS39 6UB
01761 452266
www.farringtons.co.uk
Products include traditionally-
reared meat, locally-baked bread
and fresh fruit and vegetables.
Includes Farrington's farm-
grown vegetables.

Frome Valley Farm Shop,
Poplars Farm,
Frampton Cotterell BS36 2AR
01454 773964
www.fromevalleyfarmshop.co.uk
Own beef and lamb, free-range
eggs, plus soft fruit, honey and
local cheeses.

Hobbs House Bakery,
Unit 6 Chipping Edge Estate,
Hatters Lane,
Chipping Sodbury BS37 6AA
01454 321629
www.hobbshousebakery.co.uk
Large variety of breads including
sourdough.

Jekka's Herb Farm,
Rose Cottage,
Shellards Lane,
Alveston BS35 3SY
01454 418878
www.jekkasherbfarm.com
Organically-grown herbs. Mail
order available.

BUCKINGHAMSHIRE

Aylesbury
Hunters Farm and Country
Shop,
Fleet Marston Farm HP18 0PZ
01296 651314
Home-made dishes using local
meat – casseroles, hotpots, fish
pies. Also makes fruit pies using
local fruit. Jams, pickles, local
free-range eggs and local honey.

Beaconsfield
Windsor End,
Old Town
01628 670272
www.tvfm.org.uk
Fourth Saturday of the month,
09.00 to 12.30

Chesham

High Street
01895 632221
www.wendyfairmarkets.com
Last Wednesday of the month,
09.00 to 14.00

Manor Farm Game,
96 Berkeley Avenue HP5 2RS
07778 706179
www.manorfarmgame.co.uk
Game.

Rowan Tree Goat Farm,
Ley Hill HP5 1UN
01494 793259
www.rowantreegoats.co.uk
Sells milk and cheese from
British Alpine, Toggenburg and
British Toggenburg goats. Will
supply unpasteurised milk.

Iver

Calves Lane Farm,
Bellswood Lane
01753 652727
www.copasfarms.co.uk
Pick-your-own fruit farm with
kiosk selling local vegetables and
honey.

Wingrove's Farm Shop,
Shredding Green Farm,
Langley Park Road SL0 9QS
01753 653209
Shop selling seasonal, home-
grown vegetables. Also local milk
and a selection of English
cheeses.

Milton Keynes
Fuller's Farm Shop,
Beachampton MK19 6DT
01908 562412
Free-range, native breed lamb,
beef, pork and poultry are
produced on the farm and sold in
the shop. Also organic fruit and
vegetables.

Newport Pagnell

Lodge Farm,
Cranfield Road,
North Crawley MK16 9HW
01234 391250
Milk and cream from Friesian
cross cattle, grass-fed in summer,
silage in winter. Unpasteurised
milk available.

Wolverton
Market Halls Car Park,
Stratford Road
07801 368027
Third Saturday of the month,
09.00 to 13.00

CAMBRIDGESHIRE
Cambridge
Rectory Farm Shop,
Milton
01223 860374
www.rectoryfarmshop.co.uk
Local fruit and veg. Also fresh
bread, free-range eggs and
outdoor free-range meats.

Ely
La Hogue Farm Shop and
Delicatessen,
Chippenham
01638 751128
www.lahogue.co.uk
Noted for its home cooking. Also
sells local free-range meat and
game in season. Specialities
include summer pudding ice
cream from a small fruit farm
nearby.

Huntingdon

 Broody Hen Organics,
Buckworth PE28 5AP
01480 891363
Quality vegetables, fruit and
honey supplied through local
farmers' markets.

Peterborough

 City Market (near Passport
Office),
Northminster
01733 343 358
Every day except Sunday and
Monday, 08.00 to 15.00

St Ives

Sheep Market
01480 388929
First and third Saturday of the
month, 08.30 to 14.30

St Neots

Market Square
01480 388 912
www.stneots-tc.gov.uk
Second and fourth Saturday of
the month, 09.00 to 13.00
Selling fresh local produce and
specialities

CHESHIRE

Chester

 Town Hall Square
01244 402340
First Wednesday of the month,
09.00 to 16.30

Congleton

 The Bridestones Centre (next to
Safeways)
07739 529225
First and third Tuesday of the
month, 09.00 to 14.00

Kelsall

Eddisbury Fruit Farm,
Yeld Lane CW6 0TE
01829 759157 / 0845 094 1023
www.eddisbury.co.uk
Fresh asparagus and soft fruit
from farm shop or pick-your-
own.

Lymm

 Cheshire Organics,
5 Booths Hill Road WA13 0DJ
01925 758575
Box scheme delivering mostly
local organic fruit and vegetables.
Also many other product lines
including eggs, milk and meat.

Malpas

Oakcroft Organic Gardens,
Oakcroft,
Cross O'th Hill SY14 8DH
01948 860213
www.oakcroft.org.uk
Local organic vegetable box
scheme. Customers offered a real
choice for each box.

Nantwich

 The Great Tasting Meat
Company,
Gate Farm Shop,
Poole CW5 6AL
01270 625781
www.greattastingmeat.co.uk
Free range beef, pork and lamb
reared and butchered on the
farm.

Northwich

 The Green Kitchen Garden,
1 Hodge Lane,
Gorstage Green,
Weaverham CW8 2SF
07950 916832
Vegetables, cut flowers and
bedding plants.

 Stockley Farm Organics,
Smithy Farmhouse,
Arly CW9 6LZ
01565 777492
www.stockleyfarm.co.uk
Box scheme delivering organic
fruit, vegetables and salads. Most
produce fresh off the farm.

Sandbach

 Steve Brooks Butchers,
25 High Street CW11 1AH
01270 766577 / 882248
www.qualitycuts.co.uk
Fresh seasonal game. Frozen
when not in season.

Warrington

 Northern Harvest,
Kenyon Hall,
Croft WA3 7ED
01942 608299
www.northernharvest.co.uk
Box scheme delivers organic or
locally-sourced fruit, vegetables,
salads, meat and many other
products.

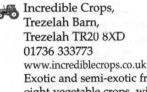

CORNWALL

Falmouth

 The Moor
01326 376244
www.trurofarmersmarket.co.uk
Every Tuesday, 09.00 to 13.00

Gulval

 Incredible Crops,
Trezelah Barn,
Trezelah TR20 8XD
01736 333773
www.incrediblecrops.co.uk
Exotic and semi-exotic fruit plus
eight vegetable crops, winter
salads and field main crop
potatoes.

Helston

 Tregoose Farm,
Treloquithack TR13 0NX
01326 565452
www.tregoosefarm.co.uk
Naturally-reared beef, lamb and
pork.

Isles of Scilly

Town Hall or on Holgates Green (depending on weather)
01720 424355
www.ios-aonb.info
First Thursday of every month (March to October but Christmas markets held in December), 15.00 to 18.00

Lanteglos by Fowey

Churchtown Farm PL23 1NH
01726 870375
www.riverfordfarmshop.co.uk
Organic lamb and beef.

Launceston

P Warren and Son,
1 Westgate Street PL15 9QT
01566 772089/777211
www.philipwarrenbutchers.co.uk
Farmers and butchers specialising in traditional British breeds.

Liskeard

Higher Redwood Farm,
Golberdon Road,
Pensilva PL14 5RL
01579 363275
Free-range eggs from Black Rock and Speckledy hens in small flocks.

Keyes Cottage Produce,
Keyes PL14 3QE
01579 342938
Members of the Rare Breed Survival Trust producing Ryeland lamb and Dexter beef. Mostly grass-fed. Small selection of vegetables.

Plumtree Farm,
Scawn,
St Keyne PL14 4QS
01579 326044
Free-range eggs, rare breed pigs, geese, ducks and guinea fowl. Also a wide range of vegetables plus small vineyard.

Looe

Keveral Veggie Boxes,
Keveral Farm,
St Martins PL13 1PA
01503 250135
Vegetable box scheme.

Lostwithiel

Trewithen Farm Foods,
Greymare Farm PL22 0LW
01208 872214
www.cornishfarmdairy.co.uk
Clotted cream from the farm's own cows. These are fed on traditional feeds.

Mevagissey

Boddington's Berries,
The Ashes,
Tregony Hill PL26 6RQ
01726 842346
www.boddingtonsberries.co.uk
Strawberry specialists growing different varieties to give a long season. Farm shop and pick-your-own.

Penzance

 Keigwin Natural Growers,
Keigwin,
Morvah TR19 7TS
01736 786425
www.yewtreegallery.com
Sculpture gardens with organic
potager beyond. Grows salads,
herbs and vegetables for sale.

 Lamorna Fayre,
Logan Cottage,
Treen,
St Levan TR19 6LF
01736 811285
Seasonal vegetable boxes and
sausages, bacon and pork from
Large Black pigs. Everything
home grown.

St Austell

 Colna Barton,
Gorran PL26 6LG
01726 843732
Beef, pigs, geese, duck, chickens,
eggs, vegetables and fruit.

 Lobbs Farm Shop
Heligan
St Ewe PL26 6EN
01726 844411
www.lobbsfarmshop.com
Locally sourced meat, poultry
and game; fresh fruit and
vegetables; traditional
delicatessen.

Truro

 Cusgarne Wollas,
Cusgarne TR4 8RL
01872 865922
www.cusgarne.org
Organic farm running box
scheme. Offers organic
vegetables, beef, eggs and fruit.

 Lemon Quay Piazza
01326 376244
www.trurofarmersmarket.co.uk
Every Saturday, 09.00 to 16.00

Brampton

 Eva's Organics,
Medburn,
Milton CA8 1HS
01697 741906
www.evabotanicals.co.uk
Box scheme serving north
Cumbria and a bit of Scotland.
Organic fruit and vegetables,
locally sourced where possible,
plus own salad crops.

Brough

 Brough Memorial Hall,
Brough-under-Stainmore
01768 342135
freespace.virgin.net/brough.farmers
market
Third Saturday of the month,
09.30 to 14.00 (13.00 from January
to March)

Carlisle

 Borderway Mart,
Rosehill
01228 590490
www.livestock-sales.co.uk/
produce/farmers_market.html
Second Saturday of the month,
09.30 to 13.00

Grange-over-Sands

 Higginsons Butchers,
Keswick House,
Main Street LA11 6AB
01539 534367
Local meat, poultry and game
including Holker Estate salt-
marsh lamb, rare breed, free-
range pork and organic, free-
range chicken.

 Howbarrow Organic Farm,
Cartmel LA11 7SS
01539 536330
www.howbarroworganic.co.uk
Box scheme delivering organic
and whole foods. Boxes contain
own soft fruits, salads and
vegetables plus other locally
sourced produce.

Holmbrook

Country Cuts Organic Meats,
Bridge End Farm,
Santon Bridge CA19 1UY
01946 726256
www.country-cuts.co.uk
Organic rare breed meats plus
non-organic free range meats.
Includes fell-croft mutton and
lamb.

Kendal

 Sillfield Farm,
Endmoor LA8 0HZ
01539 567609
www.sillfield.co.uk
Free-range wild boar, rare breed
pigs and Herdwick sheep.

Lindal in Furness

Farmer Sharp,
Diamond Buildings LA12 0LA
01229 588299
www.farmersharp.co.uk
Group of Lake District farmers
specialising in naturally reared
Herdwick lamb and mutton,
Galloway beef and pink veal.

Millom

 Richard Woodall,
Lane End,
Waberthwaite LA19 5YJ
01229 717237/717386
www.richardwoodall.co.uk
Traditional Cumbrian air dried
ham.

Penrith

Greystone House Farm Shop
and Tearoom,
Stainton CA11 0EF
01768 866952
www.greystonehousefarm.co.uk
Sells home reared, free-range
beef and lamb plus local meats.
Also seasonal local fruit and veg,
plus ice cream, cheese, fresh
bread and local beers. Kitchen
makes soup, scones and cake.

The Lakes Free-Range Eggs
Company,
Stainton CA11 0EE
01768 890460
www.lakesfreerange.co.uk
Free-range eggs direct from the
farm.

 The Village Bakery,
Melmerby CA10 1HE
01768 898437
www.village-bakery.com
Fully organic bakery with wide
range of breads.

Sedbergh

 Steadman's,
2 Finkle Street LA10 5BZ
01539 620431
www.steadmans-butchers.co.uk
Mostly Cumbrian meat,
including Cumbrian fell-bred
meat. Pork includes Garsdale
pork.

DERBYSHIRE

Bakewell

Chatsworth Farm Shop,
Stud Farm,
Pilsley DE45 1UF
01246 583392
www.chatsworth.org
Free-range beef, lamb and pork
mostly reared on the estate and
grazed on parkland.

Buxton

 Lower Hurst Farm,
Hartington SK17 0HJ
01298 894900
www.lowerhurstfarm.co.uk
Home-bred organic Hereford
beef and lamb.

Chesterfield

 Central Pavement
01246 345999
Second Thursday of the month,
09.00 to 16.00

Derby

Market Place
01332 255 802
Third Thursday of the month,
09.00 to 15.00

Kings Newton

 Chantry Farm,
Kings Newton Lane
01332 865698
www.chantryfarm.com
Sources rare breed beef and pork
locally as well as producing its
own traditional breeds meat.
Sells from farm shop.

DEVON

Abbotsham

The Big Sheep,
Bideford EX39 5AP
01237 472366
www.thebigsheep.co.uk
Shop sells local beef, lamb and
pork plus vegetables, eggs and
dairy cream.

Barnstaple

 Exmoor Naturals,
Voley Bungalow,
Parracombe EX31 4PG
01598 763385
In-season fruit and vegetables.

Bovey Tracey

 Ullacombe Farm,
Haytor Road TQ13 9LL
01364 661341
Sells local free-range and organic
eggs, jams, apple juices, lamb,
beef and pork. Also home-grown
organic vegetables and salad
leaves.

Buckfastleigh

 Riverford Organic Vegetables,
Wash Barn TQ11 0LD
0845 6002311
www.riverford.co.uk
Britain's largest box scheme
offers organic vegetables, fruit,
eggs, dairy, juices, wines and
chocolates. Most home-grown
and the rest sourced locally from
farming co-operative.

 Well Hung Meat,
Tordean Farm,
Dean Prior TQ11 0LY
0845 230 3131
www.wellhungmeat.com
Locally sourced organic beef,
lamb, pork and poultry.

Chagford

 Wild Beef,
Hillhead Farm TQ13 8DY
01647 433433
Organic, native breed beef reared
on unimproved Dartmoor
pastures.

Christow

 Teign Valley Community
Centre
07799 534974 / 01769 573656
www.devonfoodlinks.org.uk
Every Wednesday, 09.00 to 13.00

Crediton

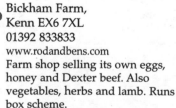 Linscombe Farm,
Newbuildings EX17 4PS
01363 84291
www.linscombe.co.uk
Local organic box scheme offers
wide variety of vegetables, all
home-grown.

Cullompton

Little Pirzwell Natural Meats,
Kentisbeare EX15 2AH
01884 266250
Naturally-grown beef and lamb
from native breeds.

Exeter

Bickham Farm,
Kenn EX6 7XL
01392 833833
www.rodandbens.com
Farm shop selling its own eggs,
honey and Dexter beef. Also
vegetables, herbs and lamb. Runs
box scheme.

Darts Farm,
Topsham EX3 0QH
01392 875587
www.dartsfarm.co.uk
Farm shop selling home-
produced local produce. Also
regional cheeses and locally-
caught fish.

 Kenniford Farm Shop,
Clyst St Mary EX5 1AQ
01392 875938
www.kennifordfarm.com
Shop sells the farm's own pork
and free-range eggs. Also locally
sourced Red Ruby Devon beef,
chicken, lamb and locally-grown
organic vegetables.

 Pipers Farm Shop,
27 Magdalen Road EX2 4TA
01392 881380
www.pipersfarm.com
Beef, pork, lamb and poultry
supplied from traditional family
farms.

 West Country Organics,
Oak Farm,
Tedburn St Mary EX6 6AW
0845 349 7420
www.westcountryorganics.com
Home delivery of organic, native
breed beef and lamb. Also cheese
and other products.

Hemyock

 Wallace's of Hemyock,
Hill Farm EX15 3UZ
01823 680307
www.welcometowallaces.co.uk
Shop sells the meat of home-
produced red deer, Highland
cattle and bison. Also a box
scheme with a range of natural
meats.

Holsworthy

 Providence Farm
EX22 6JW
01409 254421
www.providencefarm.co.uk
Home-reared organic pork,
chicken, beef and lamb.

Newton Abbot

 Happy Hens,
Sandy Meadow,
Manaton TQ13 9UN
01647 221263
Eggs produced from hens in
grassy paddock and fed locally
sourced foods.

Okehampton

 Eversfield Organic,
Bratton,
Clovelly EX20 4JF
0845 603 8004
www.eversfieldorganic.co.uk
Organic beef, lamb, pork and
poultry.

Ottery St Mary

 Blacklake Farm,
East Hill EX11 1QA
01404 812122
www.blacklakefarm.com
Organic meats from traditional
breeds of cattle, sheep and pigs.

Paignton

 Occombe Farm Project,
Preston Down Road TQ3 1RN
01803 520022
Organic farm with its own shop,
bakery, butcher, café and nature
reserve. Most foods sourced
locally.

Plymouth

Sundial,
Armada Way,
City Centre
01752 306552
Second and fourth Saturday of
the month, 08.00 to 16.00

West Country Well Hung
Lamb,
Carswell, Holbeton PL8 1HH
0845 230 3131
www.lambs.future.easyspace.com
Organically reared and processed
locally to minimize stress.

Pyworthy

Holsworthy Organics,
Ceridwen,
Old Rectory Lane EX22 6SW
01409 254450
Home-grown organic fruit and
veg offered in box scheme.

Sidmouth

Hayman's,
6 Church Street EX10 8LY
01395 512877
www.haymansbutchers.co.uk
Locally sourced meat.

Tavistock

Arthur Cameron,
Stenhouse,
1 Beera Cottage,
Milton Abbot PL19 8PL
01822 870632
Eggs, seasonal vegetables and
soft fruit. Vegetable plants in
season.

 Bedford Square
01822 820360
www.tavistockfarmersmarket.com
Second and fourth Saturday of
the month, 09.00 to 13.00

Tiverton

Little Turberfield Farm Shop,
Sampford Peverell EX16 7EH
01884 820908
Shop sells own free-range beef,
lamb, pork, turkey, sausages,
bacon, eggs, pies and local
cheeses, fruit, juice, cakes,
preserves, wines and ice cream.

Totnes

Nature's Round,
Broad Hempston TQ9 6BQ
07810 127376
Vegetables, fruit, spring water,
eggs, tofu, fruit juices and pies.
Runs vegetable box scheme.

Riverford Farm Shops,
Riverford Farm,
Staverton TQ9 6AF
01803 762523
www.riverfordfarmshop.co.uk
Long established farm shops
selling additive-free and organic
produce including meat, cooked
meats and vegetables. Also shops
at Kitley, Yealmpton, Plymouth
and in Totnes.

Umberleigh

Heal Farm,
Kings Nympton EX37 9TB
01769 574341
www.healfarm.co.uk
Rare-breed meats, beef, lamb,
pork, poultry, deli, dairy.

Higher Hacknell Farm,
Burrington EX37 9LX
01769 560909
www.higherhacknell.co.uk
Organic beef, lamb, pork and
poultry.

DORSET

Blandford

Home Farm Shop,
Tarrant Gunville DT11 8JW
01258 830083
www.homefarmshop.co.uk
Farm has traditionally-reared
free-range livestock. Shop sells
home-grown and local products
including sausages and burgers.

Bridport

 Denhay Farms,
Broadoak DT6 5NP
01308 458963
www.denhay.co.uk
Speciality foods including dry-
cured bacon and air-dried ham,
dairy, (cheddar and butter).

Washingpool Farm Shop and
Restaurant,
Dottery Road DT6 5HP
01308 459549
www.washingpool.co.uk
Family mixed farm rearing pork,
Devon beef, salads and seasonal
fruit and vegetables. Produce
sold in the shop.

Broadstone

Market Place
01258 455117
Third Saturday of the month,
09.00 to 13.00

Christchurch

Owls Barn,
Derritt Lane,
Sopley BH23 7AZ
01425 672239
www.owlsbarn.com
Farm shop sells free-range
chickens, lamb, game and
venison from Poll Dorset and
Llanwenog sheep. Most produce
organic.

Dorchester

 Green Valley Farm Shop,
Longmeadow,
Godmanstone DT2 7AE
01308 341779
Organic farm shop also running
a local box scheme. Vegetables
and fruit from Orgarden
Produce.

 Tamarisk Farm,
West Bexington DT2 9DF
01308 897781
www.tamariskfarm.co.uk
Organic mixed farm producing
beef, lamb and mutton plus fruit,
veg and organic wool.

Lyme Regis

Heritage Prime,
01308 482688
www.heritageprime.co.uk
Biodynamically-produced beef,
lamb and pork.

Sherborne

 Cheap Street
01963 210758
www.dorsetforyou.com
Third Friday of the month, 09.00
to 13.00

Wareham

Pampered Pigs,
Rye Hill Farmhouse,
Rye Hill,
Bere Regis BH20 7LP
01929 472327
www.organic-pork.co.uk
Naturally-reared lamb, beef and
pork from native breeds.

Weymouth

 Westham Bridge
01258 881274
www.bestindorset.co.uk
Second Sunday of the month,
10.00 to 15.00

Wimborne

 Holt Vale Farm Shop,
Holt BH21 7DL
01202 881525
Farm shop selling the farm's own
produce only, including eggs
from free-range hens.

DURHAM

Barnard Castle

Thorpe Farm Peel Centre,
Greta Bridge DL12 9TY
01833 627242
www.thorpefarm.co.uk
Shop sells cheese, honey, jams,
chutney, ice cream, asparagus,
free-range eggs and some organic
and gluten free produce. Bakes
own bread. Coffee shop serves
local dishes and fresh coffee.

Chester-le-Street

Market Place
0191 387 1805
www.northumberlandfarmersmarkets
.org.uk
Second Friday of the month,
09.00 to 15.00

Croxdale

Butterby,
Low Butterby Farm DH6 5JN
0191 378 9193
www.butterby.co.uk
Box scheme delivering fruit and
organic vegetables. Can also
provide free-range eggs, organic
milk and home-made honey.

Durham

Market Place
0191 384 6153
www.northumberlandfarmersmarkets
.org.uk
Third Thursday of the month,
10.00 to 16.00

Shildon

Low Deanery Farm Vegetables,
Adelaide Bank DL4 1BQ
01388 777417
Mixed vegetables, eggs, local box
delivery scheme.

Stanhope

Durham Dales Centre
Fourth Saturday of the month,
10.00 to 15.00

EAST SUSSEX

Forest Row

Cyrnel Bakery,
Lower Road RH18 5HE
01342 822283
Wide variety of breads made
with local flour. Some organic.

Tablehurst Farm,
London Road RH18 5DP
01342 823173
Biodynamic organic beef, pork,
lamb and poultry reared on the
farm. Also fruit and juices.

Hastings

Holly Park Organics,
Hollypark North Lane
TN35 4LX
01424 812229
Home produced organic meat,
veg and dairy.

Lewes

Ashurst Organics,
The Orchard,
Ashurst Lane,
Plumpton BN7 3AP
01273 891219
Organic vegetables, bread, eggs
and local honey.

Boathouse Organic Farm Shop,
Uckfield Road,
Clay Hill BN8 5RX
01273 814188
www.boathouseorganicfarmshop.
co.uk
Own or local organic beef, lamb,
mutton, fruit and vegetables.
Also sausages and locally-baked
bread.

Cliffe Pedestrian Precinct
01273 470900
www.commoncause.org.uk/farmers
market
First Saturday of the month,
09.00 to 13.00

Holmansbridge Farm,
Townlittleworth Road,
Cooksbridge BN8 4TD
01273 400679
Free-range eggs.

 Middle Farm,
Firle
01323 811411
www.middlefarm.com
Home of the English Farm Cider
Centre. Shop sells its own
organic beef and sweet apple
chutney. Also locally sourced
vegetables, free-range eggs,
pickles, jams and jellies.

Newick

Little Warren Farm,
Fletching Common BN8 4JH
01825 722545
Organic, humanely raised veal.
Totally free range.

Robertsbridge

Simply Wild,
Scragoak Farm,
Brightling Road TN32 5EY
01424 838420
Wide range of vegetables with
many varieties of each. Organic
market garden, farm shop and
box scheme. Soil Association
certified.

Rye

Ashbee and Son,
100 High Street TN31 7JN
01797 223303
www.rye-tourism.co.uk/ashbee/
Local pheasant, grouse, duck,
pigeon, rabbit and lamb plus
English pork and beef.

 Strand Quay
01797 280282
www.ryemarket.org.uk
Every Wednesday, 10.00 to 13.00

Ticehurst

Norwoods Farm
TN5 7HP
01580 200340
Apples, apple juice, lamb and
wool.

Uckfield

 Weald Hall,
Civic Centre
November to March
(undercover)
Luxford Car Park
April to October
01825 760646
First Saturday of the month,
09.00 to 13.00

Winchelsea

J Wicken's Family Butchers,
Castle Street TN36 4HU
01797 226287
Locally produced organic poultry
and free-range beef, lamb and
pork.

EAST YORKSHIRE

Driffield

 Barmston Organics,
Allison Lane End Farm,
Lissett YO25 8PS
01262 468128
Mixed organic farm delivering
vegetables, dairy foods, bread,
eggs and groceries plus organic
beef, lamb and pork.

Driffield Showground,
Kelleythorpe
01377 257494
www.driffieldshow.co.uk/farmers_
market.php
First Saturday of the month (plus
extra Christmas market dates),
09.00 to 13.00

Green Growers,
1 Station Cottages,
Wansford Road,
Nafferton YO25 8NJ
01377 255362
Flexible box scheme supplying
home-grown and locally sourced
organic vegetables, fruit and
whole foods. Fresh salads and
herbs a speciality.

Hull

Arthur Street Trading
Company,
Unit 2,
23 Arthur Street HU3 6BH
01482 576374
www.arthursorganics.com
Workers' co-op delivering locally.
Organic bread, eggs, wine and
home-made fresh hummus.
Locally-sourced fruit and veg.

Slater Organics,
16 Cross Street,
Aldbrough HU11 4RW
01964 527519
Box scheme offering organic
vegetables from four local farms.
Soil Association certified.

South Cave

Market Place
HU15 2AT
01430 421044
www.southcavepc.gov.uk/market/m
ain.html
Second Saturday of the month,
09.00 to 13.00

ESSEX

Billericay

Barleylands Farm Museum
01268 532253
www.barleylands.co.uk/museum
Every day, 10.00 to 17.00 (16.00
November to February)

Burnham-on-Crouch

Wrekin Farm Shop,
Burnham Road,
Althorne CM3 6DT
01621 786785
Sells own and locally sourced
free-range geese, turkey and
pork. Also ready meals, pies and
cakes. Has a range of 40 cheeses.

Chelmsford

Upsons Farm,
Ivy Barns Farm,
Hatfield Peveril CM3 2JH
01245 380274
www.upsonsfarm.co.uk
Farm shop selling local fruit,
vegetables and meat, free-range
eggs, cheese, ice cream, preserves
and juices. Also hens for your
garden.

Colchester

Hall Farm Shop,
The Hall,
Stratford St Mary CO7 6LS
01206 322572
www.hallfarmshop.co.uk
Shop sells its own beef and lamb,
plus organic or free-range meat
from local farms. Range of local
seasonal fruit and vegetables
plus local cheeses.

Danbury

Kelly Turkey Farms,
Springate Farm,
Bicknacre Road CM3 4EP
01245 223581
www.kellyturkeys.com
Uses traditional natural methods
to produce quality turkeys and
chicken.

Frinton-on-Sea

Park Fruit Farm,
Pork Lane,
Great Holland CO13 0ES
01255 674621
www.parkfruitfarm.co.uk
Many varieties of apple, plum,
pears and raspberries. Also
walnuts, honey and vegetables
grown on the farm or locally.

Great Bromley

Gourmet Mushrooms (UK) Ltd,
Morants Farm,
Colchester Road CO7 7TN
01206 231660
More than 20 different varieties
of organic mushrooms.

Hainault

Forest Farm Shop,
Forest Road IG6 3HQ
020 8500 2221
Farm shop selling own potatoes
plus a range of fruits, vegetables
and salads.

Halstead

Organic Choice,
60 High Street CO9 2JG
01787 478471
www.organicchoice.net
Wide variety of organic fruit,
vegetables, meat and dairy
delivered to the whole of Essex.

Spencers Farm Shop,
Wickham Fruit Farm,
Wickham St Pauls CO9 2PX
01787 269476
www.spencersfarmshop.co.uk
The farm's own traditional apple
varieties plus seasonal fruit. Also
local meat and free-range eggs,
plus home-made fruit pies and
ice cream.

Ongar

Ashlyns Organic Farm Shop,
North Weald CM16 6RZ
01992 525146
www.ashlyns.co.uk
Seasonal fruit and vegetables
plus organic meat and milk from
this farming co-operative. Also
freshly baked bread.

Romford

Market Square
01277 362414
www.essexfarmersmarkets.com
Second and fourth Sunday of the
month, 10.00 to 15.00

Saffron Walden

Graces Fruit Farm,
Causeway End,
Thaxted Road,
Wimbish CB10 2XP
01371 830387
Sells own fruit in season plus
locally-baked pies and cakes.

Southend-on-Sea

High Street
01277 362414
www.essexfarmersmarkets.co.uk
Second and fourth Saturday of
the month, 09.00 to 16.00

GLOUCESTERSHIRE

Cambridge

Wharf Farm Dairy,
Wharf Farm,
Bristol Road GL2 7AL
01453 890383
www.wharffarmdairy.co.uk
Goat milk and cheese; duck eggs.

Cheltenham

Hayles Fruit Farm,
Winchcombe GL54 5PB
01242 602123
www.hayles-fruit-farm.co.uk
Farm produces a range of
orchard fruits and soft fruit. Shop
sells meat from local farms
including outdoor reared, free-
range pork. Local dairy produce
plus chutneys, marmalades, local
bread and cakes.

Slipstream Organics,
Unit 2,
Ullenwood Court,
Ullenwood GL53 9QS
01242 227273
www.slipstream-organics.co.uk
Box scheme offering organic
fruit, eggs and vegetables mostly
sourced from local farms.

Chipping Sodbury

High Street near clock tower
(in the Town Hall during the
winter months)
01454 321010
Second Saturday and last
Thursday of the month, 09.00 to
13.00

Cirencester

The Butts Farm Shop,
South Cerney GL7 5QE
01285 862224
www.thebuttsfarmshop.com
Traditional and rare breed beef,
pork and lamb sourced from the
Cotswolds.

Chesterton Farm Shop,
Cranhams Lane,
Chesterton GL7 6JP
01285 642160
www.chestertonfarm.co.uk
Local rare breed meats, plus
fruits, veg, eggs, ice cream and
preserves. Bacon is cured on site.

The Organic Farm Shop,
Abbey Home Farm,
Burford Road GL7 5HF
01285 640441
www.theorganicfarmshop.co.uk
Mixed organic farm with shop
and cafe offering beef, lamb,
pork, sausages, bacon, eggs, pies,
prepared dishes and honey. Sells
its own seasonal veg when
available.

Downend

Christchurch Hall,
North Street
01453 890383
Fourth Friday of the month, 08.30
to 12.00

Gloucester

Stroud Community
Agriculture,
1 The Bungalow,
Brookthorpe GL4 0UN
01452 810763
www.stroudcommunityagriculture.
org
Sustainable farming co-operative
offering veg box scheme to pick
up for members.

Over Farm Market,
Over, GL2 8DB
01452 521014
www.over-farm-market.com
Range of fruit and vegetables
grown on site along with beef.
Pork and cheese from local
suppliers together with other
produce. Shop also stocks free-
range eggs and local Maizemoor
honey.

Kingham

Daylesford Organic Farm Shop,
Daylesford GL56 0YG
01608 731700
Farm shop specialising in fresh,
organic, seasonal and locally
produced food. Includes home-
grown vegetables, hand-made
cheese and breads. Organic meat
from linked estate in
Staffordshire.

Moreton-in-Marsh

Longborough Farm Shop,
Longborough GL56 0QZ
01451 830469
www.longboroughfarmshop.com
Farm grows a range of orchard
fruits and soft fruit. Shops sells
its own and locally grown fruit
and vegetables, home-made
frozen meals, bread, cheese, meat
from the Dexter herd, Jacob lamb
and Old Spot pork.

Newent

The Authentic Bread Company,
Strawberry Hill GL18 1LH
01531 828181
Organic, traditionally baked
bread including rye and spelt
loaves. Dough is allowed to
ferment naturally twice.

South Cerney

The Cotswold Gourmet,
The Butts Farm GL7 5QE
01285 862224
www.buttsfarmshop.com
Free-range, traditionally reared
chickens, Gressingham ducks
and rare breed beef, pork and
lamb plus local eggs, bacon
(home cured and smoked) and
sausages.

Stroud

Cornhill Market Place
01453 758060
www.fresh-n-local.co.uk/
markets/stroud.php
Every Saturday, 09.00 to 14.00

Tetbury

Duchy Home Farm Organic
Vegetables,
Broadfield Farm GL8 8SE
01666 503507
Range of organic vegetables from
the Prince of Wales' estate. Local
box scheme and farmers'
markets.

Wotton under Edge

Whitfield Farm Organics,
Whitfield Farm,
Falfield GL12 8DR
01454 261010
www.whitfieldfarmorganics.co.uk
Organic beef from home bred,
Aberdeen Angus cross cattle.
Raised entirely on grazed grass,
hay or silage.

GREATER LONDON

Abel and Cole
16 Waterside Way,
Plough Lane SW17 0HB
08452 626262
www.abel-cole.co.uk
Large organic delivery service.
Box scheme supplies organic fruit
and vegetables. Also offers dairy,
bread, meat and fish.

Baker and Spice,
69 St Marks Road W10 6JG
020 8960 6567
www.bakerandspice.com
Traditional breads baked the old-
fashioned way.

Borough Market,
8 Southwark SE1 1TL
020 7407 1002
www.boroughmarket.co.uk
Every Thursday, 11.00 to 17.00,
every Friday, 12.00 to 18.00, and
every Saturday, 09.00 to 16.00
Organic and whole food market.

Chadwick's Organic Butchers,
208 Balham High Road SW12
020 8722 1895
Organic meat from Dorset, the
Orkneys and Wales.

Chiswick Market
Car Park Pavilion Dukes
Meadows,
off Edensor Road,
Chiswick
020 8742 2225
www.dukesmeadowtrust.org/
farmersmarket.html
Every Sunday, 10.00 to 14.00

Coyles of Richmond,
23 Friar's Style Road TW10
020 8940 0414
www.coylesofrichmond.com
Organic beef, lamb, pork, chicken
and seafood from Wales and
Dorset.

A Dove and Son,
71 Northcote Road SW11
020 7223 5191
Free-range and organic meat
from Scotland, Wales and
Yorkshire.

James Elliott,
96 Essex Road N1
020 7226 3658
Free-range meats including
Lincolnshire lamb, Scottish beef
and seasonal game.

Everybody Organic,
110 East Duck Lees Lane,
Enfield EN3 7SR
0845 345 5054
www.everybodyorganic.com
Box scheme delivers organic
vegetables, fruit, eggs, pies, oils,
soups, dried fruit and preserve.
Delivers nationwide by courier.

Finchley Road Market
O2 Centre Car Park,
near Homebase,
Finchley Road
020 7833 0338
www.lfm.org.uk
Every Wednesday, 10.00 to 15.00

Ginger Pig,
8-10 Moxon Street,
Marylebone Lane W1U 4EW
020 7935 7788
Free-range meat from own farm
in North Yorkshire including
Longhorn beef, Tamworth and
Old Spot pork and Blue-faced
Leicester lamb.

Frank Godfrey,
7 Highbury Park N5
020 7226 2425
www.fgodfrey.co.uk
Free-range, grass-fed beef and
mutton from Orkney.

Grahams,
134 East End Road N2 0RZ
020 8883 6187
Organic Herefordshire chicken
and beef and lamb from
Yorkshire and Wales.

Growing Communities,
The Old Fire Station,
61 Leswin Road N16 7NY
020 7502 7588
www.growingcommunities.org
London's first social enterprise
group running organic box
scheme. Sources locally when
possible. Also runs the all-
organic Stoke Newington
farmers' market.

 Hammersmith Market
Lyric Square
01689 860840
Every Thursday and first and
third Saturdays of the month,
11.00 to 16.00

 Hussey's,
64 Wapping Lane E1W 2RL
020 7488 3686
Free-range beef from Scotland,
Sussex pork and Gloucestershire
chicken.

 Freemans,
9 Topsfield Parade N8
020 8340 3100
Welsh organic lamb and pork;
organic chicken from Surrey.

 Highlanders Organics,
14 Bittacy Hill NW7 1LB
020 8346 1055
www.organicbutcher.net
Organic beef, lamb, pork and
poultry reared on farms in the
Black Mountains. Soil
Association certified.

 Just Organic,
113 Wilberforce Road N4 2SP
07986 345219
www.justorganic.org.uk
London-based organic box
scheme offering fruit and
vegetables. Sourced locally where
possible from Riverford Farm in
Devon.

 Kent and Sons,
59 St Johns Wood High Street
NW8 7NL
020 7722 2258
www.kents-butchers.co.uk
Welsh organic beef, lamb, veal,
poultry, pork and speciality oils
and vinegars.

 Elizabeth King Butcher & Deli,
30-34 New Kings Road SW6
020 7736 2826
Mainly free-range Scottish beef,
Norfolk pork, Plymouth lamb
and Suffolk chickens.

 Kingsland,
140 Portobello Road W11 2DZ
020 7727 6067
Scottish free-range beef and
organic pork, chicken and lamb
from Dorset plus homemade
pies.

 C Lidgate,
110 Holland Park Avenue
W11 4UA
020 7727 8243
This famous butcher supports
small producers. Stocks organic
lamb and pork from Highgrove,
organic beef from Sussex and
Shetland Island lamb.

Meat City,
507 Central Markets,
Smithfield EC1A 9NL
020 7253 9606
www.meat-city.co.uk
Free-range Scottish beef, pork
from Gloucestershire, and
Northampton chicken.

The Meat Like It Used To be
Company,
50 Cannon Lane,
Pinner HA5 1HW
020 866 4611
Traditional butcher's shop selling
high quality meats including
free-range, traditional breed pork
and beef.

W J Miller,
14 Stratford Road W8 6QD
020 7937 1777
Organic butcher selling Welsh
organic beef and lamb.

Old Spitalfields Organic
Market,
65 Brushfield Street E1 6AA
020 7247 8556
www.visitspitalfields.com
Wide range of organic produce.
Wednesdays and first and third
Sundays of the month.

The Organic Delivery
Company,
Unit A59,
New Covent Garden Market
SW8 5EE
020 7739 8181
www.organicdelivery.co.uk
Box scheme delivers in and
around London.

Organiclea Community
Growers,
Hornbeam Environmental
Centre,
458 Hoe Street,
Walthamstow E17 9AH
0845 458 1726
Vegetables, fruit and herbs.

Pedestrian High Street,
Bromley
020 8466 0719
Every Friday and Saturday, 09.00
to 17.00

Pethers of Kew,
16 Station Parade,
Kew Gardens TW9 3PZ
020 8940 0163
Free-range butchers and award
winning pie makers.

A S Portwine and Sons,
24 Earlham Street WC2H 9LN
0207 836 2353
Highly respected traditional
butcher selling a selection of free-
range, organic and rare breed
meats.

Pure Meat Company,
258 Kentish Town Road
NW5 2AA
020 7485 0346
Organic beef, pork, lamb and
chicken from Cornwall plus a
range of organic sausages and
fresh fish.

Randalls Butchers,
113 Wandsworth Bridge Road,
Fulham SW6 2TE
0207 736 3426
Wide selection of game birds
from local shoot.

Sheepdrove Organic Farm
Family Butcher
5 Clifton Road,
Maida Vale W9 1SZ
020 7266 3838
www.sheepdrove.com
Organic beef, lamb, mutton, pork
and poultry reared on one farm.

G G Sparkes Organic Butchers,
24 Old Dover Road,
Blackheath SE3 7BT
020 8355 8597
www.ggsparkesorganicbutchers.co.uk
Sussex organic lamb, beef and
pork from south Devon, Kent
and Sussex, and Welsh chickens.

H G Walter,
51 Palliser Road W14
020 7385 6466
Organic chicken from the Welsh
borders, beef and lamb from
Yorkshire and Wales. Also
organic cheese.

Wyndham House Poultry,
2-3 Stoney Street SE1 9AA
020 7403 4788
Poultry specialists. Specialises in
Label Anglais chicken from
traditional, free-range farm in
Essex. Chicken burgers and
sausages made in-house.

GREATER MANCHESTER

Ashton under Lyne

Ashton Market Ground,
Bow Street
0161 342 3268/9
Last Sunday of the month, 09.00
to 15.00

Manchester
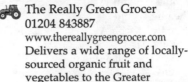
The Really Green Grocer
01204 843887
www.thereallygreengrocer.com
Delivers a wide range of locally-
sourced organic fruit and
vegetables to the Greater
Manchester area.

Piccadilly Gardens
0161 234 7357
www.manchester.gov.uk/visitorcentre
/events/markets/farmers.htm
Second and fourth Friday and
Saturday of the month, 10.00 to
18.00

Prestwich
Fetish For Food
430 Bury New Road M25 1BD
0161 7985558
www.fetishforfood.com
Sells a wide variety of organic
produce and products which sit
along side a gourmet and fine
food Delicatessen. Choose from
award winning small artisan
suppliers and own label
products. Free box delivery
within a three-mile radius of the
shop.

Ramsbottom

Ramsbottom Civic Hall,
Market Place
0161 253 5111
Second Sunday of the month,
10.00 to 16.00

Stockport
Foodlife Doorstep Deliveries,
68 Buckingham Road,
Cheadle Hulme,
Cheadle SK8 5NA
0161 486 1173
Box scheme delivering the
produce of a local growers' co-
op. Organic fruit, vegetables,
dairy, bread and meat.

Limited Resources,
Unit 3 Brook Street,
Higher Hillgate SK1 3HS
0161 477 2040
www.limited-resources.co.uk
Wide range of organic fruit and
vegetables delivered through a
box scheme. Sourced mainly
from growers in the north-west.

HAMPSHIRE

Alresford
Alre Watercress,
3 Woodlark Cottage,
Bighton SO24 9RE
01962 735608
Watercress.

West Lea Farm Shop,
Lady Croft SO24 0QP
01962 732476
Sells freshly harvested
watercress.

Andover
High Street
01420 588671
www.hampshirefarmersmarkets.co.uk
Third Sunday of the month, 10.00
to 14.00

Basingstoke
Hampshire Chilli Growers,
Herriard Nursery,
Scrathface Lane RG25 2TX
01256 464731
www.hampshirechilligrowers.co.uk
Supply 15 varieties of chilli plus
English and Oriental herbs.

Manydown Farmshop,
Upper Farm,
Wooton St Laurence RG23 8PE
01256 781145
www.manydown.co.uk
Own free-range game, beef,
chicken and lamb produced on
the farm.

Beaulieu
Countryside Education Trust,
Palace Lane SO42 7YG
01590 612401
www.cet.org.uk
Farm and gardens providing
educational facilities for young
people. Sells Christmas turkeys
and eggs all year round.

Bordon

 Blackburne & Haynes,
Meadow Cottage Farm,
Churt Road,
Headley GU35 8SS
01428 712155
Milk and cream from Jersey
cows, mostly grass-fed in
summer. Also ice cream.

Emsworth

 Southbourne Farm Shop,
Main Road,
Southbourne PO10 8AP
01243 377521
www.southbournefarmshop.co.uk
Home cooked cheesecakes and
quiches, local fruit and
vegetables, dairy produce, eggs,
bread, own honey.

Fareham

Town Centre
01329 824474
www.fareham.gov.uk/council/depar
tments/planning/markets.asp
First Saturday of the month,
09.00 to 14.00

Fordingbridge

 Pigs Direct,
The Moon and Sixpence,
Midgham SP6 3BY
01425 650237
www.pigsdirect.com
Free-range Gloucester Old Spots
reared in woodland on natural
diet.

Heckfield

 Park Farm Shop,
Near Hatchgate Pub RG27 0LD
0118 932 6650
www.pfo-shop.co.uk
Organic beef, pork and lamb,
plus fish, organic poultry and
organic fruit and vegetables.

Hook

 Holly Bush Farm,
Hollybush Lane,
Eversley RG27 0NH
0118 932 8816
www.hollybushfarm.com
Organic free-range Dexter beef
and rare breed pork and poultry.

Lymington

 Mrs Tee's Wild Mushrooms,
Gorse Meadow,
Sway Road SO41 8LR
01590 673354
www.wildmushrooms.co.uk
Specialist in wild mushrooms
most of which are organic. Box
scheme delivers within the M25
and south and west.

 Warborne Organic Farm,
Warborne Lane,
Boldre SO41 5QD
01590 688488
www.warbornefarm.co.uk
Range of organic vegetables,
organic soft fruit, top fruits, herbs
and flowers, mostly own
produce. Box scheme delivers to
New Forest area.

Overton

Laverstoke Park Butcher's Shop,
Southley Farm RG25 3DR
01256 771571
www.laverstokeparkbutchersshop.co
.uk
Biodynamic and organic, free-range, rare breed beef, pork, poultry, wild boar, water buffalo and game.

Petersfield

Durleigh Marsh Farm Shop,
Durleigh Marsh Farm,
Rogate Road GU31 5AX
01730 821626
Farm shop and pick-your-own soft fruit and asparagus.

Southampton

Chalcroft Farm Shop,
Chalcroft Farm,
Burnetts Lane,
West End SO30 2HU
02380 601154
New Forest venison, pigeon and pheasant from the farm's own land.

Sunnyfields Organic Farm,
Jacobs Gutter Lane,
Totton SO40 9FX
023 8086 1266
www.sunnyfields.co.uk
Sells over 1,000 organic products including its own fruit, locally sourced meat, dairy produce and organic eggs.

Stockbridge

Dairy Barn Farm Shop,
North Houghton SO20 6LF
01264 811405
www.dairybarn.co.uk
Native and rare breed meats from livestock used in conservation grazing projects. Meat delivery box scheme.

Titchfield

Garsons,
Fontley Road PO15 6QX.
01329 844336
www.garsons.co.uk
Farm shop selling English truffles, local apple juices, preserves, cheeses, chicken, duck and quail's eggs. Also meats and dairy produce, vegetables and fresh fruit. Also at Esher in Surrey.

Winchester

Middle Brook Street
01420 588671
www.hampshirefarmersmarkets.co.uk
Second and last Sunday of the month, 09.00 to 14.00

Upton House Farm,
Wonston SO21 3LR
01962 760219
Organic free-range chicken, wild rabbit and pigeon.

HEREFORDSHIRE

Almeley

New House Farm
HR3 6LT
01544 327561
Milk and cream from Holstein
Friesian cows, mostly grass-fed
in summer. Organic beef also
available plus unpasteurised
milk, local cider and honey.

Bosbury

Beaconhill Farm,
Nash End Lane HR8 1JY
01531 640275
www.beaconicecream.com
Milk, cream and ice cream from
organic Jersey cows.
Unpasteurised milk also
available.

Bromyard

Outside Bromyard Leisure
Centre
01886 821237
Fourth Thursday of the month,
09.00 to 13.00

Hereford

Golden Valley Organics,
Bali-Hai,
Dinedor HR2 6PD
01432 870646
www.goldenvalleyorganics.co.uk
Organically-farmed meat and
other produce.

Court Farm,
Tillington,
Burghill HR4 8LG
01432 760271
www.courtfarmleisure.co.uk
Soft fruit, ready-picked or pick-
your-own.

High Town
01873 890675
www.hfmg.org
First Saturday and Thursday of
the month, 09.00 to 14.00

Hope-under-Dinmore

Wynne's of Dinmore
HR6 0PX
01568 797314
www.wynnes.co.uk
Eggs from hens allowed to roam
freely outside all day.

Ledbury

Flights Orchard Organics,
Unit 5,
Lynden Business Park,
New Hills,
Leadon Way HR8 2SR
0845 658 9808
www.flightsorchardorganics.co.uk
Organic vegetables and fruit
grown on own farm and by a
group of local growers. Vegetable
box scheme delivered throughout
the West Midlands.

Llandinabo Farm Shop,
21 The Homend HR8 1BN
01531 632744
www.llandinabofarmshop.co.uk
Traditional, free-range, rare breed
beef such as Belted Galloway and
Dexter. Pork from Gloucester Old
Spots and British Saddleback.

Leominster

Corn Square
01568 616348
www.hfmg.org
Second Saturday of the month,
09.00 to 13.00

Ross on Wye

Pengethley Farm Shop,
Pengethley Garden Centre,
Peterstow HR9 6LN
01989 730430
Locally sourced fresh meat
including Hereford beef, Lleyn
lamb, Gloucester Old Spot pork
and free-range organic chickens.
Also vegetables and cheeses.

Soilmates,
PO Box 67 HR9 5ZA
01989 767444
www.soilmates.com
Wide range of rare and unusual
chillies and sweet peppers. Also
collections of heirloom tomatoes,
cucurbits and speciality fruits.

HERTFORDSHIRE

Barnet
Arkley Natural Veg,
92 Galley Lane, Arkley
07962 983131
Variety of vegetables.

Berkhamsted
Eastwoods Butchers,
15 Gravel Path HP4 2EF
01442 865012
Supplies organic and free-range
meat source from small
producers, free range organic
eggs, game, rare breeds plus pies.

Hertford

Market Place
01992 531 610
www.growninherts.com
Second Saturday of the month,
09.30 to 13.00

Letchworth
Leys Square
01462 486 999
www.growninherts.com
Third Saturday of the month,
09.00 to 13.00

St Albans
Willows Farm Shop,
Coursers Road,
London Colney AL2 1BB
0870 129 9718
www.willowsfarmvillage.com
Sells locally sourced rare breed
meat including Longhorn beef
and boar, plus traditionally bred
pigs and sheep. Locally baked
cakes and a local goat's cheese.

Tring
Old Cattle Market,
Brook Street
01442 842252
www.tringfarmersmarket.co.uk
Every other Saturday, 09.00 to
12.15

ISLE OF WIGHT

Arreton

Isle of Wight Tomatoes
Hale Common PO30 3AR
01983 866907
www.isleofwighttomatoes.co.uk
Wide range of tomatoes
including many organically
grown varieties.

Bathingbourne

Chinashop Rare Breeds,
Brandywell PO36 0LU
01983 840917
www.rarebreeds.org
Rare breed beef and lamb raised
on National Trust land.

The Isle of Wight Bacon
Company,
Moor Farm PO38 3JG
01983 840210
www.isleofwightbacon.co.uk
Free-range pork, dry cured bacon
and ham, plus sausages.

Newchurch

Isle of Wight Garlic,
The Garlic Farm PO36 0NR
01983 865378
www.thegarlicfarm.co.uk
Garlic.

Newport

St Thomas Square
01983 865720
www.islandfarmersmarket.co.uk
Every Friday, 09.00 to 14.00

KENT

Ashford

Bank Farm Produce,
Bank Farm,
Bank Road,
Aldington TN25 7DF
0800 587 4999
www.bankfarm.co.uk
Free-range eggs. Also quail, duck
and goose eggs.

Perry Court Farm Shop,
Bilting TN24 4EP
01233 812302
www.perrycourt.com
Sells its own fruit and vegetables.
Locally sourced bread, meat and
dairy produce, free-range-eggs
and home-made pear and apple
juice.

Potten Farm Shop,
Main Road,
Sellindge TN25 6EQ
01303 814804
Fresh fruit and vegetables,
cheeses, meat, local cream and
strawberries plus local honey
and free range eggs.

Bexley

Dennis of Bexley,
21 Naplehurst Close DA2 7WX
01322 522126
www.dennisofbexley.co.uk
Traditional butcher selling local
pheasant, rabbit and wild
venison.

Canterbury

 Perry Court Farm,
Garlinge Green,
Chartham CT4 5RU
0800 083 5942
www.perrycourtfarm.com
Biodynamic and organic fruit
and vegetable box scheme. Most
produce is home-grown.

 Yew Tree Farm,
Chillenden CT3 1NY
01304 840214
Sells its own fruit, vegetables and
free-range meat, including
Aberdeen Angus beef.

Deal

Town Hall,
High Street
01304 361999
Every Wednesday, 09.00 to 13.00

Horsmonden

Simply Wild Food Company,
The Oast,
Pullens Farm,
Lamberhurst Road TN12 8ED
0845 658 6142
www.simplywild.co.uk
Organic box scheme offering fruit
and vegetables as well as meat,
bread, dairy and eggs. Most
produce is local.

Sevenoaks

The Hop Shop,
Castle Farm,
Shoreham TN14 7UB
01959 523219
www.hopshop.co.uk
Shop sells its own beef and apple
juice. Also local cheeses and
honey plus free range eggs, pies,
cakes, bread.

Sittingbourne

The Barn Yard,
Gore Farm,
Upchurch ME9 7BE
01634 235059
www.the-barnyard.co.uk
Fruit farm with award-winning
farm shop, delicatessen,
restaurant and PYO enterprise.

Tunbridge Wells

Civic Way,
outside the Town Hall
01892 554244
www.tunbridgewells.gov.uk
Second and fourth Saturday of
the month, 09.00 to 14.00

Whitstable

Artisan Bread,
Units 16-17,
John Wilson Business Park
CT5 3QZ
01227 771881
www.artisanbread.ltd.uk
Mill own grain to make flour
from unusual grain varieties. A
biodynamic bakery that takes
account of human health and the
affect of ingredients on the
environment.

LANCASHIRE

Blackburn

Fairfield Farm Shop,
Longsight Road,
Clayton-le-Dale BB2 7JA
01254 812550
www.fairfieldfarm.co.uk
Pig farm supplying the shop
with sausages, dry cure bacon,
ham and fresh pork. Local
supplies beef, chicken, lamb,
cheese and milk. Free-range eggs,
and ready meals, soups and
puddings made on site.

Burnley

Styberry Pig Herd,
6 Pendle View,
Higham BB12
01282 772628
Stephen.green@tc.lancscc.gov.uk
Pork from rare breed pigs and
home produced lamb. Can be
purchased from Higher White
Lee Farm, Barrowford Road,
Fence, Burnley BB12 9ET. Phone
01282 772436 or e-mail
david.nutter4@btinternet.com

Chorley

Cockers Farm Shop,
Limbrick PR9 9EE
01257 260743
www.cockersfarm.com
Sells own or local produce,
organic or using minimal
chemicals. Fresh meat and
poultry, pies, home-made meals,
some fruit and veg.

Clitheroe

Cowmans Famous Sausage
Shop,
13 Castle Street BB7 2BT
01200 423842
www.cowmans.co.uk
Long established butchers using
local meats to make more than 70
types of fresh sausage.

Market Square
01200 443012
First and third Tuesday of the
month, 09.00 to 16.00

Downholland

Mossland Pure Breeds,
Hesketh Farm,
Station Road,
Barton LS9 7JW
07989 459650
www.muleskinner.nik@virgin.net
Texel sheep, pure and rare breed
poultry and eggs, herbs, baked
goods, preserves.

Kirkham

Cunliffe Fold Farm,
Salwick
01772 690622
Every Saturday, 10.00 to 14.00

Lancaster

Ellel Free Range Poultry,
The Stables,
Ellel Grange,
Galgate LA2 0HN
01524 751200
www.ellelfreerangepoultry.co.uk
Free range Poulets de Bresse and
Sasso chickens and guinea fowl,
geese reared on farm.

Growing With Grace,
Clapham Nursery,
Clapham LA2 8ER
01524 251723
www.growingwithgrace.co.uk
Farm shop and organic box
scheme run by Quakers. Boxes
contain a range of vegetables
grown on the farm. Other
produce sourced locally where
possible.

Mawdesley

Cedar Farm Galleries,
Back Lane
01257 515151
First Saturday of the month,
10.00 to 15.00

Ormskirk

The Worrall House Farm
Larder,
Flatman's Lane,
Downholland L39 7HW
0151 527 1210
www.worrallhousefarmlarder.com
Sells beef from its own Aberdeen
Angus herd along with locally
sourced pork, lamb, free-range
chicken and eggs. Also
Lancashire cheeses, ready meals
and puddings.

Pilling

Growing With Nature,
Bradshaw Lane Nursery
PR3 6AX
01253 790046
www.madeinpreston.co.uk/general/
food.html
Box scheme run by nursery
growing around 35 different
vegetables every year. All are
organic.

Preston

Farmhouse Direct,
Long Ghyll Farms,
Brock Close,
Bleasdale PR3 1UZ
01995 61799
www.farmhousedirect.com
Highland beef raised on species-
rich upland grazings. Also
Bleasdale lamb grazed on upland
pastures plus venison, poultry
and game.

Silverdale

Silverdale Vegetables,
Oaktree Barn,
Bottoms Lane LA5 0TN
01524 702891
gailran@onetel.com
Potatoes, beans, brassicas, sweet
corn, salad, carrots, strawberries,
raspberries, eggs, honey and
wax.

LEICESTERSHIRE

Billesdon

Seldom Seen Farm,
Green Lane LE7 9FA
0116 259 6742
www.seldomseenfarm.co.uk
Free range poultry including
goose, Norfolk bronze turkey,
pheasants and partridges.

Castle Donington

St Edward's School
01530 261379
Second Saturday of the month,
09.00 to 14.00

Cold Overton

Northfield Farm,
Whissendine Lane LE15 7QF
01664 474271
www.northfieldfarm.com
Free-range traditional and rare
breed beef, lamb and pork. All
sourced locally or from its own
farm.

Leicester

Market Place
0116 273 1170
Last Wednesday of the month,
09.00 to 15.00

Loughborough

Growing Concern Organic
Farm,
Home Farm,
Woodhouse Lane,
Nanpantan LE11 3YG
01509 239228
www.growingconcern.co.uk
Family farm producing
traditional British Hereford beef,
Dorset Down lamb and free-
range poultry and pork.

Manor Farm Shop,
77 Main Street,
Long Whatton LE12 5DF
01509 646413
www.manororganicfarm.co.uk
Organic Longhorn beef and
lamb. The farm has a bakery as
well as a farm shop.

Market Harborough

Farndon Fields Farm Shop,
Farndon Road LE16 9NP
01858 464838
Sells own soft fruits and many
vegetables. Also jams, chutneys,
pickles using own produce.
Home-made cakes, fresh bread
and home-reared beef.

Melton Mowbray

 Brocklebys Farm Shop,
Brocklebys,
Melton Road,
Asfordby Hill LE14 3QU
01664 813200
www.brocklebys.co.uk
Sheep farm selling rare breed lamb. Also Longhorn beef, Middlewhite pork plus some organic veg and beef. Free-range and rare breed eggs, honey and dairy, all locally sourced where possible.

Cattle Market,
Scalford Road
01664 562971
Every Tuesday and Friday, 08.00 to 13.00

LINCOLNSHIRE

Boston

Abbey Parks Asparagus,
Park Farm,
East Heckington PE20 3QG
01205 821154
www.abbeyparksaparagus.co.uk
Asparagus and rhubarb by mail order.

Country Meadows,
Marjon,
Southfield Lane,
Fishtoft PE21 0SJ
01205 302930
Chicken and duck eggs, Ryeland lamb, rare breed pigs and turkeys.

 Peter's Eden,
Lenick Mill Hill,
Friskney PE22 8NG
01754 820733
www.peterseden.com
Jams, chutneys and cordials made with local produce.

F C Phipps,
Osborne House,
Mareham-Le-Fen PE22 7RW
01507 568235
www.britainsbestbutcher.co.uk
Free-range and organic native breed beef, salt marsh lamb, pork and game.

Woodlands Farm,
Kirton House,
Kirton PE20 1JD
01205 722491
www.woodlandsfarm.co.uk
Organically reared Lincoln Red cattle, Lincoln Longwool sheep, organic vegetables and salads plus a bronze turkeys at Christmas.

Brigg

Market Place
01652 657053
Fourth Saturday of the month, 09.000 to 15.00

Gainsborough

East Farm,
Normanby By Stow DN21 5LQ
01427 788629
www.wholesome-
food.org.uk/EastFarm.html
Grass-fed traditional Lincoln Red
cattle. Meat sold in box scheme.
Also fruit, seasonal vegetables
and free-range eggs.

Grantham

W E Botterill and Son,
Lings View Farm,
10 Middle Street,
Croxton Kerrial NG32 1QP
01476 870394
Free-range geese and Bronze
turkeys. Also seasonal game.

Horncastle

Shottons Farm,
Church Lane,
Minting LN9 5RS
01507 578606
Wide range of organic seasonal
vegetables plus some soft fruit.
Leeks, onions and eggs usually
available all year.

Lincoln

City Square,
near Waterside Centre
01522 545 2333
First Friday of the month, 09.00
to 16.00

Market Rasen

Sunny Side Up,
Poplar Farm,
Tealby Road LN8 3UL
01673 844736
www.sunnyside-up.co.uk
Free-range eggs direct from the
farm, locally produced ready
meals and fresh meats.

Scunthorpe

The Pink Pig,
Holme Hall,
Holme Lane,
Bottesford DN16 3RE
01724 844466
www.pinkpigorganics.co.uk
Mixed organic farm with shop
selling its own organic pork,
chicken, eggs and veg. Also
stocks cured bacon, sausages,
organic milk, yogurts, organic
lamb and local beef.

Spalding

Fenleigh Farm Produce,
Fenleigh,
Broad Drove,
Gosberton Clough PE11 4JS
01775 750478
Wide variety of vegetables, soft
fruit and free range eggs. Also a
box scheme.

Stamford

Red Lion Square
01476 406080
Every other Friday, 08.30 to 15.00

MERSEYSIDE

Birkenhead

Next to Indoor Market Hall
0151 666 3914/5
www.birkenheadmarket.co.uk
Last Friday of the month, 10.00 to
15.00

Liverpool
Hope Street
0151 233 2165
Third Sunday of the month, 09.00
to 14.00

Lark Lane
0151 233 2165
Fourth Saturday of the month,
09.00 to 14.00

Woolton Village
0151 233 2165
Second Saturday of the month,
09.00 to 14.00

Southport
King Street & Market Street
0151 934 4283
Last Thursday of the month,
10.00 to 15.00

Wirral
Church Farm Organics,
Church Lane,
Thurstaston CH61 0HW
0151 648 7838
www.churchfarm.org.uk
Organic farm with shop selling
fresh vegetables, fruit and a
range of traditional meats
including lamb and pork.

Edge and Son,
61 New Chester Road,
New Ferry CH62 1AB
0151 645 3044
www.traditionalmeat.com
Organic, free range and rare
breed beef, lamb and pork. Sells
a range of burgers and 20 types
of sausage.

NORFOLK

Attleborough
Great Grove Poultry,
Whews Farm,
Caston NR17 1BS
01953 483808
chick-man@hotmail.co.uk
Free-range chickens all year.
Free-range Bronze turkeys and
geese at Christmas.

Aylsham
Samphire Farm Shop,
The Estate Barn,
Blickling Hall NR11 6NF
01263 734464
www.samphireshop.co.uk
All food locally made or locally
sourced. Includes rare breed
meats, venison, pork sausage,
fresh bread, cheeses and milk.
Also chicken, seasonal fruit and
veg, pork pies, sausage rolls and
cakes.

Burnham

Carnival Hall
07932 627574
Third Sunday of the month, 09.00
to 12.00

Dereham

Railway Station
01362 693821
Second Saturday of the month,
09.00 to 12.00

Diss

Goodies Farm Shop,
French's Farm,
Wood Lane,
Pulham Market IP21 4XU
01379 676880
www.goodiesfarmshop.co.uk
Rare breed pork plus locally
sourced lamb, beef and chicken.
Local dairy produce and Norfolk
jams. Café serves homemade
breakfasts, sandwiches, cakes,
soups as well as coffee and
speciality teas.

Town Council
01379 643848
Second Saturday of the month,
09.00 to 12.00

Downham Market
Dent's of Hilgay,
Hilgay PE38 0QH
01366 385661
www.dentsofhilgay.co.uk
Own and locally sourced meat
includes Aberdeen Angus beef.
Also many Norfolk seasonal
foods plus local produce, cakes,
biscuits and cheese.

Holt

H V Graves,
Inside Larners,
Market Place NR25 6BW
01263 710000
Free range beef and pork reared
on its own farm plus locally
produced lamb and poultry. Also
fruit and veg.

Hunstanton

Courtyard Farm,
Ringstead
Norfolk PE36 5LQ
01485 525251
Organic, rare breed beef, lamb
and pork reared on the farm.

King's Lynn

Abbey Farm Organics,
Flitcham PE31 6BT
01485 609094
www.abbeyfarm.co.uk
Box scheme offering organic
vegetables and fruit, home-
grown or from a co-operative of
local growers.

Castle Acre Organic,
Manor Farm,
Castle Acre PE32 2BJ
01760 755380
www.castleacreorganic.co.uk
Box scheme offering home-grown
organic vegetables and fruit plus
home produced meat.

Nar Hideaway,
Saddlebrow PE34 3AP
01553 617730
www.wholesome-food.org.uk/burr.html
Vegetables, fruit, pork, lamb and chickens.

Melton Constable

M and M Rutland,
13 Briston Road NR24 2DG
01263 860562
www.rutland-butchers.co.uk
Traditional family butchers selling local, free range meat. Produces traditional smoked bacon and ham as well as haggis and a range of sausages.

North Walsham

Tavern Tasty Meats,
The Farm Store,
The Street,
Swafield NR28 0PG
01692 405444
www.taverntasty.co.uk
Rare breeds butcher specialising in gourmet sausages.

Norwich

Barker Organics,
The Walled Garden,
Wolterton Hall NR11 7LY
01263 768966
Box scheme selling biodynamic and organic fruit and vegetables in the local area.

Harvey's Pure Meat,
63 Grove Road NR1 3RL
01603 621908
www.puremeat.org.uk
Organic butcher and game dealer. Locally sourced organic beef, lamb and pork; free range poultry and local game. Certified by the Organic Food Federation.

HFG Farm Shop,
Old Yarmouth Road,
Blofield NR13 4LQ
01603 424608
Family-run co-operative selling own Aberdeen Angus beef and free-range pork. Farm's own flour milled in nearby water mill. Also fruit, veg, local venison and meat pies. Pick-your-own at White House Farm in Sprouston.

 Peeles' Norfolk Black Turkeys,
Rookery Farm,
Thuxton NR9 4QJ
01953 860294
Naturally reared Norfolk Black, Bronze and Boubon red turkeys plus beef.

Rectory Field Smallholding and Nursery,
The Old Rectory,
Aslacton NR15 2JN
01379 677362
Seasonal vegetables, soft fruit, chickens and pigs.

Station Bungalow,
Thorpe Market NR11 8UE
01263 833406
Seasonal vegetables and eggs
through Sheringham Country
Market.

Shelton
 Oaktree Farm Partnership,
Oaktree Farm,
The Common NR15 2SH
01508 536549
Wide variety of products
including vegetables, fruit, Soay
lamb and mutton. From pedigree
Large Black pigs there are pork,
ham, sausages and bacon.

Stalham
Town Hall
01692 670 992
First and third Saturday of the
month, 09.00 to 12.00

NORTH YORKSHIRE

Bishopthorpe
 Brunswick Organic Nursery,
Appleton Road YO23 2RF
01904 701869
www.brunswickyork.org.uk
Sheltered workplace for adults
with learning difficulties. Sells
plants plus organic fruit and
vegetables.

Darlington
 Pepperfield Farm Produce,
Pepperfield Farm,
Dalton-on-Tees DL2 2NS
07849 026561
www.pepperfieldfarm.co.uk
Sausages and pork from farm
raised, free-range Gloucester Old
Spot and Tamworth pigs.
Wiltshire Horn mutton and
Orpington chicken. Member of
the Wholesome Food
Association.

Harrogate
 Market Place
01423 556761
Second Thursday of the month,
09.00 to 15.00

Leeming Bar
 Low Leases Farm,
Low Street DL7 9LU
01609 748177
www.lowleasesorganicfarm.co.uk
Farm-run box scheme offering
organic vegetables, fruit, chicken,
sausages, beef and lamb, plus
Shorthorn beef reared on the
neighbouring farm.

Leyburn
The Market Place
01748 884414
www.ndfm.co.uk
Fourth Saturday of the month,
08.00 to 15.00

Malton

The Market Place
01751 473780
Second Saturday of the month,
09.00 to 14.00

Northallerton

Hook House Farm,
Low Street,
Kirkby,
Fleetham DL7 0SS
01609 748977
Organic farm selling its own
lamb, beef and bronze turkeys.
Also its own honey.

Spring House Farm Shop,
Scruton DL7 9LG
01677 422212
www.springhouse-farmshop.co.uk
Sells pork, vegetables and free-
range eggs from the farm. Also
sells local produce including
cheese, beef and lamb. Shop
known for its home baked meat
and fruit pies, cakes and
puddings.

Pickering

Organic Farm Shop,
Standfield Hall Farm,
Westgate Carr Road YO18 8LX
01751 472249
Farm shop delivering home-
grown vegetables, home
produced beef, whole foods and
a range of fruit and meats.

Richmond

Bluebell Organics,
Forcett Hall Walled Garden,
Forcett DL11 7SB
01325 718841
www.bluebellorganics.co.uk
Box scheme delivery service for
mostly home-grown organic fruit
and vegetables. Also at local
farmers' markets.

Farmaround Organic,
The Old Bakery,
Mercury Road DL10 4TQ
01748 821116
www.farmaroundnorth.co.uk
Organic and vegetarian,
Farmaround supplies locally-
sourced vegetables and fruit in
bag scheme. Also salad boxes
and groceries. Café serves
organic, locally produced snacks,
soups, sandwiches and sweets.

Hazelbrow Visitor Centre,
Hazel Brow Farm,
Low Row DL11 6NE
01748 886224
www.hazelbrow.co.uk
Organic working farm in
Yorkshire Dales national park.
Shop sells lamb and cheese from
the farm's own cows.

Tadcaster

 The Organic Pantry,
St Helen's Farm,
Newton Kyne LS24 9LY
01937 531693
www.theorganicpantry.co.uk
Organic shop selling fruit,
vegetables, meat, dairy, bread
and whole foods. Also runs a box
scheme.

Warmfield Farm,
Green Lane,
Stutton LS24 9BW
01937 835039
www.warmfieldfarm.co.uk
Quail eggs, pedigree beef, pigs,
ducks, guinea fowl and turkeys.

Thirsk

The Smithy Farm Shop,
Baldersby YO7 4PN
01765 640676
Shop sells organic beef, lamb and
pork plus ready meals. Also
stocks organic bread, organic
milk and a variety of organic
fruit juices, plus organic eggs and
fruit and veg.

Yorkshire Farmhouse Freedom
Eggs Ltd,
Village Farm,
Catton
01845 577355
www.yorkshirefarmhouse.co.uk/eggs
.asp
Organic free range eggs from
hens roaming freely outside.

Towthorpe

The Farmer's Cart,
Towthorpe Grange,
Towthorpe Moor Lane
YO32 9ST
01904 499183
Shop selling its own fruit,
vegetables and meats. Also a
pick-your-own enterprise and
tearoom.

Whitby

Pasture Cottage Organics,
Pasture Cottage,
Bog House Farm,
Mickleby TS13 5NA
01947 840075
Home-grown or locally sourced
organic seasonal vegetables. Eggs
also available.

York

Alligator,
104 Fishergate YO10 4BB
01904 654525
www.alligatorwholefoods.com
Organic grocer, greengrocer and
whole food vegetarian shop.
Organic fruit, veg and groceries
plus locally-grown soft fruits.
Home delivery in York area.

NORTHAMPTONSHIRE

Daventry

One (Organic, Natural and
Ethical) Food,
19 Austin Way,
Royal Oak Trading Estate
NN11 5QY
0870 871 1112
www.onefood.co.uk
Box scheme of organic fruit,
vegetables, meat, sustainable
fish, dairy products, prepared
meals and range of health foods.

Higham Ferrers

Market Square
01933 312075
Last Saturday of the month, 09.00
to 14.00

Northampton

The Guildhall,
St Giles Square
01604 837837
Third Thursday of the month,
09.00 to 13.00

Towcester

Richmond Road car park
01327 351848
Second Friday of the month,
09.00 to 13.00

Wellingborough

Market Place
01933 231915
Last Thursday of the month,
09.00 to 14.00

NORTHUMBERLAND

Alnwick

Roseden Farm Shop,
Roseden,
Wooperton NE66 4XU
01668 217271
www.roseden.com
Shop sells farm's own beef and
lamb as well as baked goods
(savoury pies, cakes and
biscuits). Also stocked are
sausages, local free-range eggs
and organic milk.

Town Square
0794 732 3396
www.northumberlandfarmersmarkets
.org.uk
Last Friday of the month, 09.00 to
14.00

Bedlington

North East Organic Growers,
Earth Balance,
West Sleekburn Farm,
Bomarsund NE22 7AD
01670 821070
www.neog.co.uk
Box scheme run by organic
vegetable grower. Offers range of
vegetables plus organic eggs.

Berwick-upon-Tweed

Whistlebare,
Bowsden TD15 2TG
01289 388777
www.whistlebare.co.uk
Rare breed farm in organic
conversion. Pedigree Aberdeen
Angus cattle, Large Black pigs
and Light Sussex and Maran
chickens.

Corbridge

 Brocksbushes Farm Shop
NE43 7UB
01434 633100
www.brocksbushes.co.uk
Specialises in pick-your-own
raspberries, strawberries and
asparagus. Shop sells fruits,
organic vegetables, free-range
eggs and preserves. Also local
sausages and fish. Tea room
makes quiches, pies, ready meals
and is licensed to serve alcohol.

Greenhead

 Hadrians Wall Market
off the A69
01697 747448
www.northumberlandfarmersmarkets
.org.uk
Second Sunday of the month,
10.00 to 14.00

Hexham

 Jo's Home-baked Bread,
33 Rye Terrace NE46 3DX
01434 608456
Wide variety of home-baked
breads using local and organic
ingredients when possible.
Available at Hexham Farmers'
Market.

 Kielder Organic Meats,
Dunterley Farm,
Bellingham NE48 2JZ
01434 220435
www.kielderorganicmeats.co.uk
Organic, free-range, rare breed
pigs, venison, Hexham black-
faced sheep, laying hens and
Angus and Galloway cattle.

 Market Place
07963 426932
www.hexhamfarmersmarkets.co.uk
Second and fourth Saturday of
the month, 09.00 to 13.30

 Northumbrian Quality Meats,
Monkridge Hill Farm,
West Woodburn NE48 2TU
01434 270184
www.northumbrian-organic-
meat.co.uk
Organic, traditionally-farmed
Scottish Blackface sheep,
Aberdeen Angus and Galloway
cattle.

Morpeth

 Moorhouse Farm Shop and
Café,
Station Road,
Stannington NE61 6DX
01670 789016
www.moorhouosefarmshop.co.uk
All pigs and lambs born and
reared on the farm. Shop has its
own butchery and delicatessen.
Also sells local fruit and
vegetables.

 New Barns Farm Shop,
New Barns Farm,
Warkworth NE65 0TR
01665 710035
Shop sells the farm's own
Northumbrian beef and rare
breed pork. On site bakery makes
cakes, pies, ready meals and
patties. Also restaurant and tea
room.

Otterburn

 Haven Organics,
Havens Farm,
Heatherwick NE19 1LY
01830 520806
Box scheme delivering all own
organic vegetables. Also
premium organic beef from own
Dexter herd.

Stamfordham

 Gilchesters Organics,
Gilchesters Organic Farm,
Hawkwell NE18 0QL
01661 886119
www.gilchesters.com
Organic traditional English and
Scottish cattle. Also its own beef
burgers and organic stoneground flour from rare-variety
wheats.

NOTTINGHAMSHIRE

Cossall

Trinity Farm,
Awsworth Lane NG16 2RZ
0115 944 2545
www.trinityfarm.co.uk
Shop sells its own organic fruit
and veg. Organic meat and dairy
produce is sourced from local
farms. Box scheme delivers fruit,
veg and salads.

Gonalston

 Gonalston Farm Shop,
Southwell Road NG14 7DR
0115 966 5666
www.gonalstonfarmshop.co.uk
Sells free-range beef reared on its
own farm and sources lamb and
pork from local farmers. Also
new fishmongery, locally
produced fruit and veg, free-
range eggs, jams, cakes and pies.

Mansfield

 The Buttercross Market
01623 463470
Third Tuesday of the month,
09.00 to 15.00

Newark

Barn Bacon Farm,
Hardy's Farmshop,
Farndon NG24 3SD
01636 610700
www.barnbacon.co.uk
Beef, lamb and free-range poultry
plus its own traditional bacon
and hams.

Church Farm Shop,
Main Street,
South Scarle NG23 7JH
01636 892003
www.churchfarmshop.co.uk
Shop sells the farm's own
produce including asparagus,
apples and free-range eggs. Local
farmers supply rare breed meat
such as Dexter beef. Also local
dairy produce.

Nottingham

 Spring Lane Farm Shop,
Spring Lane Farm,
Maperley Plains NG3 5RQ
0115 926 7624
www.springlanefarmshop.co.uk
Farm grows potatoes and a range
of other vegetables. Shop also
sells home-reared meat and the
farm's own free-range eggs. Also
stocked: blue stilton cheese,
cured bacon and ham, local
cordials.

West Brigford

Main Shopping Precinct,
Central Avenue
01664 822 114
Second and fourth Saturday of
the month, 09.00 to 14.00

Worksop

Bridge Street
01909 533533
Second Friday of the month,
08.30 to 14.30

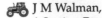
OXFORDSHIRE

Abingdon

Millets Farm Centre,
Millets Farm,
Kingstone Road,
Frilford OX13 5HB
01865 392200
www.milletsfarmcentre.com
Shop sells apples, gooseberries,
currants and strawberries
supplied by the farm. Also
vegetables and fresh herbs.
There's a cheese counter plus
fresh meat, free-range and
organic eggs and bread.

Banbury

 Wykham Park Farm Shop,
Wykham Park Farm OX16 9UP
01295 262235
www.wykhampark.co.uk
Home produced beef and lamb,
home-grown seasonal fruit and
vegetables. Plus farmhouse
cheeses and home-made cakes.

Bicester

J M Walman,
1 Station Road,
Launton OX26 5DS
01869 252619
Traditional breed butchers with
wide variety of locally produced,
rare breed meats.

Brize Norton

Foxbury Farm Shop,
Foxbury Farm,
Burford Road OX18 3NX
01993 844141
www.foxburyfarm.co.uk
Gloucester Old Spot pork, lamb
and beef produced on the farm.
Ready meals a speciality, plus a
range of local foods.

Deddington

 Market Place
01869 337904
www.deddington.org.uk/community
/farmersmarket.html
Fourth Saturday of the month
(except 16 December), 09.00 to
12.30

Oxford

 M Feller, Son and Daughter,
54-55 The Oxford Covered
Market OX1 3DY
01865 251164
www.mfeller.co.uk
Organic butcher selling organic
free-range chicken and organic
beef, lamb, pork, bacon and
sausages.

 Gloucester Green Open Market
01789 267000
First and third Thursday of the
month, from 08.30

Spelsbury

 Coldronbrook Meats,
Glebe Farm OX7 3JR
01608 811118
www.coldronbrookmeats.co.uk
Direct sales of free-range Dexter
beef.

Thame

 Upper High Street Car Park,
Near Retail Market
0118 984 3114
www.tvfm.org.uk
Second Tuesday of the month,
08.30 to 13.30

Wallingford

 Bridge House,
72 Wallingford Road,
Shillingford OX10 7EU
01865 858540
www.bridge-house.org.uk
Christian community offering
free-range eggs.

Wantage

 Real Farm Foods,
Blandys Farmhouse,
Letcombe Regis OX12 9LJ
0808 006 7426
www.realfarmfoods.com
Organic beef, lamb, pork and
poultry. Also delivers organic
fruit and vegetables.

RUTLAND

Oakham

 Ashwell Farm Shop,
Rutland Garden Centre,
Ashwell LE15 7QN
01572 759492
Organic poultry and eggs
(Rutland Organic Poultry);
Bassingthorpe Beef and Lamb; as
well as other local suppliers'
produce.

 Gaol Street
01780 722009
Third Saturday of the month,
09.30 to 12.30

 Northfield Farm Ltd,
Cold Overton LE15 7ER
01664 474271
Meat and preserves.

Uppingham

 The Deli,
Printers Yard LE15 9RA
01572 822588
Delicatessen products

 Mercers Yard
01780 722009
Second Friday of the month,
09.30 to 12.30

SHROPSHIRE

Church Stretton
Market Square
01694 722113
Second and fourth Friday of the
month, 09.00 to 13.00

Ludlow
Upper Wood Farm,
Hopton,
Cangeford SY8 2GF
01584 823319
Vegetables and fruit.

Market Drayton
Ben's Eggs,
Heathcote Avenue,
Hookgate,
Loggerheads TF9 4QF
01530 673218
www.foodconnection.co.uk/rheas
Naturally produced eggs.

Fordhall Organic Farm,
Ternhill Road TF9 3PS
01630 638696
www.fordhallorganicfarm.co.uk
Free-range Hereford and
Aberdeen Angus beef grazing
species-rich pastures all year
round. Also organic lamb and
pork, dry cured bacon, free-range
eggs, fresh local vegetables,
Shropshire honey and jams.

Park Hill Farm,
Park Hill,
Hales TF9 2QA
01630 652178
www.parkhillfarm.co.uk
Slow maturing beef allowed to
range freely on long-established
grassland.

Much Wenlock
Guild Hall
01952 727509
www.shropshirehillsaonb.co.uk/
thingstodo/market.htm
First and third Friday of the
month, 09.00 to 13.00

Rodington
Boxfresh Organics in
Shropshire,
Unit 5c, Rodenhurst Business
Park SY4 4QU
01952 770006
www.boxfreshorganics.co.uk
Box scheme offering organic fruit
and vegetables in Shropshire, the
west midlands and mid Wales.
Aims to source locally where
possible.

Shrewsbury
Hollies Farm,
16 Valeswood,
Little Ness SY4 2LH
01939 261046
Supplies raspberries, potatoes,
beans and cabbage.

Telford

Live Organic,
Food for Thought,
Unit 3, Heath Hill Industrial
Estate,
Dawley TF4 2RH
01952 630145
www.liveorganic.com
All organic produce delivered
locally in a box scheme. Includes
organic dairy products, meats,
vegetables, fruits and salads.

Wellington

Market Square
01952 240192
Third Saturday of the month,
09.00 to 12.30

SOMERSET

Bath

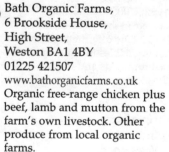

Bath Organic Farms,
6 Brookside House,
High Street,
Weston BA1 4BY
01225 421507
www.bathorganicfarms.co.uk
Organic free-range chicken plus
beef, lamb and mutton from the
farm's own livestock. Other
produce from local organic
farms.

Ivy House Farm,
Beckington BA3 6TF
01373 830957
Produces unpasteurised cream
from Jersey cows. The milk is
pasteurised.

Bridgwater

Quantock Traditional Pork,
Martindale,
Aisholt TA5 1BD
01278 671467
Hand-made sausages, dry cured
bacon, gammon steaks, gammon
hams and roasting joints.

Bruton

Somerset Organics,
Gilcombe Farm BA10 0QE
01749 813710
www.somersetorganics.co.uk
Organic beef, lamb, pork and
chicken. Also cheese and other
products.

Chard

Swaddles Green Farm,
Hare Lane,
Buckland St Mary TA20 3JR
0845 456 1768
www.swaddles.co.uk
Organic beef, lamb, pork and
poultry sourced from local farms.

Crewkerne

Falkland Square
01373 812757
www.somersetfarmersmarkets.co.uk
Third Saturday of the month,
09.00 to 13.00

Fuzzy Ground Produce,
46 Hermitage Street TA18 8ET
01460 74690
Chickens, waterfowl, orchard
and soft fruits, vegetables.

Frome

Barrow Farm,
Rode Hill,
Rode BA11 6PS
01373 830841
www.barrowfarm.com
Seasonal vegetables and apples
plus pick-your-own soft fruits.

Whiterow Farm Shop,
Whiterow Country Foods,
Beckington BA11 6TN
01373 830798
Shop sells the farm's own
produce including pork,
vegetables and salads. Also
organic cream and milk from a
local farmer, plus locally sourced
eggs.

Glastonbury

St John's Car Park
01458 830801
www.somersetfarmersmarkets.co.uk
Fourth Saturday of the month,
09.00 to 13.00

Langport

Merricks Organic Farm,
Park Lane TA10 0NF
01458 252901
www.merricksorganicfarm.co.uk
Superb quality organic fruit and
vegetables offered in a box
scheme.

Pitney Farm Shop,
Glebe Farm,
Woodsbirdshill Lane,
Pitney TA10 9AP
01458 253002
www.pitneyfarmshop.co.uk
Shop sells organic pork, lamb,
beef and free-range eggs from its
own farm. Also home-made
sausages and burgers, fresh
vegetables, home-made pies and
pasties, smoked and dry cured
bacons and hams.

Milverton

Spring Grove Market Garden
TA4 1NW
07956 429531
Seasonal box scheme offering
vegetables, fruit and eggs.

Minehead

Exmoor Organic Farmers,
Hindon Organic Farm,
Exford TA24 7JY
01643 705244
www.exmoororganicmeat.co.uk
Organic beef, pork and lamb.

Shepton Mallet

Brown Cow Organics,
Perridge Farm,
Pilton BA4 4EW
01749 890298
www.browncoworganics.co.uk
Organic vegetables grown on-
farm or by local growers. Also
pasture-fed dairy products and
award-winning beef.

John Thorner's Ltd,
Bridge Farm Shop,
Pylie BA4 6TA
01749 830138
Full range of local game. Fresh in
season, otherwise frozen.

Somerton

Merryacre,
The Old Dairy,
Ersome TA11 6JD
01458 272859
Chicken, eggs, turkeys, geese,
lamb and beef.

Olive Farm,
Babcary TA11 7ES
Milk, cream, yogurt and butter
from Guernsey cows, grass-fed in
summer, home-made silage in
winter. Sold at farmers' markets
in London, Guildford, Henley,
and Wallingford.

Taunton

Dykes Farm,
Slough lane,
Stoke St Gregory
01823 490349
Organic dairy farm selling
unpasteurised milk.

Rumwell Farm Shop
TA4 1EJ
01823 461599
Shop sells home produced free-
range chickens, eggs and pork.
Also fresh fruit and vegetables,
fruit juices and preserves.

Somerset Country Produce,
Prockters Farm,
West Monkton TA2 8QN
01823 413427
Sells own organic beef and lamb
plus free-range pork and many
local foods.

Somerset Farm Direct,
Bittescombe Manor,
Upton TA4 2DA
01398 371387
www.somersetfarmdirect.co.uk
Direct sellers of lamb, mutton,
beef, pork and poultry.

Stoneage Organics,
Stoneage Farm,
Cothelstone TA4 3ED
01823 432488
Home-grown organic vegetables
offered in box scheme.

Wellington

The Bell and Bird Table,
Runnington TA21 0QW
01823 663080
Smallholding selling 47 tomato
varieties grown organically. Also
soft fruit.

West Quantoxhead

Woodside Orchard,
Woodside Staple Lane TA4 4DE
01984 633060
Vegetables, chickens and duck
eggs.

Weston Super Mare

Town Square (Rear of Winter Gardens)
01934 417117
www.n-somerset.gov.uk/Business/Food/Farmers+markets
Second Saturday of the month, 09.00 to 14.00

Yeovil

Barrow Boar,
Fosters Farm,
South Barrow BA22 7LN
01963 440315
www.barrowboar.co.uk
Traditional meats, game and exotic meats.

Goose Slade Farm,
East Coker BA22 9JY
01935 863735
Farm shop with its own free-range geese and lamb plus locally-sourced products such as Blue Vinny cheese.

SOUTH YORKSHIRE

Doncaster

Goose Hill,
Doncaster Market
01302 886479
First and third Wednesday of the month, 10.00 to 16.00

Penistone

Market place
S366DY
01226 766202
www.penistonefarmersmarket.co.uk
Second Saturday of the month, 09.00 to 13.00

Sheffield

Heeley City Farm,
Richards Road,
Heeley S2 3DT
0114 258 0482
www.heeleyfarm.org.uk
Community project on organic inner city educational farm. Grows fruit and vegetables.

Roney's Traditional and Free Range Butchers,
276 Sharrowvale Road,
Hunters Bar S11 8ZH
0114 266 0593
www.freerangebutchers.co.uk
Specialises in traditional and rare breed meats.

Wentworth

Wentworth Garden Centre
S62 7TF
01909 567 588
Second Sunday of the month

STAFFORDSHIRE

Cannock

The Market Place,
Town Centre
01384 440059
www.lsdpromotions.com
Third Friday of the month, 09.00 to 15.00

Lichfield

 The Old Stables Farm Shop and
Bakery,
Packington Moor Farm
WS14 9QB
01543 481223
www.packingtonmoor-events.co.uk
Shop sells a wide variety of fruits
plus cheeses and other dairy
products, free-range eggs,
poultry, meat and locally baked
bread. Farm has a PYO fruit
enterprise.

Newcastle-under-Lyme

Brookfields Farm Shop,
Stone Road,
Blackbrook ST5 5EG
01782 680833
Shop sells home-grown potatoes
and locally sourced produce.
Also eggs, pork products, fruit
and vegetables. Local turkeys at
Christmas.

Penkridge

Pinfold Lane
01785 714221
www.southandstubbs.co.uk/
Penkridgemarket/
FarmersMarketsgeneral.htm
Third Saturday of the month,
09.00 to 15.00

Rudyard

Daisy Bank Farm,
Rudyard Road ST13 8PE
01538 306267
Free-range eggs and some
vegetables.

Stafford

Market Square
01785 245935
www.staffordbc.gov.uk/static/
page998.htm
Second Saturday of the month,
09.00 to 16.00

Stoke-on-Trent

Jacobs Fold,
18 Sutherland Road,
Tittensor ST12 9JQ
jacobsfold@aol.com
Produce includes vegetables and
salads, Jacobs lamb and
Tamworth bacon, pork and
sausages.

SUFFOLK

Beccles

Beccles Heliport,
Ellough Airfield
01502 476 240
First and third Saturday of the
month, 09.00 to 13.00

Bungay

Eden Organics and Whole
foods,
Southview,
165 Yarmouth Road,
Broome NR35 2NZ
07789 965904
www.edenorganics.co.uk
Box scheme offering organic,
fruit, vegetables, eggs and whole
foods from a local growers co-
operative.

Bury St Edmunds

 Longwood Farm,
Tuddenham St Mary IP28 6TB
01638 717120
www.longwoodfarm.co.uk
Organic chicken, beef, lamb and
pork reared on the farm.

Eye

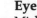 Michael Knights,
Daganya Farm,
Nuttery Vale,
Hoxne IP21 5BB
01379 668060
www.eostreorganics.org/mknights.
html
Box scheme delivering a range of
vegetables from the local
farmers' co-operative, Eostre
Organics.

Felixstowe

Goslings Farm Shop,
High Road,
Trimley St Martin IP11 0RJ
01394 273361
www.goslingsfarm.co.uk
Shop stocks own fruit and veg
plus meat from local suppliers
and fresh bread from local
bakery. Own potatoes all year
round.

Hadleigh

Hollow Trees Farm Shop,
Semer IP7 6HX
01449 741247
www.hollowtrees.co.uk
Award-winning shop sells own
meat plus local bread, preserves,
wines and honey. Own
vegetables when available.

Ipswich

Alder Carr Farm Shop,
Alder Carr Farm,
Creeting St Mary IP6 8LX
01449 720820
www.aldercarrfarm.co.uk
Seasonal fruit and vegetables,
plus Highland beef, all grown on
the farm. Local free-range
chickens and home-made ice
cream using the farm's own fruit.

The Essex Pig Company,
Pannington Hall Farm,
Wherstead IP9 2AR
01473 601770
www.essexpigcompany.com
The famous Jimmy's Farm. Rare
breed beef, lamb and poultry
sourced from local, free-range
farms.

Hillside Nurseries,
Hintleham IP8 3NJ
01473 652682
Box scheme from a nursery
grows full range of organic
vegetables. Fruit and organic
eggs sourced locally.

Rookery Farm Shop,
Rookery Farm,
Tattingstone IP9 2LU
01473 327220
Locally produced foods
including smoked fish, meat
preserves, honey and ice creams.
Seasonal foods include salads,
sweetcorn, purple sprouting and
broad beans.

Laxfield

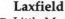 Little Meadows Farm,
Banyards Green IP13 8EU
01986 798138
Smallholding selling seasonal
vegetables and herbs plus free-
range eggs. Also lamb, pork and
Shetland wool.

Needham

 Alder Carr Farm
01449 720820
www.aldercarrfarm.co.uk
Third Saturday of the month,
9.00 to 13.00

Saxmundham

Emmett's Stores,
Peasenhall IP17 2HJ
01728 660250
www.emmettsham.co.uk
Traditional Suffolk ham and
bacon sourced from local free-
range farms.

Friday Street Farm Shop,
Farnham IP17 1JX
01728 602783
Locally sourced, home-grown
meat, fruit and vegetables, plus
many organic foods.

Snape Maltings
01728 688 303
First Saturday of the month,
09.30 to 12.30

Sudbury

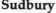 Assington Farm Shop,
Willow Tree Farm CO10 5LW
01787 211610
Home-made apple juice from
own fruit, local free-range eggs,
local sweetcorn and locally
sourced cheeses. Also vegetables,
locally-baked bread, cream and
ice cream.

Woodbridge

Grange Farm Shop,
Grundisburgh Road,
Hasketon IP13 6HN
01473 735610
Sells local produce including
meat, fruit and veg, preserves,
juices, ice cream and groceries.
Apples in season.

SURREY

Betchworth

In A Crystal Garden,
Gatton Point,
Leigh Road RH3 7AW
01306 611499
www.inacrystalgarden.com
Seasonal garden produce
including vegetables, free-range
eggs, jams, chutneys and cooked
products.

Cranleigh

Food Revolution,
Freepost (SCE10589) GU6 8BR
0800 169 6673
www.foodrevolution.com
Nationwide delivery of organic
groceries and fresh meat, locally
sourced where possible.

Sunshine Organics,
2 Knowle Cottages,
Knowle Lane GU6 8JL
01483 272209
www.sunshine-organics.co.uk
Box scheme started for mums of
young children who wanted a
variety of fruit and vegetables.
Sourced from two local growers.

Dorking
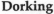 Kingfisher Farm Shop,
Abinger Hammer RH5 6QX
01306 730703
Based on a watercress farm, the
shop's speciality is watercress.
Also fruit and vegetables plus
meat and dairy products from
local farms.

Effingham
Badgers Farm,
High Barn Road KT24 5PP
01372 450046
Farm shop selling home-reared
beef, pork, lamb and goat.

Egham
Green Landscape Nurseries,
Hurst Lane TW20 8QJ
01784 435545
Variety of quality vegetables
including peppers, aubergines,
Borlotti beans and many tomato
varieties.

Epsom
Market Place,
High Street
01372 732562
First Sunday of the month, 09.30
to 13.30

Esher
 The Game Larder,
24 The Parade,
Claygate KT10 0NU
01372 462879
Game and free-range poultry.

Ewell
Kenneth J Eve Butchers,
9 Corner House Parade,
Epsom Road KT17 1NX
020 8393 3043
www.kjeve.co.uk
Traditionally reared beef from
Orkney and lamb from the South
Downs.

Farnham
Cucumber Field,
Greenacres,
Dippenhall,
Crondall GU10 5PE
01252 850335
Vegetable box scheme plus eggs.

Godalming
C H Wakeling Ltd,
41 Farncombe Street GU7 3LH
01483 417557
www.wakelings.co.uk
Aberdeen Angus beef from a
local farm with pastures
receiving no sprays or chemical
fertilizers.

Lightwater
 George Arthur Ltd,
70 Guildford Road GU18 5SD
01276 472191
www.georgearthur.com
Locally sourced game.

Milford

Secretts Farm,
Chapel Lane
01483 520500
www.secretts.co.uk/markets.htm
Third Sunday of the month, 10.00
to 14.00

Redhill

Fanny's Farm Shop,
Markedge Lane RH1 3AW
01737 554444
www.fannysfarm.com
Farm shop specialising in honey,
home-made marmalades, bacon,
sausages and local cheeses.

Wallington

Old Town Hall & Library
Gardens,
Woodcote Road
020 8770 5668
www.sutton.gov.uk/environment/
farmersmarket.htm
Second Saturday of the month,
09.30 to 13.30

TEES VALLEY

Darlington

Market Place
01325 388691
Third Friday of the month, 09.00
to 17.00

Hartlepool

Quay Car Park
01748 884965
www.ndfm.co.uk
Second Saturday of the month,
08.30 to 15.30

Guisborough

Market Square
01287 651601
www.ndfm.co.uk
Second Saturday of the month,
10.00 to 15.00

Larberry Pasture Farm,
Long Newton TS21 1BN
01642 583823
Shop sells own home reared beef,
lamb, pork and organic free-
range eggs. Cakes and bread
supplied by local baker.

TYNE AND WEAR

Newcastle upon Tyne

Blagdon Farm Shop,
Milkhope Centre,
Seaton Burn NE13 6DA
01670 789924
www.theblagdonfarmshop.co.uk
Sell rare-breed beef and pork
from the Blagdon estate. Also
free-range chickens, quail, turkey
and duck. Honey from the farm
plus a range of fruit and veg.

George Payne Butchers,
27 Princess Road,
Brunton Park,
Gosforth NE3 5TT
0191 236 2992
www.georgepaynebutchers.co.uk
Rare breeds butcher whose meat
comes from trusted local
Northumberland farmers who
practise traditional, non-intensive
farming.

Grey's Monument
0191 211 5533
www.newcastle.gov.uk/core.nsf/a/
marketfarmers
First Friday of the month, 09.30
to 14.30

Wallsend

Rising Sun Farm,
Kings Road North NE28 9JL
0191 234 0114
www.northtyneside.gov.uk/
environment/risingsun/contact.htm
Organic farm producing seasonal
fruit and vegetables.

WARWICKSHIRE

Kenilworth

Talisman Square
01789 267000
www.sketts.co.uk/farmersmarkets.
html
Second Saturday of the month,
09.00 to 14.00

Leamington

Aubrey Allen Direct,
108 Warwick Street CV32 4QP
01926 311208
www.aubreyallen.co.uk
Guinea fowl, Gressingham duck
and free-range, corn-fed
chickens. Other meats include
free-range pork and Cornish
lamb.

Meriden

Berkswell Traditional
Farmstead Meats,
Larges Farm,
Back Lane CV7 7LD
01676 522409
www.farmsteadmeats.co.uk
Traditional and rare-breed meats
from around Warwickshire.

Rugby

Clock Tower,
Market Place
01608 664659
www.warwickshirefarmersmarkets.
co.uk
Last Thursday of the month,
09.00 to 14.00

Stratford upon Avon

Talton Mill Farm Shop,
Talton Mill,
Newbold on Stour CV37 8UG
01789 459140
www.talton-mill.co.uk
Shop sells only meat produced
on the farm. Includes beef, pork
(bacon and sausages) and
chicken. Also seasonal
vegetables.

Warwick

Market Square
01789 267000
www.sketts.co.uk/farmersmarkets.
html
Third Friday of the month, 09.00
to 14.00

Wellesbourne

 Hunscote Farm,
Stratford Road CV35 9ES
01789 840240
Farm shop sells own lamb,
potatoes and other vegetables.
Also home-made jams, cakes and
pies, local cheeses and free-range
eggs.

WEST MIDLANDS

Birmingham

 R Brown,
6 Northfield Road B17 0SS
0121 427 2057
Organic beef, free-range Welsh
salt marsh lamb, free-range
Gloucestershire chickens and
free-range pork from Shropshire.

 Organic Roots,
Crabtree Farm,
Dark Lane,
Kings Norton B38 0BS
01564 822294
www.organicroots.co.uk
Organic shop selling beef, lamb,
pork and chicken as well as
seasonal meats such as rabbit,
mutton and venison.

Coventry

 Ryton Organic Gardens,
Ryton on Dunsmore CV8 3LG
02476 303517
www.hdra.org.uk
National Centre of Organic
Gardening. Hundreds of
different apple varieties plus
locally produced fruit and
vegetables.

 Spon Street
01789 267000
www.sketts.co.uk/farmersmarkets.
html
Second Thursday of the month,
09.00 to 14.00

Halesowen

 The Square,
Cornbow Centre
01384 440059
www.lsdpromotions.com
Second and fourth Saturday of
the month, 09.00 to 15.00

Solihull

 Hopwood Organic Farm,
Bickenhill Lane,
Catherine-de-Barnes B92 0DE
0121 711 7787
www.hopwoodorganic.co.uk
Organic vegetable box scheme
run by small family farm. Most
produce home-grown with some
sourced from local farms.

Stourbridge

 High St/Coventry Street
01384 440059
www.lsdpromotions.com
First and third Saturday of the
month, 09.00 to 15.00

Wolverhampton

 Essington Fruit Farm,
Bognop Road,
Essington WV11 2BA
01902 735724
Farm shop sells soft fruit and
some vegetables. Also pick-your-
own.

WEST SUSSEX

Billinghurst

 Lee House Farm,
Plaistow RH14 0PB
01403 753311
www.leehousefarm.co.uk
Organic farm with a range of
products including organic eggs,
rare breed pork, bacon and
sausages; lamb, beef, casserole
chickens and a variety of
seasonal vegetables.

Chichester

East Street & North Street,
Chichester City Centre
01243 785166
www.chichester.gov.uk/
First and third Friday of the
month, 09.00 to 14.00

Wayside Organics,
Wayside,
Oving PO22 2BT
01243 779716
Organic box scheme using
mostly home-grown produce.
Fresh vegetables and fruit.

East Grinstead

Old Plaw Hatch Farm,
Sharpthorne RH19 4JL
01342 810201
Partner to Tablehurst Farm (see
below). A biodynamic farm
making raw milk cheeses. Also
breads, raw milk cream and
butter, live yogurt, organic fruit
and vegetables.

Horsham

Carfax Centre
01403 215549
www.horsham.gov.uk
Every Saturday, 09.00 to 17.00

Selham

Farm Fresh Express,
GU28 0PJ
0845 612 4040
www.farmfreshexpress.co.uk
Online home delivery service
offering local produce. Includes
meat, game, fish, dairy,
vegetables and fresh-baked
bread.

Shoreham by Sea

East Street
01273 263152
www.adur.gov.uk/markets
Second Saturday of the month,
09.00 to 13.00

Steyning

Chanctonbury Butchers,
51 High Street BN44 3RE
01903 813239
Local meat from the South
Downs area.

WEST YORKSHIRE

Addingham

Beanstalk Organix,
Unit 9, Townhead Trading
Centre,
Main Street LS29 0PD
01609 748177
www.beanstalkorganix.co.uk
Home delivery offering fruit,
vegetables, milk, meat, eggs, fish
and range of groceries.

Bingley

Bingley Local Produce Market
Chapel Lane Market
BD16 1NN
01535 670950
Fourth Saturday of the month,
09.00 to 13.00

Bradford

The Farm Shop,
Keelham Hall Farm,
Thornton BD13 8XC
01274 833472
www.thefarmshop.net
Sells lamb from the farm plus
locally sourced beef, pork and
chicken. Also free-range eggs,
Yorkshire yogurts, local jams and
special breads.

Chapel Allerton

Mustard Pot,
20 Stainbeck Lane LS7 3QY
07982 445 047
www.organicleeds.co.uk
First Sunday of the month, 09.00
to 17.00

Halifax

Far Barsey Farm Shop,
Barkisland, HX4 0BG
01422 371287
Sells a variety of local produce
including own beef and ready
meals plus products from other
regional food producers.

Ingfield Farm Shop,
Law Farm, Law Lane,
Southowram HX3 9UG
01422 330333
www.ingfieldfarmshop.co.uk
Farm has its own beef herd. Pork,
lamb, fruit and veg are sourced
from local farms. Shop has deli
selling cooked meats and other
products. Also sells farm's own
free-range eggs.

Osbourns Organics,
1A Bracken Farm,
Priestley Green HX3 8RQ
01422 205578
Box scheme delivering organic
foods in West Yorkshire. Most
vegetables and soft fruit grown
on the farm.

Huddersfield

Hinchcliffes Farm Shop and
Butcher,
Sunny Side Farm,
Netherton Moor Road
HD4 7LE
01484 661231
Free-range and rare breed pork,
reared by the butcher and local
farmers. Also free-range organic
poultry and Morecambe Bay salt-
marsh lamb.

Thorncliffe Farm Shop,
West Field Lane,
Emleymoor HD8 9SZ
01924 848171
Large shop selling mainly
produce from Thorncliffe Grange
farm. Includes beef, pork, lamb,
and free-range eggs. Also locally
sourced vegetables and milk.

Ilkley

Lishman's of Ilkley,
25 Leeds Road
01943 609436
Maker of award-winning
sausages. Pork is reared by the
butcher using Saddleback pigs
fed on a natural grain diet.

Keighley

Cranswick Gourmet Bacon,
Mill Lane,
Oakworth BD22 7QH
01706 216439
www.cranswick.co.uk
Traditional dry cure bacon. Also
ham, sausages and black
pudding from free-range
traditional pig breeds.

Leeds

Kirkgate Market
0113 214 5162
First and third Sunday of the
month, 09.00 to 14.00

Swillington House Farm,
Garden Cottage,
Coach Road,
Swillington LS26 8QA
0113 286 9129
www.swillingtonhousefarm.co.uk
Organic farm producing lamb,
pork, chicken and eggs.

Otley

George Middlemiss and Sons,
3 Market Street LS21 3AF
01943 462611
www.dalesnet.co.uk
Traditionally-fed beef, pork and
lamb reared locally. Home-cured
ham plus pies and sausages.

Rigton Wholesome Foods,
6 St Clair Terrace LS21 1JA
01943 461102
Seasonal outside vegetables plus
polytunnel grown tomatoes,
peppers, chillies, cucumbers and
aubergines.

Pontefract

Brickyard Farm Shop,
Badsworth WF9 1AX
01977 617327
Organic home-grown fruit and
vegetables picked fresh daily.
Farm sales plus box scheme.

Wetherby

Goosemoor Organics,
Warfield Lane,
Cowthorpe LS22 5EU
01423 358887
www.goosemoor.co.uk
Box scheme delivering local and
home-grown organic produce.
Range of fruit and vegetables,
specialising in protects crops
such as salads.

WILTSHIRE

Chippenham

 Market Place
01249 446699
www.chippenham.gov.uk/about/
market.htm
Alternate Tuesdays, 09.00 to 13.30

Cholderton

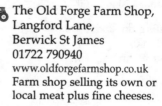 Source at Cholderton
SP4 0DR
01980 629745
www.sustainable-cholderton.co.uk
Farm shop selling organic meat
from the Cholderton Estate. Also
home-made gluten-free sausages,
ready meals and cakes.

Devizes

Chestnuts Farm,
Dairy Cottage,
Little Horton SN10 3LH
01380 860214
Vegetables, sheep, chickens,
geese, ducks, eggs and goats.

Lacock

Whitehall Garden Centre,
Corsham Road SN15 2LZ
01249 730204
www.whitehallgardencentre.co.uk
Farm shop and restaurant
supplied by nearby Whitehall
Farm and other local farmers.
Free-range organic eggs, local
milk and dairy produce and on-
site bakery. All meat grass-fed
outdoors.

Purton House,
Church End SN5 4EB
01793 770219
www.purton-house.co.uk
Locally-delivered box scheme
provides home-grown organic
vegetables and fruit, plus beef.
Also locally-sourced chicken and
pork.

Malmesbury

 The Market Cross
01453 758060
www.fresh-n-local.co.uk/
markets/Malmesbury.php
Second and fourth Saturday of
the month, 09.00 to 14.00

Salisbury

Market Square
07775 614790
www.wiltshirefarmersmarkets.org.uk
First and third Wednesday of
month, 10.00 to 14.00

The Old Forge Farm Shop,
Langford Lane,
Berwick St James
01722 790940
www.oldforgefarmshop.co.uk
Farm shop selling its own or
local meat plus fine cheeses.

Pigman,
86 Longford Park,
Bodenham SP5 4EG
01725 513929
www.pigman.co.uk
Bacon, gammon and other
products from British Saddleback
pigs.

Swindon

Coleshill Organics,
59 Coleshill SN6 7PT
01793 861070
Fruit, herbs and vegetables sold
from the farm and by box
scheme.

Eastbrook Farm,
Bishopstone SN6 8PW
01793 790460
www.helenbrowningorganics.co.uk
Organic beef, lamb, pork and
poultry.

Warminster

John Herd's Organic
Watercress,
Stonewold,
Hill Deverill BA12 7EF
01985 840260
Grown to maturity for strong
taste and traditionally bunched.
Farmgate sales and local box
scheme.

The Real Meat Company
BA12 0HR
01985 840562
www.realmeat.co.uk
High animal welfare standards
and genuinely free range.
Animals have natural diet and
stress-free lives.

West Knoyle

Bush Farm Bison Centre
BA12 6AE
01747 830263
www.bisonfarm.co.uk
Supplies bison meat. Also elk
and red deer.

WORCESTERSHIRE

Broadway
Kites Nest Farm
WR12 7JT
01386 853320
Organically-grown, free-range
Welsh Black and Lincoln Red
beef available only from the
farm shop.

Bromsgrove

High Street
07795 656148/9
www.worcestershirefarmersmarkets.
net
Second Saturday of the month,
09.00 to 17.00

Defford
Hopyard Farm,
Bourne Road WR8 9BS
01386 750902
www.hopyardfarm.co.uk
Eggs from small flock of hens
allowed to roam outdoors.

Great Witley
Mill Orchards,
Stourport Road WR6 6JP
01299 896222
www.millorchards.co.uk
Apples are the speciality, but in
the farm shop you'll find other
prepared fruits and soft fruits.
Also a variety of juices, pickles,
home-made jams and local
honey.

St Michael's Farm
WR6 6JB
01299 896608
Unpasteurised goats' milk and
cheese from British Toggenburg
and British Saanen dairy goats.

Kidderminster

Augernik Fruit Farm,
Hopton Wafers DY14 0HH
01299 272870
Soft and top fruits, nuts and free-
range eggs.

Tony's Bakery,
1 Peel Street DY11 6UG
01562 636463
Hand-made bread from recipes
over a century old.

Knightwick

Teme Valley Market,
The Talbot at Knightwick
01886 821235
Second Sunday of the month,
11.00 to 13.30

Malvern

Malvern Country Meals,
37 Church Street WR14 2AA
01684 568498
Award-winning butchers whose
meat is mainly sourced locally
and free-range.

Stanford Bridge

Happy Meats,
Bank House Farm WR6 6RU
01886 812485
www.happymeats.co.uk
Rare breed beef including Dexter
and Longhorn, plus Gloucester
Old Spot pork.

Mill Farm and Garden Shop
WR6 6SP
01886 853267
Shop sells home-grown potatoes,
local traditional meats and local
vegetables. Also home-made
jams and milk from local
supplier, free-range eggs, duck
eggs, quail eggs and goose eggs.

Upton Upon Severn

Clive's Fruit Farm,
Upper Hook Road WR8 0SA
01684 592664
www.clivesfruitfarm.co.uk
Sells its own large range of fruit
and vegetables, fruit juices, perry
and cider. Also stocks ice cream,
local beers, free-range eggs,
organic meat and bread baked on
site.

Worcester

Broomfields Farm Shop,
School Plantation,
Holt Heath WR6 6NF
01905 620233
www.broomfieldsfarmshop.co.uk
Sells own fresh fruit and juices
plus organic and locally
produced cheeses. Fresh local
vegetables, meat, jams and
pickles.

Farm Direct Produce,
10 Beckett Close,
Northwick WR3 7NL
01905 356068
www.farmdirectproduce.co.uk
Box scheme delivering a variety
of fresh vegetables to the local
area.

 Goodman's Geese,
Walsgrove Farm,
Great Witley WR6 6JJ
01299 896272
www.goodmansgeese.co.uk
Traditionally reared free-range
geese and bronze turkeys, fed
only on natural foods.

 Gwillams Farm Shop,
Ombersley Road,
Claines WR3 7RH
01905 756490
Farm grows its own seasonal
vegetables. Milk and dairy
produce supplied by local
producers. Also local pickles,
beers and ciders.

 Roots at Rushwick,
Bransford Road,
Rushwick WR2 5TD
01905 421104
Shop sells the farm's own organic
seasonal veg, organic beef, lamb.
Chicken and eggs, plus its own
soft fruit. Also local dairy
products and fresh baked organic
bread.

 Royal Worcester,
Severn Street
01789 267000
www.sketts.co.uk/farmersmarkets.
html
First Sunday of the month, 10.00
to 14.00

CO ANTRIM

Antrim
Maze Organics,
Lisburn
028 9262 1771
Offers organic vegetable box
scheme.

Ballyclare
Ballylagan Organic Farm Shop,
12 Ballylagan Road,
Straid BT39 9NF
028 9332 2867

Ballymena
Dundermotte Farmhouse Ice
Cream,
30 Station Road,
Glarryford BT44 9RA
028 2568 5357
Cheese and dairy products.

O'Kane Poultry Ltd,
170 Larne Road BT42 3HA
028 2564 1111
A major supplier of poultry to
supermarket and food outlets.

Belfast
St Georges Market,
Oxford Street
028 3834 9100
www.belfastcity.gov.uk/
stgeorgesmarket/citymarket.asp
Every Saturday, 09.00 to 15.00

CO ARMAGH

Armagh
McArdle Mushrooms,
Knockaconey,
Allistragh
028 3889 1506
Manufacturers and distributors
of quality mushroom compost,
organic mushrooms and casings.

Loughgall
Gilpins Farm,
72 Drumilly Road BT61 8JJ
028 3889 1528
Grows organic fruit such as
apples, pears and plums and also
finisher of beef cattle.

Portadown
Barnhill Farm,
23 Drumanphy Road BT62 1QX
028 3885 1190
Apple juice including new
flavours created by blending
apple with the juice of other
whole fruit such as raspberry,
blackcurrant and blackberry.

Irish Certified Organic
Nutrients (ICON),
20 Maghery Road,
Portadown BT62 1SZ
028 3885 1055
Farm sales offering organic
vegetables, potatoes, strawberries
and soup vegetables.

CO DOWN

Downpatrick

Churchtown Farm,
30 Churchtown Rd BT30 7AT
028 4488 1686
Farm shop offering organic beef,
lamb and chicken.

Finnebrogue Venison
Company,
20 Finnebrogue Road BT30 9AB
028 4461 7525
www.finnebrogue.com
Specially selected from the prime
deer herd that roam freely in the
rolling parkland, raised on
natural feed, free from
genetically modified material
and without the use of growth
promoters or antibiotics.

Helens Bay
Helens Bay Organic Gardens,
Coastguard Ave
028 9185 3122
An organic market garden
producing and packing fresh
organic vegetables and fruit for a
box scheme delivery service for
the greater Belfast area. Other
organic products also available.

Hillsborough
Secret Garden,
22 Moira Rd BT26 6DU
028 9268 8886
Farm shop offering organic
vegetables, soft fruit, apples and
pears (when in season).

Holywood
Camphill Holywood,
8 Shore Road BT18 9HX
028 9042 3203
Organic bakery, cafe and shop
offering a range of baked goods
and other organic and local
produce.

CO FERMANAGH

Enniskillen
O'Doherty's Fine Meats,
Belmore Street
028 6632 2152
Organic bacon and other
speciality meat products in select
stores across Northern Ireland,
including own butchers shop in
Enniskillen

Irvinestown

The Orchard,
4 Mill Street BT94 1GS
028 6862 1533
Organic greengrocers.

Tickety-Moo,
Oghill,
Killadeas BT94 1RG
028 6862 8779
www.tickety-moo.com
Cheese and dairy products,
including ice creams made from
the milk of award-winning Jersey
cows.

CO LONDONDERRY

Coleraine

Culdrum Organic Farm,
31a Ballylintagh Road,
Aghadowey BT51 3SP
07764 638356
Organic farm sales and delivery
service offering organic
vegetables, herbs, potatoes, beef,
pork, poultry and eggs. Box
scheme as well.

Lundy Fruit Markets,
Long Commons BT52 1LB
028 70343044
Organic fruit and vegetables.

Garvach

Arkhill Farm,
25 Drumcroone Road BT51 4EB
028 2955 7920
www.arkhillfarm.co.uk
Offers organic produce including
duck and hen eggs, pork,
sausages, bacon, ham, fillets,
chops, roasts, lamb, turkeys and
chickens.

CO TYRONE

Castlederg

Organic Doorstep,
125 Strabane Road BT81 7JD
028 8167 9989
www.organicdoorstep.net
Delivers a large selection of food
directly to the doorstep. As well
as the organic fruit and veg, the
weekly boxes also include
organic milk, free-range eggs,
and juices.

Dungannon

Cloughbane Farm Shop,
160 Tanderagee Road BT70 3HS
028 8775 8246
www.cloughbanefarm.co.uk
Own beef and lamb as well as
locally produced pork and
chicken.

Down-to-earth,
6 The Linen Green,
Moygashel BT71 7HB
028 8772 2006
www.downtoearthni.co.uk
Organic whole food store.

Pat Corr Farm Meats,
20 Dernanaught Road
BT70 3BX
028 8775 8072
Good quality meats.

Strabane

Canal Basin
028 71880680
Last Saturday of the month, 10.00
to 14.00

ABERDEEN

Belmont Street
01224 649000
First and last Saturday of the
month, 08.30 to 16.30

Easter Anguston,
Peterculter AB14 0PL
01224 733627
Farm shop selling local fruit and
produce.

Strawberry Grange,
Wood End,
Peterculter AB14 0NS
01224 735699
Home grown fruit, veg, herbs, in
shop bakery.

Terroir (Bellentot Ltd),
22 Thistle St AB10 1XD
01224 623262
Cheese, olives. meats and
preserves.

ABERDEENSHIRE

Banchory
Scott Skinners Square
01330 825895
www.aberdeenshire.gov.uk/support
/agriculture/markets/index.asp
Third Saturday of the month,
11.00 to 15.00

Inverurie

Donald Russell Direct,
Harlaw Road AB51 4FR
01467 629666
www.donaldrussell.co.uk
Grass-fed, traditionally reared
beef and lamb, free-range
poultry, welfare friendly veal,
fish and game.

Lenshaw Organic Produce,
Upper Lenshaw Farm,
Rothienorman AB51 8XU
01464 871243
Wide variety of vegetables. Also
organic, free-range Gloucester
Old Spot pork and free-range
chicken. Local box scheme.

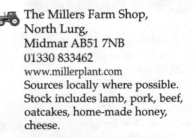
The Millers Farm Shop,
North Lurg,
Midmar AB51 7NB
01330 833462
www.millerplant.com
Sources locally where possible.
Stock includes lamb, pork, beef,
oatcakes, home-made honey,
cheese.

Peterhead
Drummers Corner
01771 622594
www.aberdeenshire.gov.uk/support
/agriculture/markets/index.asp
First Saturday of the month,
10.00 to 15.00

Stonehaven

 Lembas,
Lorieneen,
Bridge of Muchalls AB39 3RU
01569 731746
Organic box scheme offering
fruit, vegetables, eggs, cheeses
and preserves. Mostly home-
grown or from local growers.

 Charles McHardy,
11 Market Square AB39 2BT
01569 762693
Free-range beef and pork sourced
from north-east Scotland. Also
farm reared chicken and organic
eggs.

ANGUS

Arbroath

Milton Haugh Farm Shop,
Carmyllie DD11 2QS
01241 860579
www.miltonhaugh.com
Shop stocks free-range eggs, free-
range chicken and home grown
veg. Also Highland beef and Fife
pork. The dairy sources local
butters and Scottish cheeses.

Forfar

Myre Park
01382 370203
www.scottishfarmersmarkets.co.uk
Second Saturday of the month,
09.00 to 13.00

Kirriemuir

 Angus Organics,
Airlie Estate Office,
Cortachy DD8 4LY
01575 570103
www.angusorganics.com
Beef and lamb produced from
animals grazing clover-rich
pastures.

Montrose

Charleton Farm
01674 830226
www.charleton-fruit-farm.co.uk
Soft fruit farm selling PYO and
ready picked during season.

Town House Car Park
01307 464392
www.gable-enders.co.uk/
show.php?contentid=78
First Saturday of the month,
09.00 to 13.00

ARGYLL AND BUTE

Ardfern

 Highland Geese,
Corranmor Farm PA31 8QN
01852 500609
www.highlandgeese.co.uk
Natural seasonal production of
free-range geese.

Ardrishaig

Chalmers Street
01586 554510
www.scottishfarmersmarkets.co.uk
Second Saturday of the month,
10.00 to 14.00

Cardross

 Ardardan Estate and Farm Shop,
Ardardan Estate G82 5HD
01389 849188
www.ardardan.co.uk
Shop sells home-grown soft fruits and vegetables plus locally reared meats. Also Scottish cheese, ham and salmon, Fife dairy cream and locally sourced organic ice cream.

Isle of Mull

Ardalanish Organic Farm and Weaving Mill,
Bunessan PA67 6DR
01681 700265
www.ardalanishfarm.co.uk
Organic Highland beef, locally slaughtered, and Hebridean mutton. Wool used to make organic tweed.

Lochgilphead

Ormsary Farm
PA31 8PE
01880 770700
Scottish beef including sirloin steak.

Oban

The Cured Pig,
Corachie Farm,
Taynuilt PA35 1HY
01866 822564
Free-range Tamworth pork, bacon and sausages.

Kintaline Farm Plant and Poultry Centre,
Benderloch PA37 1QS
01631 720223
www.kintaline.co.uk
Eggs from Black Rock hens roaming all day on permanent pasture. Also duck eggs and fresh herbs.

Saulmore Farm Shop,
Connel PA37 1PU
01631 710247
www.saulmore.com
Free-range Highland and Aberdeen Angus cattle, Blackface sheep grazed on heather hills and pastured Texel sheep.

CLACKMANNANSHIRE

Alloa

 Gartmorn Farm
FK10 3AU
01259 750549
www.gartmornfarm.co.uk
Turkeys and chickens reared in open barns and given free access to surrounding orchards and fields.

DUMFRIES & GALLOWAY

Castle Douglas

Buccleuch Scotch Beef,
Cotton St DG7 1AH
0800 587 5011
www.scotchbeef.com
Traditionally-reared, grass fed beef from some of the best farms in Scotland.

Scottish Organic Lamb,
Knockreoch,
St Johns Town of Dairy
DG7 3XS
01644 430354
www.scottishorganiclamb.com
Organic Blackface lamb naturally
reared on local grazings.

 Sunrise Wholefoods,
49 King Street,
Parkhead Farm DG7 1AE
01556 504455
Sells pork, lamb, eggs,
vegetables, honey and fleeces for
hand-spinners. All local and high
quality.

Irongray

 Blackface,
Weatherall Foods,
Crochmore House DFG2 9SF
01387 730326
www.blackface.co.uk
Lamb, haggis, iron-age pork,
grouse, turkeys and venison
sourced from hill farms and local
producers in south-west
Scotland.

Newton Stewart

 Garrocher Market Garden,
Garrocher Sand Pit,
Creetown DG8 7EU
07944 080335
Range of salads and vegetables
plus top fruit, tomatoes, melons
and herbs.

DUNDEE

 Reform Street
01382 434548
Third Saturday of the month,
09.00 to 16.00

EAST AYRSHIRE

Kilmarnock

 Foregate (by bus station)
01655 770217
www.ayrshirefarmersmarket.co.uk
Third Saturday of the month,
09.00 to 14.00

Mauchline

 Corrie Maines Farm KA5 5DT
01290 550338
Free-range Isa Brown hens eggs
plus free-range quail, goose and
duck eggs.

EAST DUNBARTONSHIRE

Kirkintilloch

The Precinct
Third Wednesday of the month,
10.00 to 14.00

Milngavie

Douglas Street
01436 679882
First Wednesday of the month,
10.00 to 14.00

 The Mill House,
Dowan Road,
Baldernock G62 6HB
01419 562577
www.wholesome-food.org.uk/
directory.htm
Eggs, relishes and chutneys.

EAST LOTHIAN

Dunbar

The Crunchy Carrot,
43 High Street EH42 1EW
01368 860000
www.crunchycarrot.co.uk
Box scheme providing locally-grown fruit and vegetables.
Organic milk and organic free-range eggs also available.

Knowes Farm Shop,
Knowes,
East Linton EH24 1XJ
01620 860010
Shop stocks a variety of potatoes,
free-range eggs, dry-cured bacon,
sausages, fruit puree, organic
milk and a variety of vegetables.
On site kitchen makes a variety
of soups and ready meals.

Haddington

Outside Corn Exchange,
Court Street
01368 863593 / 01620 823964
www.scottishfarmersmarkets.co.uk
Last Saturday of the month, 09.00
to 13.00

Pencaitland

East Coast Organics,
24 Boggs Holdings EH34 5BD
01875 340227
www.eastcoastorganics.co.uk
Biodynamic farm running box
scheme. Home-grown fruit and
vegetables make up 80 per cent
of the produce in summer, but
some veg locally sourced.

Tranent

Elvingston Farm,
Elvingston,
By Gladsmuir EH33 1EH
01875 408000
www.elvingstonfarmproduce.co.uk
Products include: pedigree rare-breed pork, pedigree Highland
beef, Southdown and Jacob lamb
& mutton, healthy goat meat,
free-range Christmas geese, free-range hen, duck and goose eggs,
as well as dry-cured bacon and
traditional recipe butcher's
sausages.

EAST RENFREWSHIRE

Clarkston

Station Car Park
01555 771757
www.lanarkshirefarmersmarket.co.uk
Fourth Saturday of the month,
09.00 to 13.00

EDINBURGH

Castle Terrace
0131 6525940
www.edinburghcc.com/
farmersmarket
Every Saturday, 09.00 to 14.00

George Bower,
75 Raeburn Place,
Stockbridge EH4 1JG
0131 332 3469
Wide variety of organic, rare
breed and speciality meats.

Findlays,
116 Portobello High Street
EH15 1AL
0131 669 2783
www.findlayofportobello.co.uk
Free-range meat from border
farms and farms in Angus.
Widely famed haggis.

 Grow Wild,
Unit 10 New Lairdship Yards,
Broomhouse Road EH11 3UY
0131 443 7661
Supply organic produce such as
meats and cheeses, wines, dairy
and store-cupboard goodies, fruit
& veg boxes, delivered
throughout Central Scotland.

 Main Street,
Balerno
01738 449430
www.scottishfarmersmarkets.co.uk
Second Saturday of the month,
10.00 to 13.00

FALKIRK

 High Street
01324 611293
www.falkirkinspired.com/second.
html
Second Sunday of the month,
12.00 to 16.00

FIFE

Auchtermuchty

 Fletchers of Auchtermuchty,
Reediehill Deer Farm
KY14 7HS
01337 828369
www.seriouslygoodvenison.co.uk
Slow Food award nominees
producing superb, stress-free
venison.

Crossford

 Overton Farm
01555 771757
www.scottishfarmersmarkets.co.uk
First Saturday of the month,
10.00 to 15.00

Kirkcaldy

 Town Square
01383 730811
www.scottishfarmersmarkets.co.uk
Last Saturday of the month, 09.00
to 13.00

Newburgh

 Jamesfield Organic Centre,
Jamesfield Farm KY14 6EW
01738 850498
www.jamesfieldfarm.co.uk
Organic beef, lamb, pork, bacon,
sausages and burgers. Free-range
poultry. Organic shop.

Pittenweem

 Adamson's Bakery,
29 High Street KY10 2LA
01333 311336
Traditional Scottish oatcakes.

St Andrews

Allanhill Farm,
Grange Road KY16 8LJ
01334 473244
www.allanhill.co.uk
Farm shop stocks free-range
eggs, some local veg and home-
made jams. Local bakery supplies
fresh bread.

GLASGOW

Grassroots,
20 Woodlands Road,
Charing Cross G3 6UR
0141 353 3278
Organic food, ecological beauty,
household products, vitamins &
supplements. The vast majority
of organic vegetables are grown
specially at a local farm.

Mansfield Park,
Partick
0141 287 2500
www.glasgow.gov.uk/en/Business/
Markets/glasgowsfarmersmarkets.
htm
Second and fourth Saturday of
the month, 10.00 to 14.00

Queen's Park
0141 287 2500
www.glasgow.gov.uk/en/Business/
Markets/glasgowsfarmersmarkets.
htm
First and third Saturday of the
month, 10.00 to 14.00

HIGHLANDS

Achasheen

Good For Ewe,
Inverasdale,
Poolewe,
Wester Ross IV22 2LW
01445 781331
www.goodforewe.org
Range of vegetables through
local market in Poolewe,

Beauly

Wild Boar from Scotland,
Convinth Steading,
Kiltarlity IV4 7HT
01463 741807
www.scottishwildboar.co.uk
Wild boars range free in over 200
acres of Scottish hillside, and
mature in natural family
groupings.

Inverness

Eastgate Shopping Precinct
01463 723531
First Saturday of the month,
08.30 to 15.00

Isle of Skye

Glendale Salads,
19 Upper Fasach,
Glendale IV55 8WP
01470 511349
Range of organic vegetables,
salads, herbs and soft fruit.

Lairg

Croft 338,
Drumbeg IV27 4NW
croft338@virgin.net
Range of vegetables.

Greenock

Clyde Square
01505 503 553
www.scottishfarmersmarkets.co.uk
Third Saturday of the month,
09.00 to 14.00

Dalkeith

Malt Kiln Farm Shop
Campend Fruit Farm EH22 1RS
0131 6602128
Pick-your-own fruit and
vegetables.

Loanhead

Bonaly Farm Dairy
8 Dryden Rd EH20 9LZ
0131 440 0110
Dairy products.

Simply Organic,
21 Dryden Vale,
Bilston Glen EH20 9HN
0131 448 0440
Producer of fresh organic soup,
pasta sauce, baby food, kids
meals and dips.

Aberlour

Speyside Organics,
Knockanrioch,
Knockamdo AB36 7SG
01340 810484
www.speysideorganics.com
Home-reared, naturally matured
organic beef and lamb. Speciality
is smoked beef.

Elgin

Easterton Farm Venison
Easterton Farm Birnie IV30 8SP
01343 860294
Locally-farmed venison.

Plain Stones
Last Saturday of the month plus
extra dates June to September,
09.00 to 16.00

Forres

Macbeth's Butchers,
11 Tolbooth Street IV36 1PH
01309 672254
www.macbeths.com
Highland, Shorthorn and
Aberdeen Angus beef from
Edinvale Farms. Pasture-fed in
summer and naturally fed in
winter. Also pork, lamb, venison,
game and a variety of meat
products.

Fairlie

Fencefoot Farm
01475 568918
Last Sunday of the month, 10.00
to 15.00

NORTH LANARKSHIRE

Kilsyth

Kilsyth Main Street
01236 823167
www.northlan.gov.uk
First Saturday of the month,
09.00 to 14.00

ORKNEY ISLANDS

Orkney

Broad St
01856 831537
Last Saturday of the month
(except January to March), 09.00
to 13.00

Orkney Organic Meat,
New Holland Farm,
Holm KW17 2SA
01856 872417
www.orkneyorganicmeat.co.uk
Organic suckler beef and sheep
raised on grassland and heather
hills.

PERTH AND KINROSS

Blairgowrie
Wellmeadow (Community
Market)
01828 640763
www.strathmoreglens.org
Fourth Saturday of the month,
10.00 to 15.00

Bridge of Earn

Brig Farm Shop,
Gateside Home Farm PH2 8QR
01738 813571
Shop sells beef from the farm's
own herd of Highland cattle.
Also mutton from another local
farm. Shop emphasises local
produce.

Dunkeld

Kirk Park,
Easter Dalguise Farm PH8 0JU
01350 727118
Seasonal vegetables and flowers.

Perth

Hugh Grierson,
Newmiln Farm,
Tibbermore PH1 1QN
01738 730201
www.the-organic-farm.co.uk
Home-reared organic beef and
lamb. Also supplies organic pork
from a local farm.

King Edward Street
01738 450417
www.perthfarmersmarket.co.uk
First Saturday of the month,
09.00 to 14.00

Pitlochry
Atholl Glens,
Mains of Killiechangie Farm
PH16 5NB
01796 481482
www.athollglens.co.uk
Organic Scottish beef and lamb
from a small co-operative of
Scottish farms.

RENFREWSHIRE

Erskine

 Aberdeen Angus Direct,
Linburn Farm PA8 6AW
01418 120220
Prize-winning herd, sells from
farm shop.

Lochwinnoch

 Castle Semple VC
01505 614791
www.scottishfarmersmarkets.co.uk
First Sunday of March, June and
December, 11.00 to 14.30

Paisley

County Square,
outside Gilmour St Station
01655 770217
www.paisley.org.uk/todo/
farmersmarket.php
Last Saturday of the month, 09.00
to 13.00

SCOTTISH BORDERS

Hawick

Kershope Farm,
18 Bourtree Place TD9 9HL
01450 372072
Free-range organic chicken and
turkeys. Also traditional Scottish
steak pies made from local beef.

Kelso

Town Square
01573 470263
Fourth Saturday of the month,
09.30 to 13.30

Peebles

 East Station Car Park
01890 870370
www.scottishfarmersmarkets.co.uk
Second Saturday of the month,
09.30 to 13.30

West Linton

Acme Organics,
Blyth Bridge EH46 7DH
01721 788178
www.acmeorganics.co.uk
Organic fruit and veg delivery
service, home-grown or from
local growers.

SHETLAND ISLANDS

The Handmade Fish Company,
Bigton ZE2 9JF
01950 422214
Fresh and smoked fish.

SOUTH AYRSHIRE

Ayr

Ayrshire Farmers Co-op Farm
Shop,
SAC,
Auchincruive KA65HW
01292 521 765
Fresh local seasonal produce
from 20 suppliers.

River Street
01655 770217
www.ayrshirefarmersmarket.co.uk
First Saturday of the month,
09.00 to 14.00

Tarbolton

Stair Organic Growers,
11 The Yetts KA5 5NT
01292 541369
Home delivery of organic fruit,
vegetables and a box scheme to
Glasgow, Ayrshire and
Renfrewshire.

SOUTH LANARKSHIRE

Biggar

Black Mount Foods,
8 The Wynd ML12 6BU
01899 221747
Products include organic beef,
lamb, pork, poultry, sausages and
bacon. Wholesale and mail order
(to anywhere in the UK)
available.

Carmichael Estate Meats,
Carmichael Estate Office,
Westmains,
Carmichael ML12 6PG
01899 308336
www.carmichael.co.uk
Oldest single estate (family
owned) producer business in
Scotland (est 1292). All venison,
beef and lamb is born, reared and
slaughtered on the farm. Outlets
include farm shop, farmers'
markets, mail order and
distribution to some delis.

Hamilton

New Cross,
Top of Quarry Street
01555 771757
www.lanarkshirefarmersmarket.co.uk
Third Saturday of the month,
09.00 to 13.00

Organic Cakes by Ann,
6 Carron Court ML3 8TD
01698 336448
Offer organic cakes for all special
occasions and events including
weddings, created using 100%
organic ingredients.

STIRLING

Blairmains Farm Shop,
Manor Loan,
Blairlogie FK9 5QA
01259 762266
Local and Scottish products.

Maxwell Place
01877 330151
www.scottishfarmersmarkets.co.uk
Second Saturday of the month,
09.00 to 14.00

WEST DUNBARTONSHIRE

Alexandria

Lomond Organics,
207 Main Street,
Jamestown G83 8PW
07916 193 992
Organic shop & box scheme
using local produce.

Balloch

Loch Lomond Shores
01436 679882
www.scottishfarmersmarkets.co.uk
First and third Sunday of the
month, 10.00 to 15.00

WEST LOTHIAN

Bathgate

 Grow Wild,
Unit 8, Block 3, Whiteside
Industrial Estate EH48 2RX
0845 2263393
www.growwild.co.uk
Box scheme offering organic fruit
and vegetables, locally grown
where possible.

Linlithgow

Pardovan Farm Shop
Pardovan Holdings,
Philpstoun EH49 7RX
01506 834470
Farm shop with home produced
beef and lamb.

South Queensferry

West Craigie Farm
0131 319 1048
www.thejamkitchen.com
Fruit farm with pick-your-own.
Attends local farmers markets
with own jams, chutneys &
vinegars.

WESTERN ISLES

Benbecula

West Minch Salmon Ltd,
Gramsdale Factory,
Gramsdale HS7 5LZ
01870 602081
Produce organic farmed Atlantic
Salmon.

Harris

 Tarbert Market
07810 603188
www.scottishfarmersmarkets.co.uk
Every second Saturday from June
until the end of September, 09.00
to 13.30

Lewis

Point Street,
Stornoway
07810 603188
www.scottishfarmersmarkets.co.uk
Every Saturday, 09.00 to 13.30

BLAENAU GWENT

Tredegar

 Mr A Vowells Butchers,
88 Commercial Street
NP22 3DN
Butcher and game dealer

BRIDGEND

Gellifeddgaer

C & G Morgan & Son
CF356EN
01443 672357
Lamb, beef & pork. All good
quality home produced.

Pencoed

Pencoed Growers,
Felindre CF35 5HU
01656 861956
Home grown vegetables to
collect from the farm.

Porthcawl

 Awel y mor
CF36 5TS
01656 058963
www.bridgendfarmersmarket.co.uk
Fourth Saturday of the month,
10.00 to 13.00

CAERPHILLY

The Source,
26 Cardiff Road CF83 1JP
029 2088 3236
Offering fresh organic fruit and
veg box scheme with delivery
service. Health foods,
wholefoods, organic ranges,
dairy and meat alternatives.
Wheat/gluten free ranges,
organic food supplements.

 Twyn Community Centre
CF83 1JL
01656 658963
www.caerphillyfarmersmarket.co.uk
Second Saturday of the month,
09.30 to 13.30

CARDIFF

 Fitzhammon Embankment
Riverside CF11 7BE
02920 190036
www.riversidemarket.org.uk
Every Sunday, 10.00 to 14.00

The Fruit Garden,
Groesfaen Road,
Peterston-Super-Ely
01446 760358
Soft fruit growers with many
varieties of strawberry. Ready
picked and pick-your-own.

Green Cuisine Organic Food,
Unit 2, Taff Workshops,
Tresillian Terrace CF10 5DE
029 2039 4321
www.greencuisineorganics.net
Box scheme delivering organic
fruit and vegetables in Cardiff
area. Produced sourced mainly
from local small suppliers.

Thornhill Farm Shop,
New House Farm,
Capel Gwilym Rd CF14 9UB
029 2061 1707
Own meat, fresh veg & fruit.
Also a coffee shop.

CARMARTHENSHIRE

Carmarthen

 S and J Organics,
Llwyncrychyddod,
Llanpumsaint SA33 6JS
01267 253570
www.sjorganics.co.uk
Golden Welsh chickens and other
poultry. Plus a range of organic
chicken pies. Phone first for
farm-gate sales.

 Town Centre
SA31 3DX
01550 777244
www.fmiw.co.uk
First Friday of the month, 09.00
to 13.00

Lampeter

 May Organic Farms,
Panteg,
Cellan SA48 8HN
01570 423080
www.themay.co.uk
Organic upland beef, lamb and
mutton produced by a group of
collectively farmed
smallholdings.

Pencader

Blossom Farm,
New Inn SA39 9BA
01559 384621
Organic, grass-fed Welsh Black
beef and lamb.

St Clears

Eynon's of St Clears,
Pentre Road SA33 4LR
0800 731 5816
www.eynons.co.uk
Organic Welsh Black or Angus
beef depending on the season,
plus four types of Welsh lamb.

Whitland

Calon Wen Organic Foods,
Unit 4, Whitland Industrial
Estate,
Spring Gardens SA34 0HR
01994 241368
www.calonwen.co.uk
Box scheme delivering in south-
west Wales. Offers organic meats,
vegetables and fruit, plus
unpasteurised cheese made in
own dairy.

CEREDIGION

Aberaeron

 Alban Square Field
SA46 0AD
01970 633066
www.fmiw.co.uk
First Wednesday of the month
(June to October), 10.00 to 14.00

Aberystwyth

North Parade
SY23 2NF
01970 633066
www.fmiw.co.uk
First and third Saturdays of the
month, 10.00 to 14.00

Llandysul

 Blaensarn Produce,
Blaensarn,
Plwmp SA44 6ER
01545 580250
Vegetables, hen and duck eggs
and table chicken.

 Cambrian Organics,
Horeb SA44 4JG
01559 363151
www.cambrianorganics.com
Locally sourced organic meat
including pasture reared Welsh
Mountain lamb, pasture fed
Welsh Black beef and grass-fed
poultry.

Llwynhelyg Farm Shop,
Sarnau SA44 6QU
01239 811079
Long-established farm shop
selling more than 60 Welsh
cheeses plus locally sourced fruit
and vegetables. Also locally
produced meats, preserves and
dairy produce.

CONWY

Abergele

Farmers Garden,
Pentre Smithy,
Pentre Isa,
Llangernyw LL22 8PH
01745 860430

Colwyn Bay

Bayview Shopping Centre
LL29 9LJ
01492 680209
www.fmiw.co.uk
Every Thursday, 09.00 to 15.00

Conwy

 Conwy RSPB Reserve,
Llandudno Junction
01492 584091
www.tasteofconwy.co.uk
Fourth Wednesday of the month,
09.00 to 14.00

 Edwards of Conwy,
18 High Street LL32 8DE
01492 592443
www.edwardsofconwy.co.uk
Traditional butcher specialising
in Welsh salt marsh lamb and
mature Welsh beef.

Llanrwst

Ancaster Square
01492 651033
www.tasteofconwy.co.uk
Third Saturday of the month,
09.00 to 14.00

DENBIGHSHIRE

Bodelwyddan

Min-y-Morfa Farm Shop
LL22 9SB
01745 590524
www.minymorfa-farm-shop.co.uk
Fresh succulent Welsh lamb, beef,
pork, venison, fresh farm
chickens, bacon, gammon,
sausages.

Corwen

 Glyndwr Farmers Market,
Station Campsite,
Carrog LL21 9BD
01691 860357
www.fmiw.co.uk
First Sunday of the month (May
to October), 10.00 to 16.00

Rhug Organic,
Rhug Estate LL21 0EH
01490 413000
www.rhugorganic.com
Organic meat reared on the
estate. Sold in the farm shop and
on-line.

Llannefydd
Bryn Cocyn Organic Beef and
Lamb
LL16 5DH
01745 540207
www.bryncocynorganic.co.uk
Organic beef and lamb produced
on the farm and killed locally.

Ruthin
Old Gaol Courtyard
St Peters Square
07798 914721
www.ruthinproducemarket.co.uk
Last Saturday of the month (May
to September plus a Christmas
market), 10.00 to 15.00

FLINTSHIRE

Ewloe
Newbridge Farm,
Holywell Road,
01244 532108
Farm shop selling unpasteurised
milk and cream from Ayrshire
cows.

Eyton
Brook Cottage
01978 780852
Own lamb, beef and potatoes;
local beef, pork, speciality
sausages, dry cured bacon.

Mold
St Marys Church Hall,
King Street
01745 561999
www.celynfarmersmarket.co.uk
First Saturday of the month,
09.00 to 14.00

Northrop
Northrop Organics,
Welsh College of Horticulture,
Northrop CH7 6AA
01352 841015
www.wcoh.ac.uk
Vegan organic box scheme run
from the college. Produce is
grown at the college.

Plas Wilkin,
Coed Du,
Rhydymwyn
01352 741263
Organic raw milk, also organic
pasteurised milk and cream.
Runs local milk round.

GWYNEDD

Bala
Aran Lamb,
Cwmonnen Farm,
Llanuwchllyn LL23 7UG
01678 540603
www.aran-lamb.co.uk
Home-reared Welsh mountain
lamb and mutton.

Penrhyandendraeth

 Cig Traddodiadol,
Joli Traditional Meat,
Fferm Y Llan,
Llanfrothen LL48 6DU
01766 770399
Minority breed beef and sheep.
Also pigs and porkers.

Pwlheli

Glasfryn Parc Farmers Market
LL53 6RD
01766 810044
www.fmiw.co.uk
Second Sunday of the month,
10.00 to 16.00

Ty'n Lon Uchaf,
Llangybi LL53 6TB
01766 810915
Smallholding that produces a
wide range of seasonal, organic
vegetables, have a box scheme
available, but with no delivery,
also produce organic eggs.

Talsarnau

Griffith David Williams,
Cefn Trefor Fawr LL47 6UF
01766 770486
Farmgate sales of Harlech salt-
marsh lamb.

Amlwch

Tyddyn Mon,
Bryn Refail,
Dulas LL70 9PQ
01248 410648
www.tyddynmon.co.uk
Salad crops and a wide variety of
vegetables. Plus shrubs and
herbs.

Brynsiencyn

Hooten's Homegrown
Gwydryn Hir
LL61 6HQ
01248 430322
Farm shop selling its own pork,
bacon, sausages and other local
meats. Also home-made
preserves from its own fruit.

Corwas Amlwch

O Roberts a'i Fab
LL68 9ET
01407 830277
Game, some locally sourced.
Includes wild boar.

Tyn-Y-Gongl

Plas Llanfair,
LL74 8NU
01248 852316
Smallholding specialising in soft
and top fruit, and the production
of preserves, jams and chutneys,
also supplies a wide range of
vegetable production on a small
scale.

MERTHYR TYDFIL

Merthyr Tydfil
High Street
CF47 8AN
01685 725106
www.merthyr.gov.uk/FarmersMarket/
First Friday of the moth, 10.00 to
14.00

Treharris
Pen Rhiw Organic Meat
Pen Rhiw Farm CF46 6TA
01443 412949
Retailers of own organic lamb
and beef.

MONMOUTHSHIRE

Abergavenny
Llanthony Valley Organics,
Maes y Beran,
Llanthony NP7 7NL
01873 890701
www.llanthony-valley.co.uk
Organic, grass fed Red Ruby
cattle and Welsh Mountain lamb.

Market Hall
NP15 7EN
01873 860271
www.abergavennyfarmersmarket.co.
uk
Fourth Thursday of the month,
09.30 to 14.30

Monmouth
The Monnow Bridge,
Monnow Street NP25 3EG
0845 610 6496
www.fmiw.co.uk
Fourth Saturday of the month,
10.00 to 13.00

Raglan
N S James and Son,
Crown Square NO15 2EB
01291 690675
Meats from local Monmouthshire
farms, processed in the local
abattoir.

NEATH PORT TALBOT

Neath

Panorama Pedigree Welsh Pigs,
Panorama,
Tyla Morris,
Gardners Lane SA11 2AU
01639 644091
Produce quality free range pork,
sausages and bacon from
pedigree Welsh pigs. The UKTV
Food Local Food Hero 2007
regional finalists for Wales.

Port Talbot
Aberafon Shopping Centre
01639 882274
www.fmiw.co.uk
First and third Saturday of the
month, 09.00 to 16.00

NEWPORT

Bridge Street
01633 263 117
www.fmiw.co.uk
Second and fourth Friday of the
month, 10.00 to 14.00

Whitebrook Organic Growers,
The Old Rectory,
Llanvaches NP6 3AY
01633 400406
Organic box scheme.

PEMBROKESHIRE

Fishguard
Town Hall
SA65 9HA
01348 873004
www.fmiw.co.uk
Every other Saturday, 09.00 to
14.00

Haverfordwest
Bumpylane Rare Breeds,
Shortland Farm,
Druidstone SA62 3NE
01437 781234
www.bumpylane.co.uk
Home-reared organic beef and
lamb.

Welsh Hook Meat Centre,
Woodfield SA62 4BW
01437 768876
www.welsh-organic-meat.co.uk
Rears much of its own organic
meat in Pembrokeshire while
buying the rest from local farms.

Tenby
Ritec Valley Organics,
Robertswall Farm,
Penally Alley SA70 8NF
01834 845967
www.ritec-valley.co.uk
Vegetable box scheme running
through the winter only. All
produce is home grown. Also
offers organic free-range eggs.

POWYS

Brecon
Market Hall
LD3 7LG
01874 636 169
www.brecknockfarmersmarkets.org.
uk
Second Saturday of the month,
10.00 to 14.00

The Welsh Venison Centre,
Middlewood Farm,
Bwlch LD3 7HQ
01874 730929
Farmed Red Deer venison.

Builth Wells
Cwmchwefru Farm,
Llanafan Fawr LD2 3PW
01597 860244
www.lesleywickham.co.uk
Rears pedigree Dexter cattle and
a variety of sheep. Sells a range
of wool products.

Caersws
Jacobs' Lawn Fresh Produce,
Bronfelen SY17 5SF
07811 329765
Variety of vegetables and fruit.

Evenjobb
Castlering Organic Woodland
Pork,
Castlering Wood,
Beggars Bush LD8 2PB
01547 560231
Bacon, gammon and pork from
woodland reared, organic
Saddleback pigs.

Knighton

Community Centre
LD7 1DR
01547 520096
www.thefarmersmarket.co.uk
Fourth Saturday of the month,
09.00 to 14.00

Llanidloes

Great Oak Foods,
14 Great Oak Street SY18 6BU
01686 411128
office@lles.co.uk
Organic products include cider,
cheese, fruit and wine. Local
vegetables and fruit when
available.

Edward Hamer Ltd,
Plynlimon House SY18 6EF
01686 412209
www.edwardhamer.com
Traditional Welsh butcher
stocking Welsh Black beef.

Llandrindod Wells

Graig Farm Organics,
Dolau LD1 5TL
01597 851655
www.graigfarm.co.uk
Organic beef, lamb, mutton and
pork reared by Welsh producer
group.

Machynlleth

Dyfi Organic Vegetables.
01970 832883
Organic box scheme sourcing
from local farmers and growers.

Meifod

Cefn Goleu,
Pontrobert SY22 6JN
01938 500128
Organic, free-range turkeys and
chickens sold at the farm gate.

Rhaeaor

The Wild Carrot,
Allt Gogh,
St Harmon LD6 5LG
01597 810871
Organic farm shop and home
delivery service. Offers fruit,
vegetables, bread; dairy chilled
and frozen products, skin and
baby care products. Also pulses,
grains and flours.

Welshpool

Pentre Pigs,
Pentre House,
Leighton SY21 8HL
01938 553430
www.pentrepigs.co.uk
Traditionally produced, free-
range, rare breed pork, bacon
and gammon.

RHONDDA CYNON TAFF

Llantrisant

Gwaun Ruperra Car Park
01443 425342/01443 425431
www.fmiw.co.uk
First Friday of the month, 10.00
to 14.00

Penderyn

Penderyn Community Centre
CF44 0SX
01685 813 909
www.penderyn.net/penderyn-farmers-market/
Last Sunday of the month, 10.00 to 14.00

Pontypridd

Llantwit Fardre Sports Centre
Church Village CF38 1RJ
01443 425343
www.fmiw.co.uk
Third Thursday of the month, 10.00 to 14.00

Wally Greens,
1 Beech Villas CF372HW
01443 408355
Producer of luxury handmade chutneys and preserves, containing no artificial colourings, flavourings or preservatives.

Tonypandy

Dunravon Street
01443 425343
www.fmiw.co.uk
Second Friday of the month, 10.00 to 14.00

SWANSEA

National Waterfront Museum,
Oystermouth Road,
Maritime Quarter SA1 3RD
www.fmiw.co.uk
First Sunday of the month, 10.00 to 15.00

Penclawdd Community Centre,
Penclawdd SA4 3XN
01792 850147
www.fmiw.co.uk
Third Saturday of the month, 09.30 to 12.30

Sea Front (Oystermouth) Car Park,
Newton Road,
Mumbles SA3 4AY
01792 405169
www.fmiw.co.uk
Second Saturday of the month, 09.30 to 12.30

Sketty Parish Hall
St Pauls Church
Sketty SA2 9AR
01792 850162
www.fmiw.co.uk
First Saturday of the month, 09.30 to 12.30

The Unusual Food Company,
43-45 Commercial St,
Ystalyfera SA9 2HS
01639 849999
www.unusualfoodcompany.co.uk
Breads, sweet & savoury pastries, beef, bacon, sausages, chicken, cheeses, chutneys, jams, marmalades, honey.

TORFAEN

Cwmbran
Cwrt Henllys Farm,
Henllys NP44 7AS
01633 612349
Supplier of Premium rare and
traditionally bred meats directly
off the farm including 21 day
matured Longhorn Beef, 7 day
matured lamb, free range
Gloucester Old Spot and Middle
White pork (also hams, bacon &
sausages), Kelly Bronze turkeys
and geese.

Pontypool
The Secret Garden,
Pentwyn Farm,
Mamhilad NP4 0JE
01495 785237
Retailers of Just Green organic
garden products.

VALE OF GLAMORGAN

Bonvilston
Venison from the Vale,
Llantrithyd Park CF5 6TQ
01446 781900
www.healthyvenison.co.uk
Venison, steaks, joints, sausages,
burgers.

Cowbridge
Arthur Johns Car Park
43 High Street CF71 7AB
01656 661100
www.valefarmersmarkets.co.uk
First and third Saturday of the
month, 10.00 to 13.00

Dinas Powis
Wenvoe Stores,
Wenvoe CF5 6AL
Sells Cambrian organics products
including burgers and/or ready
meals.

Penarth

Westbourne Scool,
4 Hickman Road CF64 2EZ
01565 661100
www.valefarmersmarkets.co.uk
Fourth Saturday of the month,
10.00 to 13.00

WREXHAM

Lewis's Farm Shop,
Brook Cottage,
Eyton LL13 0SW
01978 780852
Shop sells home produced lamb,
beef and Gloucester Old Spot
pork. Home-made ready meals,
apple juice, free-range eggs and,
when available, organic eggs.

J T Vernon,
The Cross,
Holt LL13 9YG
01829 270247
www.jtvernon.co.uk
Sells 60 varieties of home-made
sausages and burgers.

Wrexham Road Farm,
Holt LL13 9YU
01829 270302
Pick-your-own blackberries,
black and red currants,
gooseberries, raspberries,
strawberries, tayberries, runner
beans and courgettes.

A Selection of National Box Schemes:

Abel & Cole
www.abel-cole.co.uk   08452 626262

Bath Organic Farms
www.bathorganicfarms.co.uk   01225 421507

Everybody Organic
www.everybodyorganic.co.uk   0845 345 5054

GoodnessDirect
www.goodnessdirect.co.uk   01327 704197

Graig Farm Organics
www.graigfarm.co.uk   01597 851655

One (Organic, Natural & Ethical) Food Ltd
www.organic-supermarket.co.uk   0870 871 1112

Organic Connections International Ltd
www.organic-connections.co.uk   01945 773374

RodandBens
www.rodandbens.com   01392 833833

Swaddles Organic
www.swaddles.co.uk   0845 456 1768

Westcountry Organics
www.westcountryorganics.co.uk   0845 349 7420

Further resources

Log on to these websites to find out more about real food and how and where to get it.

www.wewantrealfood.co.uk
The website that accompanies this book

www.seercentre.org.uk
The Sustainable Ecological Earth Regeneration Centre

www.angus-horticulture.co.uk
An associate of the SEER centre

www.seedsofhealth.co.uk
A resource that lists UK producers and suppliers of 'old fashioned traditional food'

www.wholesome-food.org
The Wholesome Food Association

www.rbst.org.uk
The Rare Breeds Survival Trust

www.wildlifetrusts.org
The Wildlife Trusts

Which Foods To Buy

What to Avoid

Most commercial growers rely heavily on chemical nitrogen fertilizers to boost their output. Chemical fertilizers disrupt soil biology and destroy many of the living communities which supply the apple tree with the nutrients it needs and which hold diseases in check. That's why chemical growers have to spray their trees so many times with pesticides to keep the fruit free of disease. The soils in commercial chemical orchards are malnourished; so are the trees that grow on them. As a result the apples they produce have fewer of the health-promoting flavenoids of fruit from fertile soils.

What to Buy

The best apples are grown on soils teeming with life. Crops such as vegetables or cereals come from soils under cultivation. The regular planting and harvesting of whole plants robs the land of nutrients and weakens the myriad communities of soil organisms. But under a mature and well-managed orchard soil organisms reach huge numbers. Populations of bacteria, nematodes and fungi can be hundreds of times larger than in cultivated crop land. It's this vast army of underground organisms that mobilizes trace elements and other soil nutrients, and makes them available to tree roots. Since the land isn't being regularly shaken and stirred about mycorrhizal fungi flourish, boosting the supply of minerals to the tree. It's the fertility and soil life of the orchard that make apples nourishing.

Benefits

Many studies have linked the consumption of apples with reduced cancer risk, especially lung cancer. Quercetin, a flavenoid abundant in apples, helps prevent the growth of prostate cancer cells, while phytochemicals found in the skin of apples inhibit the reproduction of colon cancer cells. Fibre and phytonutrients found in apples together lower blood cholesterol and are linked to a reduced risk of heart disease, stroke, prostate cancer, Type ll diabetes and asthma. Eating just two apples a day reduces the damage of 'bad' LDL cholesterol. The high antioxidant content of apples may protect against age-related memory loss.

Nutrients

Flavenoids, antioxidants that improve immune function and help prevent heart disease and cancer. Quercetin is one of the most important. Soluble fibre – especially pectin – which promotes bowel health and helps to lower blood cholesterol. Minerals, particularly potassium, calcium and magnesium. Vitamins, including vitamin C and folate. Malic and tartaric acids inhibit fermentation in the intestines.

ASPARAGUS

What to Avoid

Asparagus tips sold out of season having been flown in from some distant part of the world. Also to be avoided are stalks that are fat or twisted. Check that the cut ends are not too woody. Although they may be dry, if they're woody it's likely that much of the stalk will be too. Since this is an expensive 'gourmet' vegetable it's worth buying fresh. Pre-packed samples from supermarkets are unlikely to provide a great eating experience. Occasionally asparagus plants are earthed up to produce white shoots. These are popular in Germany, but the green, 'open air'

version is better. It's likely to be richer in vitamins.

What to Buy

Buy it in season and buy it locally if you can. Asparagus is one of those special vegetables that's often sold by small scale producers at the farm gate. If you see an 'Asparagus-for-sale' sign on the road, check it out. The chances are it'll be a specialist producer who has grown it with care and plenty of organic matter – even if the crop isn't registered organic. So the spears will be full of nutrients – and flavour. A good sample should be made up of spears with firm, thinnish stems and deep green or purple tips.

Benefits

Since earliest times Chinese herbalists have used the asparagus root to treat a range of ailments from arthritis to infertility. It contains compounds called steroidal glycosides which are thought to have anti-inflammatory properties. The fleshy green spears – the part eaten as a vegetable – are extremely rich in nutrients. The vitamin content is high, particularly for folic acid and vitamin K. Folic acid is essential for a healthy cardiovascular system. When levels are low, blood levels of homocysteine rise, a condition that greatly increases the risk of heart disease. Folic acid may also help to prevent birth defects, cervical cancer and colorectal cancer.

Asparagus is a good source of potassium and other minerals. This mineral profile – combined with the amino acid asparagine, also found in asparagus – makes the plant a natural diuretic. A compound called rutin in the plant helps prevent the fracture of small blood vessels.

Asparagus also contains a carbohydrate called inulin which promotes the development of beneficial flora in the gut. This reduces the chance of pathogenic bacteria gaining a foothold in the intestinal tract.

Nutrients

High levels of the vitamins A, C and K plus folic acid. Also good levels of the B vitamins thiamine, riboflavin, pyridoxine and niacin. A good source of the amino acid tryptophan. Useful levels of a number of minerals including manganese, copper, phosphorus, potassium, iron, zinc, magnesium, selenium and calcium. Also contains good amounts of dietary fibre.

BACON

What to Avoid

The best bacon comes from the meat of outdoor-reared, rare-breed pigs which has been traditionally cured. Bacon from intensively-reared pigs is best avoided even when cured by traditional methods. Equally bacon from outdoor-reared pigs is seldom worth eating if it has been cured using the modern method of injecting the meat with salt and preservatives. Nitrates and nitrites are commonly used in the mass manufacture of bacon. When exposed to high heat during cooking, these are converted to cancer-causing nitrosamines. Though the health risks are small they are best avoided.

Many of the practices used by the industrial bacon curers are designed to increase the water content of the meat. This allows them to sell less meat to the kilogram and results in the bacon shrinking considerably during cooking. Smoked bacon has been linked with cancer so it makes sense to choose the unsmoked variety whenever possible.

What to Buy

For many centuries bacon was the only meat to be regularly

eaten by the poor since almost every family kept their own pigs. These were killed and salted down at the start of winter, providing meat during the months when little fresh meat was available. Look for bacon that starts out as meat from slow-grown, rare-breed pigs that have spent most of their lives outdoors.

The traditional way of curing bacon is by the process of dry curing. The meat is rubbed down with a curing mixture that includes salt, brown sugar and other natural flavourings such as black pepper. There are many local and regional variations with individual curers having their own secret recipes. But the principles of dry curing are the same. They bear no resemblance to 'wet curing', the modern industrial practice of injecting the meat with brine and other preservatives.

Benefits
While well-cured bacon can provide high quality protein, it is not as beneficial as fresh meat. Whatever the curing method, the salt content is relatively high. However, bacon is a good source of B vitamins and zinc, which helps boost the immune system. Bacon can be

extremely high in fat, but surprisingly more is in the form of monounsaturated fat than saturated fat, so it can be a nutritious food, though it's best not to eat it too often. Even for those who eschew meat, the smell of grilled bacon is often enough to get your mouth watering.

Nutrients
A good source of B vitamins – thiamine, nicotinic acid, pyridoxine, vitamin B12 and pantothenic acid. Also rich in the essential minerals potassium, zinc and phosphorus.

BANANAS

What to Avoid
Any fruits that are bruised or damaged. In their tough skins bananas appear very robust. In fact they are remarkably fragile and are easily damaged. Look out for fruits with darkened areas that may suggest damage inside. This is quite distinct from the brown freckling which simply indicates that the fruit is very ripe. The ones to avoid have a slightly blackened or grey appearance. When fully ripe a good quality fruit will have a bright yellow colour with or without brown spots.

What to Buy

The banana plant grows up to eight metres high and carries the fruits in clusters of up to a hundred and fifty. As with all fruit and vegetables, the most nutrient-dense come from soils that are fertile and high in organic matter. That's why it's best to stick to organic fruit.

Bananas are picked when they're green, and many supermarket packs still have that green, unripened colour. When buying bananas it's worth thinking about when they're going to be consumed. Fruits with a lot of green colour in them will take time to ripen at home, so if the kids are going to want to eat them straight away it's worth sticking to fully ripe samples.

Bananas should be firm and bright yellow in colour. Their stems and tips should be undamaged. There's no particular flavour or nutrient benefit from either large-sized or small-sized fruits, so it's worth picking up fruits of a size that best meets your need.

Benefits

Bananas are one of nature's best sources of the element potassium, which is essential for maintaining normal blood pressure and cardiac function.

A daily banana alone can be very effective in bringing down or preventing high blood pressure. It may also protect against hardening of the arteries.

Potassium-rich foods such as bananas have been shown to reduce the risk of strokes. Fibre in bananas is also believed to protect against heart disease. Bananas have been shown to have antacid properties in the stomach, reducing the risk of ulcers and ulcer damage. They work by stimulating the cells lining the stomach to produce a thicker mucous barrier against stomach acids. Compounds known as protease inhibitors help to eliminate stomach bacteria believed to be the primary cause of ulcers. The soluble fibre pectin helps ease constipation and normalize the movement of materials through the digestive tract.

Along with other fruits, bananas are protective against age-related macular degeneration, a condition that can lead to blindness. They can also help improve the body's ability to absorb calcium. Bananas are a rich source of a compound called fructo-oligosaccharide, a substance known as a prebiotic since it nourishes beneficial bacteria in the gut. These bacteria produce vitamins and digestive enzymes which improve the body's ability to absorb nutrients in the food. Bananas are also known to promote kidney health.

Nutrients
Extremely rich source of vitamin C and vitamin B6, pyridoxine. Also contains high levels of the minerals potassium and manganese. A good source of dietary fibre with low levels of fat. Its sweet taste and moderate calorie levels make it an ideal food for between-meal snacks.

BEEF

What to Avoid
Though traditional beef used a small amount of barley to provide a 'finish' to the animal, avoid beef produced on large amounts of grain. This includes American 'feedlot' beef. In the UK, some intensive beef systems use large amounts of grain. The only way to spot these is to ask the butcher about the production method. Choose traditional British breeds such as the traditional Hereford, Welsh Black, Devon, Sussex and Angus.

What to Buy
The roast beef of old England –
and Scotland, Wales and Ireland for that matter – used to be easy to produce. You simply turned your cattle on to wild, herb-rich pastures for three or four years and that was it. Nature provided the ideal food for ruminant animals, and in the process raised some of the finest beef in the world.

Today, the evidence is piling up that this sort of grass-fed beef contains a battery of nutrients that protect against a range of diseases from cancer to heart disease. Much of the beef we eat in Europe and the United States is produced on chemically grown cereals and soya, which fill the meat with unhealthy fats and rob it of protective nutrients such as vitamin E and conjugated linoleic acid (CLA). Until the world's politicians come to their senses and axe the subsidies on grains it's well worth paying extra for the genuine grass-fed product. It's around in larger amounts, particularly if you shop online or at farmers' markets.

Benefits
Beef is a good source of high-quality protein, with many additional micronutrients. These include a number of essential trace elements such as

magnesium and zinc, together with fat-soluble vitamins and a substance called palmitoleic acid which protects against pathogenic organisms.

But the greatest health benefits are linked to pasture-fed animals. These contain a far healthier balance of omega-3 and omega-6 fats than grain-fed animals. Omega-3 levels in the grass-fed product are up to ten times higher than that in grain-fed beef. In addition, levels of the anti-cancer fatty acid CLA are three times higher, while the vitamin E content is up to three times higher. Levels of beta-carotene are up to ten times higher.

Nutrients

Complete protein, including sulphur-containing amino acids. Taurine and carnitine, required for sound vision and heart.   Co-enzyme Q10, needed for cardiovascular function. Essential minerals, including zinc. Vitamin B12, vital for healthy nervous and vascular systems. Fat soluble vitamins A and D. CLA, especially grass-fed beef. Long chain fatty acids, including EPA and DHA. Omega-3 fatty acids, especially in grass-fed beef.

BLACKBERRIES

What to Avoid

The cultivated variety. Better than nothing, but if you get the chance, go out to your local common, recreation ground or fields in September and pick the real thing. The advantage of the wild type is that they are well established on undisturbed soils. This means the root system will delve deep into soils that are rich in minerals. There will be a healthy community of soil organisms – including mycorrhiza-supplying minerals to the plant. Cultivated blackberries are likely to come from inferior, cultivated soils.

What to Buy

A truly remarkable food and one which, for generations of British people, came free. Blackberry seeds were found in the stomach of a Neolithic man dug up in the Essex clay, and ever since people have gathered the annual autumn harvest from hedgerows and commons. There's no better example of a commonplace food held in high regard by people endowed with a received wisdom of things that would protect their health. Modern science shows blackberries to be packed full of nutrients that protect against everything from common colds to cancer. It's no coincidence that in towns and villages across the land people gathered this fruit for pies and puddings, jellies and jams.

Benefits

With exceptionally high levels of antioxidants, blackberries are protective against damaging free radicals. Blackberries have been found to combat dysentery, sore throats, heart disease, colds, diarrhoea, cancer and gout. Many of the antioxidant benefits have been attributed to a particular flavenoid known as C3G. This compound has been shown to reduce cancerous tumours and prevent the spread of cancer cells.

Nutrients

Blackberries contain significant amounts of major minerals including calcium, magnesium, phosphorus, potassium and manganese. Useful trace elements include selenium, copper and zinc. Rich in vitamin C, vitamin A, vitamin K, vitamin E and folate. Other vitamins include pantothenic acid, vitamin B6 and riboflavin. Phytonutrients include lutein and zeaxanthine, ellagic acid, quercetin, anthocyanidins, proanthocyanidins. Rich source of the powerful anti-cancer compound C3G.

BLUEBERRIES

What to Avoid

Check the pack carefully for damaged fruit. Damage is likely to lead to mould in storage. Any dampness in the pack will have a similar effect. Good quality blueberries should be firm, undamaged and an even blue colour, with a lighter coloured 'bloom'. Before buying, shake the pack and make sure the individual fruits are firm and separate, and that they move about freely. Where fruits are clumped together there is the suggestion of damage or mould. Like all fruits, blueberries deteriorate when kept in storage for too long, so buy them as fresh as you can. Though they will keep for a few days in the fridge, it's far better to eat them while still fresh.

What to Buy

Blueberries are the fruits of a shrub belonging to the same plant family as the cranberry and bilberry, as well as laurel and rhododendron. They grow best in light, slightly acid soils.

Blueberries grow wild in north America where they played an important part in the diets of many tribes of native peoples. There's no doubt that the wild fruit – with its tangy, sharp flavour – is better than the cultivated variety. However for most of us the wild version is simply not available, and the health-giving properties of this fruit are so outstanding that the cultivated version remains a superb food. Choose organic when you can. Nutrient levels are likely to be highest in fruits grown on fertile soils rich in organic matter. The organic symbol provides some assurance of a reasonable level of soil fertility.

Benefits

Buy this fruit whenever you see it and throw it into fruit salads. Alternatively eat it alone with fresh dairy cream.

The list of benefits from eating blueberries is so long they could easily pass for a health tonic. Though low in calories, they are packed with nutrients and flavours. In terms of their antioxidant capability – their ability to neutralize damaging free radicals – they are among the highest performing fruits. Their rich levels of anthocyanins make them highly protective of cardiovascular health. Extracts of the related fruit bilberry have been found to promote night-time vision, and blueberries themselves have been found to protect against the vision-threatening condition, macular degeneration. Blueberries help to improve brain function and protect against oxidative damage. They also contain the health-promoting compound ellagic acid, which blocks metabolic pathways leading to cancer.

Blueberries are high in the soluble fibre pectin which helps to lower blood cholesterol. Flavonols and tannins in the fruit may help to lower the risk of colon cancer as well as reducing inflammation in the digestive system. Other compounds in the fruit have powerful anti-bacterial properties. Components of both blueberry juice and cranberry juice reduce the ability of the damaging bacterium E. coli. to stick to the gut wall.

Nutrients

Contains high levels of vitamin C. A single cup of blueberries supply almost one-third of the recommended daily allowance. An extremely valuable source of antioxidants. Also contains high levels of the essential mineral manganese. Good levels of dietary fibre and an important source of vitamin E.

BREAD

What to Avoid

It's unlikely that any of the bread in the average supermarket would fit the description of nutrient-dense. Unless it's labelled as organic it'll almost certainly have been produced from chemically grown wheat. It'll have been ground in a high-speed mill running so hot that many of the vitamins and omega-3 fats will have been destroyed. In the process of making flour for the standard white loaf around thirty essential nutrients will have been largely removed to be replaced by just four. Without any obvious irony the milling industry refers to this exchange as 'enrichment'. As if this weren't sufficient abuse, a clutch of chemical additives are put into the dough so that it performs better in the mass-production machines of the industrial bakers.

What to Buy

Only bread made from the wholewheat grain can be said to be rich in nutrients. There are three parts to the grain kernel: the fibre-rich *bran* of the outer layer; the *germ*, or inner layer, where many nutrients and essential fatty acids are found; and the starchy middle layer, or *endosperm*. Only when all three are included in the final loaf will the bread have a high nutrient density.

There's a second essential feature of truly nourishing bread; the whole grain must have been soaked for at least 12 hours before baking. In the making of cakes and pancakes pre-industrial societies invariably soaked the flour in sour milk or buttermilk first. In the slightly acid conditions phytic acid – the compound which can block the intake of essential minerals in the gut – is neutralized. Soaking enhances the vitamin content and assists nutrient absorption.

Benefits

Traditionally made wholewheat bread such as sourdough bread is one of nature's finest foods. It helps reduce the risk of many modern diseases including cardiovascular disease, diabetes and many cancers. The B vitamins in wheat play a part in the functioning of almost every body system, including the nervous and vascular systems, the skin, vision, fertility and hearing. Similarly, minerals such as potassium, iron, magnesium and zinc play a part in most metabolic systems.

Nutrients

Wholewheat bread made from stoneground flour should contain most of the nutrients in the original grains. Nutrients include the minerals potassium, iron, magnesium, zinc and selenium; vitamin E, a potent antioxidant which greatly reduces the risk of heart attack, cancer and diabetes; dietary fibre; and omega-3 fatty acids.

BREAKFAST CEREALS

What to Avoid

The world of breakfast cereals is full of fakes. Almost all the brightly coloured boxes of supposedly healthy cereals on the shelves of supermarkets are at best worthless, and may even be dangerous. This includes even those that are proclaimed to have 'all the benefits of whole grains'.

Commercial breakfast cereals are made by a process known as extrusion. Manufacturers first make a slurry of the milled grains, then force them through tiny holes at high temperatures and pressure. In this way they create the familiar flakes, shreds and shapes. Extrusion destroys most nutrients in the grain while rendering some amino acids toxic. In one experiment, rats fed on wheat grains treated this way died in two weeks. Most boxed cereal products are also high in sugar and salt.

What to Buy

Few products qualify as real food. The best by far is traditional porridge. Make it from pinhead oatmeal soaked overnight in water with a few drops of lemon juice added. This mildly acid solution neutralizes phytic acid and other 'anti-nutrients'. In the morning the pre-soaked porridge will cook quickly. Serve with cream or butter. High-quality organic muesli also qualifies as real food. This should contain things such as oat, rye and barley flakes; dried fruits and seeds, such as sunflower, sesame, linseed and pumpkin. Once again it's important to soak them overnight so as to maximize the availability of nutrients.

Benefits

Properly prepared porridge delivers the full health benefits of oats. Because of their high content of soluble fibres, oats promote healthy bowels and help to reduce blood cholesterol levels, so cutting the risks of coronary heart disease and strokes. They are low in gluten but contain more phytates than other cereals. Whole oats have a low glycaemic index (GI) and so are useful in the regulation of blood sugar. Traditionally, herbalists have used oats to induce sleep. Best used as pinhead oatmeal in which the whole grain kernel is cut in half.

Nutrients

Oats contain higher levels of protein and fat than most other grains. They are rich in the B vitamins thiamine, riboflavin and B6. Useful amounts of the minerals calcium, iron, magnesium, phosphorus and potassium. Small amount of vitamin E and folic acid. Soluble fibre.

BROCCOLI

What to Avoid

As with other vegetables, large areas of broccoli are grown with heavy inputs of chemical fertilizer. Chemicals, especially nitrogen and phosphate fertilizers, damage soil structure and reduce biological activity. Crops grown on soils damaged in this way are unable to take up the minerals they need for healthy growth. They are attacked by pests and diseases and so have to be sprayed with pesticides. They also contain fewer of the protective nutrients that should make broccoli one of the healthiest foods you can eat. Crops grown in this way are fakes and best avoided.

What to Buy

Broccoli, like other vegetables, thrives in soils with plenty of organic matter. Soil organic matter supports the biological activity which produces the best conditions for plant roots to take up minerals. Good mineral uptake is essential if the plant is to thrive and produce the range of compounds that will protect consumers against cancers and other diseases. To be sure of getting a nutrient-rich crop it's necessary to establish that it was grown in a healthy soil with high levels of organic matter and available minerals. When buying at a farmers' market check with the grower that well-prepared compost is used to maintain soil fertility. If in doubt, buy organic.

Benefits
With its numerous cancer-fighting compounds, broccoli is important in any diet designed to protect against the disease. Oxidative damage is believed to a factor in both cancer and heart disease, and both beta-carotene and vitamin C act as strong antioxidants, protecting cells against the damage caused by free radicals. Indoles and sulphoraphane provide additional protection against cancer, as do calcium, selenium and folic acid. Vitamin C also supports the immune system in fighting infection. The mineral potassium helps to regulate the normal fluid balance in cells and maintains heart function and blood pressure.

Nutrients
Carotenoids, plant pigments – including beta-carotene – which act as antioxidants, protecting human health. Indoles, compounds found in cruciferous vegetables that have powerful anti-cancer properties. Sulphoraphane, a compound that stimulates human cells to produce cancer-fighting enzymes. Minerals, particularly calcium, phosphorus, potassium and selenium, together with chromium, which protects against diabetes. Quercetin and

glutathione, antioxidants and anti-cancer agents. Vitamins C and B complex, including folic acid, which plays a major role in the synthesis of nucleic acids and many amino acids.

BRUSSELS SPROUTS

What to Avoid
Out-of-season vegetables or any that have been imported. Home-grown Brussels sprouts start appearing in September, and, with a number of new varieties on the market, can be available right through to April. Traditionally sprouts were always believed to taste better after the plant had received a dose of frost. These are wonderful winter vegetables but are best avoided in early autumn and spring. Also avoid any samples with yellowing or wilted leaves, soft patches or blackened outer leaves, which may indicate rotting on the inside. Look out for small holes or perforations in the outer leaves as this may reveal invasion by aphids.

What to Buy
Good quality sprouts should be a vivid green in colour and be firm and well-fleshed. Buy them loose rather than pre-packed, as the packaging is

certain to trap moisture and encourage mould. Handling or viewing loose sprouts will give you a better idea of their condition.

Benefits
Sprouts are a member of the cruciferous family along with kale and broccoli. And like these two vegetables they pack a powerful nutritional punch. Brussels sprouts contain a battery of health-protecting compounds including a glucosinolate phytonutrient called sulphoraphane. This stimulates the body's detoxification enzymes, helping to neutralize carcinogens and protecting against a number of cancers.

When Brussels sprouts or other cruciferous vegetables are cut or chewed, they release a sulphur-containing compound called sinigrin which stimulates the body's anti-cancer enzymes. The vegetable's arsenal of cancer-fighting compounds also includes indoles. These deactivate oestrogens that might otherwise initiate tumour growth. Brussels sprouts contain high levels of both soluble and insoluble fibre which promote colon health and protect against colon cancer and diverticulosis. High

levels of vitamin C in sprouts help to protect against inflammatory types of arthritis, while folic acid reduces the risk of birth defects in babies. The antioxidants, vitamins C and E, together with beta-carotene, protect against cancer and coronary artery disease.

Nutrients
Exceptional levels of vitamins K and C. Good levels of other vitamins including folic acid, beta-carotene, thiamine, pyridoxine, riboflavin and vitamin E. A useful source of a number of minerals including manganese, potassium, iron, phosphorus, magnesium, copper and calcium. Rich in a wide range of protective phytonutrients. Rich in dietary fibre. Contains omega-3 fatty acids and the amino acid tryptophan. Low in calories and with useful amounts of protein.

BUTTER

What to Avoid
Margarines and other non-dairy yellow fat spreads, the products of corporate agribusiness which needs markets for its pesticide-ridden industrial grain crops. Also includes the pallid butter

produced by cows fed industrial grains and soya. Sadly, the two categories include many of the products on sale at your local supermarket. But real butter is well worth a long search.

What to Buy

When the American dentist Weston Price carried out his study of the diets of pre-industrial communities, he found that butter was a valued food for some of the healthiest peoples on the planet. But it was butter produced by cows grazing fresh, herb-rich grasslands, not feeding on the industrial crops fed by many of today's dairy farmers.

New research shows that the healthiest butter is produced by cows grazing fertile pastures, especially in the spring when grass is growing at its fastest rate. Back in the 1950s and 1960s this is the very time that most butter was made in Britain. Many butter factories were operated principally to deal with the flush of milk coming from cows on spring pastures. In winter, the machinery was shut down.

Today, farmers are paid to produce milk all year round so that the processing factories can be operated more cost-effectively. To achieve this,

farmers feed their herds unsuitable rations, such as grain and soya. Our butter is the poorer for it.

Benefits

Real butter protects against a number of diseases, including heart disease and cancer, the very scourges it was once blamed for causing. Vitamin A in butter is needed by the thyroid and adrenal glands which help to maintain the normal functioning of the heart and vascular system. With other antioxidants, including vitamin E and selenium, it protects against free radical damage to arteries. Many of the short and medium chain fatty acids in butter have strong anti-cancer effects, as do its many antioxidants. Butter is also beneficial to the immune system and thyroid function. It protects against arthritis, osteoporosis and many gastro-infections.

Nutrients

Vitamins A, D and E. Lecithin, a substance that helps in the metabolism of cholesterol. Trace elements, including selenium, a powerful antioxidant, and iodine. The Wulzen factor, a nutrient which protects against degenerative arthritis as well as hardening of the arteries and cataracts. Sadly it is destroyed by pasteurization. Glycospingolipids, a group of fatty acids that protect against gastro-intestinal infection. The 'X factor' discovered by Dr Weston Price and thought to be important for healthy growth – only in butterfat of cows on pasture.

CABBAGE

What to Avoid

Non-organic cabbage. The outer leaves of the plant can have the highest content of vitamins, minerals and other nutrients. These are the very leaves that are likely to contain chemical contaminants in crops that have been sprayed. So make sure the cabbages you buy are organically-grown, unless you have access to vegetables grown in gardens or allotments where you know pesticides are not used and the fertility comes chiefly from organic sources. Choose cabbages that are firm and where the outer leaves are not heavily cracked, bruised or blemished. These outer signs may indicate worm or pest damage inside. Avoid cut, shredded or pre-prepared cabbages. As soon as they are cut or prepared in this way

they begin losing vitamins, so make sure you buy whole vegetables that look plump and fresh.

What to Buy

Cabbages come in a variety of types. Spring greens are loose-leaved, green cabbages, picked before the centres or 'hearts' have had time to fill out. White, green and red cabbages have large, tightly-packed heads. Green cabbages vary in colour from pale green to dark green types, and from smooth leaves to crinkly-leaved varieties.

Choose dark-green types rather than the 'white' or pale varieties as they're likely to be better flavoured and have a higher content of vitamins and health-giving antioxidants and other nutrients. From a health point of view the dark green, crinkly-leaved Savoy cabbage is widely considered the best.

Benefits

It would be hard to overstate the health benefits of the humble cabbage. It contains powerful antioxidants that neutralize damaging free radicals, so protecting DNA, cell membranes and fat-containing molecules such as cholesterol. It helps to lower the risk of heart disease and strokes.

There's also growing evidence that phytonutrients in cabbage – along with other members of the cruciferae family like kale, broccoli and Brussels sprouts – stimulate genes to produce enzymes that help detoxify the body. In doing so they lower the risk of prostate, colorectal and lung cancers, even compared with people who regularly eat other vegetables.

Indoles inactivate oestrogens that can promote the growth of some tumours. These compounds are thought to protect against breast cancer. Cabbage also produces a group of anti-cancer compounds called glucosinolates, formed when the vegetables are sliced or chopped. The process is halted by cooking, so for maximum benefit the vegetable should be eaten lightly-cooked or raw.

Other benefits of cabbage as a regular part of the diet include a reduced risk of spina bifida and cataracts. It's also thought to speed the healing of ulcers.

Nutrients
Rich in the vitamins C and K. Also a good source of B vitamins including pyridoxine, thiamine and riboflavin.

Contains useful amounts of folic acid plus the amino acid tryptophan. A good source of the minerals manganese, calcium, potassium and magnesium. Provides omega-3 fatty acids and vitamin A. A good source of dietary fibre.

CARROTS

What to Avoid
Poor-tasting crops are likely to be depleted in minerals and health-giving phytochemicals. The chances are they have been grown on damaged soils with an imbalance of trace elements and impaired biological activity. It's worth avoiding samples that are pale in colour. If there are tops attached, choose only those whose tops are bright and feathery. Reject those with wilted tops. When shopping in supermarkets it's best to stick with organic, but in farm shops and farmers' markets there's a chance to ask about growing methods. Buy from farms that rely on compost and other organic forms of fertilizer rather than chemicals. If the crop's from a mixed farm with plenty of livestock so much the better.

What to Buy
The best carrots come from

light, sandy soils or peaty soils with good moisture-holding capacity. Whatever the soil, it must have plenty of organic matter so the plant root can take up minerals. Without a full quota of essential minerals the plant cells cannot manufacture the hundreds of compounds that give carrots their taste and health-giving properties. A well-mineralized carrot will be full of flavour and have a bright orange colour. The deeper the colour, the higher the content of beta-carotene.

Benefits

The carrot is a power pack of disease fighting micro-nutrients. Beta-carotene and other antioxidants help to guard against cell damage and reduce the risk of a wide range of cancers. By reducing blood cholesterol, calcium pectate helps to prevent coronary heart disease and strokes. Two carrots a day have been shown to reduce cholesterol levels by up to 20 per cent, while just one a day can halve the risk of lung cancer in smokers.

Nutrients

Beta-carotene, a carotenoid with powerful antioxidant properties. Converts to vitamin A in the body. Alpha-carotene, a carotenoid with anti-cancer properties. Vitamins B1, B3, B6, C, D, E and folic acid. Calcium pectate, a pectin fibre that lowers blood cholesterol. Essential minerals potassium, manganese, molybdenum, phosphorus and magnesium. Monoterpenes, antioxidants that protect against heart disease and cancer. Polyacetylenes, compounds which may limit tumour growth. Lutein and zeaxanthine, carotenoids which reduce the risk of cataracts. Dietary fibre. Phytochemicals, plant compounds that protect against disease and slow the ageing process. They include falcarinol, which protects against colon cancer.

CAULIFLOWER

What to Avoid

Cauliflowers whose compact head, or curd, is dull in colour or is pitted with dark spots or patches. Also avoid heads that are not surrounded by thick green leaves. The leaves surrounding the curd offer protection and keep the vegetable fresher. It's also a good idea to avoid ready-prepared florets as they quickly lose their freshness.

What to Buy

Choose whole, fresh cauliflowers with a good covering of green leaves on the outside. Inside the leaves look for a firm, creamy white curd without blemishes or dark patches. Choose a size that meets your needs. There is no link between size and quality. As usual it's best to choose organic. It will be less likely to be contaminated with pesticide residues, and it will have been grown on soil rich in organic matter making it more likely to be high in minerals and protective phytonutrients.

Benefits

Cauliflowers belong to the cruciferous family, as do broccoli and Brussels sprouts. Along with these other vegetables they provide formidable health benefits. People who eat them regularly have lower rates of cancer than those who don't.

Among the chemical compounds in cauliflowers are substances called glucosinolates and thiocyanates – including sulphoraphane. These compounds stimulate the production of cancer-fighting enzymes in the body. Sulphoraphane is released when the vegetable is chopped or chewed. It then acts on the liver, stimulating it to produce enzymes which inhibit the development of cancers. When combined with the spice turmeric, phenethyl isothiocyanate – a phytonutrient in cauliflowers and other cruciferous vegetables – has been shown to destroy tumour cells in the prostate.

Quite apart from the valuable phytonutrients, cauliflowers deliver a sizeable dose of vitamin C, a powerful antioxidant, which helps protect against cancer, some forms of arthritis and coronary heart disease. Cauliflowers also contain good amounts of minerals, including potassium, which regulates heart function, helps control blood pressure and maintains normal fluid balance. Has a useful amount of dietary fibre which protects against colorectal cancer.

Nutrients

Contains exceptional amounts of vitamin C, plus good levels of other vitamins including vitamin K, folic acid and pyridoxine. Useful amounts of the vitamins pantothenic acid, riboflavin, thiamine and niacin. Contains good levels of dietary fibre. A useful range of minerals includes manganese, potassium, phosphorus and magnesium. Supplies some protein.

CELERY

What to Avoid
Avoid industrially grown crops. These are the sort you'll find in most supermarkets and will come from chemically-fertilized soils. Find a local source where this great health food is grown on an organically-rich soil.

What to Buy
Celery is a biennial – it has a two-year life cycle – belonging to the same plant family as carrots, parsley and fennel. With its origins in southern Europe and northern Africa, it was first used as a medicine and only later as a food. Growing to a height of about forty centimetres, it forms a collection of leaf-topped stalks growing from a common base. The stalks have a crunchy texture with a mild, salty taste. It grows best in a rich soil with plenty of moisture, so it benefits from large amounts of well-prepared compost.

Benefits
Celery is very rich in vitamin C, making it a powerful supporter of the immune system. Foods rich in vitamin C can help fight the symptoms of colds. They prevent free radical damage and so help protect against a range of inflammatory conditions such as asthma, osteoarthritis, and rheumatoid arthritis. Vitamin C also protects against cardiovascular disease.

Celery has long been known to help reduce high blood pressure. In the past doctors have advised patients with high blood pressure to avoid the vegetable because of its relatively high sodium content. But more recently compounds called pthalides have been found to relax muscles around the arteries, easing the flow of blood and lowering blood pressure.

Celery is also known to help lower blood cholesterol levels. Compounds called coumarins help prevent free radicals and boost the body's immune response to potentially harmful cells, while another group of compounds called acetylenics have been shown to halt tumour growth. Yet another group of compounds called psoralens may help prevent psoriasis.

Nutrients
Contains high levels of vitamin C and vitamin K. Good levels

of folate, vitamin A, vitamin B1 (thiamine), vitamin B2 (riboflavin) and vitamin B6 (pyridoxine). High levels of minerals including potassium, molybdenum, manganese, calcium, magnesium, phosphorus and iron. Contains good levels of dietary fibre. Contains the amino acid tryptophan. Phytonutrients include coumarins, acetylenics, psoralens and pthalides.

CHEESE

What to Avoid
Factory-made cheeses sourcing milk from many producers often scattered over wide geographical areas. They may include some pasture-fed herds, but will also contain milk produced on unhealthy foods such as chemically grown grain and soya. Pasteurization is essential for such milk since there are many opportunities for contamination during transport. Other fakes include processed cheese, the sort of cheese you're likely to find on your cheeseburger in the fast-food restaurant. It's made from natural cheese combined with milk solids, water and colouring additives. Emulsifiers and other chemical additives are mixed to give it a smooth texture.

What to Buy
Real cheese is made from the milk of cows grazing fertile pastures. And it's milk that has not been pasteurized. Pasteurization destroys vitamins and denatures protein in the milk. It also kills bacteria – good and bad – along with the enzymes that help the body to absorb and utilize essential nutrients such as calcium. Harmful bacteria can flourish in milk that has been pasteurized, whereas in the acid conditions produced by the ripening of unpasteurized cheese they cannot survive. Real cheese is more likely to be made by a specialist artisan cheese-maker than a factory.

Benefits
Cultured dairy products, including cheese, have been found to lower blood cholesterol levels and protect against bone loss. Fermentation helps to break down the milk protein casein, one of the hardest proteins to digest. In pasteurized milk the culturing process restores some of the enzymes destroyed by heat, including those that help the body to absorb calcium and other minerals. Both B vitamins

and vitamin C levels in the milk increase during fermentation. Cheese is a good provider of riboflavin – vitamin B2 – which helps in the metabolism of proteins, fats and carbohydrates. It is also a rich source of the essential amino acids phenylalanine and tyrosine which are converted into a brain chemical that promotes mental alertness, memory and a sense of well-being.

Nutrients

High-quality protein including the amino acids phenylalanine and tyrosine. Healthy fats. Cholesterol, needed by the body to make hormones, produce bile, synthesize vitamin D, construct cell membranes and insulate nerves. B vitamins, including riboflavin and B12 which, with folic acid, forms red blood cells in the bone marrow and helps prevent anaemia. Minerals including calcium, zinc and selenium.

CHICKEN

What to Avoid

Avoid birds raised in crowded conditions in sheds. Most broiler meat comes from operations with more than a hundred thousand birds. Broilers are slaughtered at six to eight weeks old. Their intensive, grain-based diet makes them intrinsically unhealthy and depletes the meat of many of the nutrients that could protect human health.

What to Buy

In his best-seller *The Farming Ladder*, published during the Second World War, George Henderson described keeping a profitable poultry enterprise on his mixed farm in Oxfordshire. Each day the birds were moved in their portable pens to a new patch of fresh, green grass. This was the popular way to keep poultry half a century ago, and modern science has shown that it produced meat and eggs of the highest nutritional standard.

Today, most broiler chicken are kept in large sheds and fed on chemically grown grain. Free-range birds – while they are allowed outside – are usually confined to a single patch of grass for days or even weeks on end. To produce really healthy meat, chickens need to eat fresh grass every day. Fortunately some poultry farmers in the United States have begun switching to the traditional system of 'folding' their birds over fresh pasture. In Britain real, pasture-fed poultry are still rare.

Benefits

Chicken has grown in popularity as an alternative to red meat, in part because it contains less saturated fat and more polyunsaturates. The protein of chicken meat is of high quality. The meat is also a good source of selenium, which is vital for thyroid hormone metabolism, immune function and the efficient operation of antioxidant defences.

Grass-fed chicken delivers very much more. When broiler chicken are confined to sheds and denied their daily intake of fresh grass their fats become artificially depleted in omega-3s, making the meat far less healthy. Omega-3s protect against heart disease and cancer. Grass-fed poultry meat also contains higher levels of vitamin E than meat produced inside on cereal grains alone. Given the chance chicken will take up to one-third of their calorie intake as grass.

Nutrients

B vitamins including niacin, which works with other B vitamins in carbohydrate metabolism, and pyridoxine which aids fat and nucleic acid

metabolism and helps to build body tissue. Tryptophan, the amino acid which builds niacin. Selenium and other minerals including phosphorus. Omega-3 fatty acids, high in pasture-fed birds. Vitamin E, high in pasture-fed birds.

COD

What to Avoid

As with all fish, it's best to avoid stale and old fish that has been stored for too long. Pre-packed supermarket fish is also best avoided, since there's far less chance of buying the truly fresh product. Pre-packed fresh fish – even when within its sell-by date – often smells strong, a sign that it is far from fresh. Buy from a traditional fishmonger whenever possible and ask when the fish came in. Before you pay for the fish make sure that it doesn't smell too fishy. If you can't find cod that's really fresh, you're better off buying a frozen product.

What to Buy

Because cod – like most fish – is a truly healthy food, it's worth taking the trouble to find genuinely fresh examples. Ask the fishmonger to prepare your fillets from a whole fish. Prefilleted fish that has lain on the slab for a while will never taste as fresh as newly-prepared fillets. Fresh cod has a good texture, breaking easily into milky white flakes. While not so flavoured as some other fish, cod more than compensates with its satisfying texture.

Benefits

Fish is a real health food. Traditional peoples who lived mostly on fish and seafood were among the healthiest on the planet. Today people who eat fish regularly have been found to have a far lower risk of heart disease and heart attack than those who seldom eat it. Cod is particularly beneficial in promoting cardiovascular health because as well as containing blood-thinning omega-3 fatty acids, it contains both vitamins B6 and B12, which help reduce the level of homocysteine in the blood. Homocysteine is known to damage blood vessels.

Regular fish consumption reduces the risk of strokes. It has also been linked to a lower risk of some cancers including colon cancer, probably because of useful levels of selenium, vitamin B12 and vitamin D in fish. Omega-3 fats in fish – including cod – are thought to protect against Alzheimer's

disease, depression and macular degeneration. Together selenium, vitamin D and omega-3 fatty acids in cod can reduce the inflammation that leads to asthma attacks, rheumatoid arthritis, osteoarthritis and migraines.

Nutrients

Cod – like other fish – is a good, low-calorie source of high quality protein. It also contains a variety of important nutrients. Cod is a rich source of the amino acid tryptophan which, in the body, is used in the production of the neurotransmitter serotonin, which gives feelings of well-being. Essential minerals are plentiful in cod, particularly selenium, phosphorous and potassium. Also contains useful amounts of the B vitamins pyridoxine, niacin and B12. High in omega-3 fatty acids.

DANDELION LEAVES

What to Avoid

It's worth taking care in the selection of plants. Avoid those growing near busy roads as they contain vehicle exhaust contaminants. Also avoid plants growing on cultivated land. They may have been contaminated with toxic sprays. Equally the soil may have been damaged by chemical fertilizers, restricting plant nutrient uptake. Choose plants growing on undisturbed ground such as hedgebanks or old pastures. Pick the youngest leaves and wash them well before adding them to your salads or cooking like spinach.

What to Pick

During the Second World War dandelion leaves were recommended by the BBC's Radio Doctor, Charles Hill, as a useful source of nutrients at a time of food scarcity. It was good advice. Dandelion leaves are a rich source of minerals and vitamins and have been used as a medicinal herb for centuries. Traditionally, they were used to treat liver and gall bladder conditions. They were also used as a diuretic. Their great advantage was that the plant grew almost everywhere, and the leaves are available at all times of the year.

Dandelion leaves are rich in a number of vitamins, particularly vitamin C and the vitamin A precursor, beta-carotene. This helps protect against heart disease and a number of forms of cancer. Vitamin C, a powerful anti-oxidant, also protects against heart disease, as well as strengthening the immune system. There's also evidence that the traditional use of dandelion as a treatment for liver disease may have some scientific basis. The plant has been found to be rich in lecithin, which is being investigated as a possible treatment for liver cirrhosis. Other compounds in the plant have been shown to improve liver function by stimulating the production of bile.

Nutrients

A rich source of vitamins, including vitamins A, C, D and B-complex. Contains good levels of minerals including iron, magnesium, zinc, potassium, manganese, copper, calcium, boron and silicon. Rich in lecithin. Contains tannins, some essential oils and flavenoids.

EGGS

What to Avoid

Eggs from caged birds kept in confinement. Also many so-called free-range eggs from hens that seldom tread on fresh pasture.

What to Buy

Properly produced eggs are one of mankind's finest,

nutrient-dense foods. They are rich in a wide variety of protective nutrients. But as with so many modern foods their health benefits are largely wasted in production systems that put price and profit before quality. Like poultry meat the best eggs come from hens that have daily access to fresh, botanically diverse pastures. Until the mid-twentieth century most eggs were produced by hens moved or 'folded' daily around pastures in mobile units.

Today, most are produced by hens caged in battery houses and fed chemically grown commodity grains. Sadly, not even free-range birds are given access to fresh new grassland every day. It's now possible to buy eggs from hens fed on fish meal or flax seed to boost omega-3 content. Nutritionally these are an improvement on standard battery eggs but they don't compare with proper 'pasture-fed' eggs. In the United States these healthy eggs have begun to reappear as an increasing number of poultry farmers return to the traditional 'folding' system.

Benefits

B vitamins in eggs are vital to a range of body functions including energy metabolism,

stress alleviation and the maintenance of healthy arteries. Other vitamins include A, essential for normal growth and development, vitamin E which protects against heart disease and some cancers, and vitamin D which aids mineral absorption and helps build healthy bones. Among essential minerals are iodine, needed for making thyroid hormones, and phosphorus, essential for healthy teeth and bones.

Eggs are also a good source of iron, which aids the production of red blood cells, and zinc which supports a healthy immune system. Among the special benefits of 'grass-fed eggs' are an omega-3 to omega-6 fatty acid balance close to one. This is far healthier than in battery eggs where the omega-6 content may be up to nineteen times higher than omega-3s. 'Pasture-fed eggs' also contain higher levels of folic acid, which protects against cancer, and vitamin B12, which aids red blood cell formation.

Nutrients

B vitamins. Fat soluble vitamins A, D and E. Sulphur-containing proteins needed to maintain cell membranes. Minerals including iron, zinc, iodine and selenium.

Cholesterol and lecithin, essential to cell structure and function. Lutein and zeaxanthine, powerful antioxidants protecting against macular degeneration. Essential long chain fatty acids known as EPA and DHA.

HERRINGS

What to avoid

Herrings and other oily fish are among the healthiest foods, but they are widely smoked, salted and pickled. In the smoked form – as kippers – they're best not eaten too often as the smoking process may make them carcinogenic. They are also likely to be high in salt.

Pickled herring in the form of rollmops have been a delicacy for centuries. The pickling process preserves many of the nutrients. However, for maximum benefits it's best to stick to the fresh form when possible. Despite their healthy attributes, oily fish can become contaminated with pollutants in the sea, so the UK Food Standards Agency has issued guidelines on maximum intakes – no more than two portions a week for pregnant and breast-feeding women and girls under 16, and no more than four portions a week for

everyone else.

What to Buy

As with all fish, herrings are best bought from a good fishmonger who can tell you when they were landed. Freshness is the most important characteristic. The herring has adapted to each of its major habitats in the North Sea, the north Atlantic and the Baltic, with the Atlantic herring being larger than the others, and the Baltic herring being less fatty. However all are extremely nutritious and have much to contribute to a healthy diet.

Benefits

Oily fish – including the herring – are one of the richest sources of omega-3, polyunsaturated fatty acids which help to prevent heart disease and strokes and may be protective against some cancers. Just one portion of fish per week has been shown to make a significant reduction in the risk of heart attacks. Fish may also reduce the risk of some cancers. Omega-3s have been found to reduce cholesterol in people with elevated levels and lower blood triglycerides in patients with high levels.

Herrings are a rich source of many minerals including

iodine, which maintains thyroid function and the hormones that regulate many body functions, and selenium, an important antioxidant which protects against many cancers; also a good source of B vitamins including niacin which is essential for energy metabolism, pyridoxine which is important for protein and fat metabolism, and B12 which is essential for the formation of red blood cells and for nervous function. Also a good source of vitamin D which helps build strong bones and teeth as well as protecting against cancer.

Nutrients

Good, low-calorie source of high-quality protein. A rich source of B vitamins, including niacin, pyridoxine and vitamin B12. Rich in vitamin D. A useful source of many minerals including phosphorous, iodine, selenium, potassium, calcium, iron and magnesium. Useful levels of vitamin E and one of the best sources of omega-3 fatty acids and long chain polyunsaturated fatty acids.

KALE

What to Avoid

Kale is a veritable powerhouse of health-protecting nutrients,

so it makes no sense to buy the poorly-grown 'commodity' version you'll find on the shelves of most supermarkets. Find a local grower with a dark, humus-rich soil and you're more likely to take home a food that will deliver its full nutrient potential.

What to Buy

This leafy, green vegetable is a descendant of wild cabbage and belongs to the *brassica* family, which includes cabbage and Brussels sprouts. It's a group of vegetables becoming known for their health-promoting properties, derived from sulphur-containing phytonutrients. Originating in Asia Minor, curly kale is thought to have been brought to Britain in Roman times. Kale grows to be its most nutritious on soils with plenty of organic matter and high lime content.

Benefits

Kale has powerful anti-cancer properties. Its sulphur-containing compounds, which include glucosinolates and cysteine sulphoxides, seem able to protect against a wide range of cancers. One potent glucosinolate known as sulphoraphane may offer protection to individuals with a gene making them susceptible to colon cancer. New research shows that phytonutrients in kale and related vegetables stimulate the body's own genes to produce detoxifying enzymes that will eliminate harmful toxins. Kale contains an unusually high level of the plant form of vitamin A – beta-carotene. It also contains high levels of vitamin C and vitamin E. This powerful group of anti-oxidants offers good immune protection against many different forms of cancer as well as heart disease. Calcium and potassium in kale help to maintain normal blood pressure, while the plant's good level of dietary fibre provides additional protection against colorectal cancer.

Nutrients
Contains high levels of Vitamins A, C and K. Rich in dietary fibre. Good levels of minerals including manganese, copper, calcium, potassium, iron, magnesium and phosphorus. Health-protecting phytonutrients include glucosinolates and cysteine sulphoxides. Contains useful levels of vitamins B1 (thiamin), B2 (riboflavin), B3 (niacin), B6 (pyridoxine) and folate. Contains the amino acid tryptophan. Useful amounts of omega-3 fatty acids.

LAMB

What to Avoid
British lamb is raised mainly on grassland, so it's likely to contain reasonable amounts of vitamin E, omega-3 and CLA. Unfortunately, the owners of some intensive flocks attempt to speed lamb 'finishing' by supplementing grass with high-energy grains and concentrate foods. Their meat is best avoided since it's likely to contain fewer of these protective nutrients. Avoid, too, lamb produced on pastures where large amounts of chemical nitrogen fertilizers are applied and which won't contain the diverse range of plant species necessary.

What to Buy
Sheep are ruminant animals; they're adapted to obtaining their nutrients from vegetation. Not surprisingly the healthiest lamb comes from animals that have been raised chiefly on pasture. Their meat contains more vitamin E, beta-carotene, CLA and omega-3s than the meat of animals fed on grain. There's also new scientific evidence to show that lambs raised on botanically diverse grassland such as salt marsh, heaths and moorlands contain more of these protective

nutrients than those reared on grass monocultures.

Benefits

Well-produced lamb is a nutrient-dense food. A small serving supplies many of the nutrients essential for good health. Lamb provides a range of vitamins and minerals. Among the most important is iron. Diets low in iron lead to learning problems in children and poor concentration in young adults. Iron deficiency can lead to anaemia which produces symptoms of fatigue and reduced immunity. Haem iron found in lamb and other meats is more efficiently absorbed than the iron found in plant tissues. Lamb, like other red meats, is a good source of fat-soluble vitamins such as A, D and E which help the body utilize minerals in food.

Nutrients

Iron, in the form of easily absorbed haem iron. Zinc, essential for many enzyme systems. High-quality protein, with an ideal balance of amino acids. Magnesium, the macro-mineral needed for many enzyme systems, bone formation, nerve transmission and carbohydrate metabolism. Vitamins B1, B2, B3, B6 and the essential B12, found naturally

only in animal foods. Also vitamins A, D and E. Omega-3s, the polyunsaturated fats that are important for brain function and cardiovascular health. CLA (conjugated linoleic acid), a polyunsaturated fat with powerful anti-cancer properties. Stearic acid, a saturated fat that actually lowers blood cholesterol. Selenium, the trace element vital to a healthy immune system. Palmitoleic acid, a monounsaturated fatty acid which offers protection against viruses and other pathogens.

LENTILS

What to Avoid

No real fakes. Lentils are a sustainable and nutritious food. They occur in a number of types. Best known in Britain are the red lentils that become mushy on cooking. The French prefer the green variety, which retains its shape with cooking.

What to Buy

Lentils are legumes. In association with soil bacteria they are able to 'fix' atmospheric nitrogen at their roots, naturally increasing the fertility of the soil. This gives them a key role in many sustainable farming systems. It's also the reason why they've been a popular food crop for thousands of years. Lentils are seeds that grow in pods. They are one of the world's first cultivated foods and have been consumed since prehistoric times. Traditionally they are eaten with barley and wheat, a practice that provides a balance of different amino acids. Lentils are highly regarded in traditional Indian cuisine where they form the basis of the spiced lentil dish known as dal.

Benefits

Lentils are a good source of dietary fibre which helps to lower blood cholesterol levels. They are also helpful in managing blood sugar disorders since their high fibre content prevents blood sugar levels from rising too quickly after a meal. In wide-scale trials, lentils have been found to play an important role in reducing the risk of heart disease.

Good levels of folate and magnesium also help reduce cardiovascular risk. Folate helps lower the level of blood homocysteine, a compound that damages artery walls. It also protects against some

forms of cancer and helps to prevent neural tube defects in the foetus. Magnesium strengthens artery walls and improves blood flow. As if this weren't enough, the iron in lentils helps to prevent anaemia, which is especially important for menstruating and pregnant women.

Nutrients

High levels of the minerals iron, manganese, potassium and copper. Particularly high in molybdenum, a mineral that plays a role in protein metabolism, iron absorption and normal cell function. Exceptionally rich in dietary fibre. Rich in folate. A good source of protein. Contain useful levels of vitamin B1 (thiamine) and the amino acid tryptophan.

LIVER

What to Avoid

Avoid liver – and other meats – from all animals kept in confinement, or which are fed unnatural feeds such as soya. Ideally choose the livers of cattle, lambs, pigs and poultry that have spent their lives outdoors on pasture. If you can't be sure of their history, choose only organically reared meat.

What to Buy

A couple of generations ago liver was at least an occasional dish served in every home. Along with other offal meats, it has now gone out of fashion. This is a pity. Throughout history liver has been amongst the most highly prized foods in many parts of the world. Some societies regard it more highly even than best steak, and virtually every cuisine has its liver specialities.

Dentist and nutritionist Weston Price reported on the consumption of raw liver by tribes of African hunter-gatherers. They considered the meat to be so sacred that they would only touch it with their spears, never their hands. Our modern aversion to liver is partly because of its physiological role of dealing with toxins. The fear is that the meat will be riddled with them. But the liver does not store toxins, and while it makes sense to stick to the liver of organically reared animals, the nutritional benefits far outweigh any risks.

Benefits

Helps build strength and vitality. The high vitamin A and mineral content means this food can play a big part in maintaining healthy immune function. It helps fight colds and infections, and may have some anti-cancer properties. Essential for the maintenance of normal vision. Through its store of minerals and fat-soluble vitamins, liver also helps the human body deal with toxins.

Nutrients

A good source of high-quality protein. The most concentrated source of Vitamin A found in nature. Rich in B vitamins, especially vitamin B12. Contains iron in a highly usable form. According to the Weston Price Foundation liver contains an anti-fatigue factor. A good source of folic acid. Contains a large number of essential trace elements, such as copper, zinc and chromium. Contains the nutrient CoQ10 which is important for cardiovascular function. A rich source of purines, compounds that are precursors for DNA and RNA.

MILK

What to Avoid

Skimmed and semi-skimmed milks are depleted in fat-soluble vitamins and other nutrients that are crucial to health. Too much milk comes from grass monocultures treated with chemical fertilizers. These high-tech pastures no longer contain the broad mix of grasses and herbs needed to keep the cow well-nourished and her milk full of nutrients. Cows are fed large amounts of cereal grain and soya meal, a diet regime that does nothing for the health of the cow or the human drinking the milk. Most of today's milk is pasteurized, a practice that is thought to destroy many important nutrients.

What to Buy

Despite the bad press given to today's commercial milk, the real thing is one of nature's finest foods. To produce nutrient-rich milk, cows need to graze botanically diverse pastures containing a number of different grasses and clovers, plus wild flowers and deep-rooting herbs. Ideally, cows should graze these pastures for much of the year, though limited amounts of hay, silage, and home-grown forage crops are acceptable for winter milk production. For maximum nutritional benefit, milk should be drunk whole with minimal processing. Real milk contains its natural complement of fat and has not been homogenized. The very best is raw and

unpasteurized, though it's important to make sure the herd it came from is free of *brucella* – the cause of undulant fever – and bovine TB.

Benefits

Many studies have shown that well-produced milk helps to build strong bones. Calcium from dairy sources increases bone mineral density, reducing the risk of osteoporosis and subsequent fractures in older people. Low levels of dietary calcium have been linked to an increased incidence of colon cancer. A similar relationship has been found for vitamin D. Deficiency of vitamin D is as widespread as calcium deficiency, and is chiefly obtained by exposure to sunlight. Food sources of the vitamin – offal meats, lard, egg yolks of pasture-fed hens and whole dairy foods – have largely fallen from favour. Vitamin D – like calcium – in real milk reduces the risk of both colon cancer and breast cancer.

Nutrients

Minerals, particularly calcium and phosphorus. Vitamin D and other fat-soluble vitamins including A, E and K, as well as 'activator X', the fat-soluble nutrient discovered by Weston

A. Price to aid mineral absorption. Water soluble vitamins C, B12 and B2 (riboflavin). Omega-3 fatty acids. Conjugated linoleic acid (CLA).

OATS

What to Avoid
Because they're tolerant to a range of growing conditions, oats are routinely treated with far fewer pesticides and chemical fertilizers than other cereals. Even so, they are often grown on chemically damaged soils and may be depleted in minerals as a result. Oats are mostly consumed as oat flakes, grains that have been rolled and steamed to make them softer. The process destroys some of the B vitamins that are present in pinhead oatmeal. But the biggest abuses of this food are perpetrated by the manufacturers of so-called healthy breakfast cereals. To make their fancy shapes they subject oats to high temperatures and pressures in the extrusion process. Far from being healthy, these products are nutritionally impoverished, perhaps even dangerous. Don't be fooled by the list of essential minerals and vitamins on the packet. These are mostly additives put in to make the product look good.

What to Buy
Of all the commonly grown cereal crops, oats are the hardiest. They'll grow in a range of different soils and withstand the ill-effects of cold and wet. That made them popular with farmers in the hilly areas of western Britain. The crop will ripen in limited sunshine. Traditionally some of the best crops came from the dull, rainy districts bordering the coasts of the west and north. While oats do best on heavy clay loams, they are more tolerant of acid conditions than wheat. Samuel Johnson once quipped that oats were a grain used in England to feed horses and in Scotland to feed the people.

Benefits
Because of their high content of soluble fibres, oats promote healthy bowels and help to reduce blood cholesterol levels, so cutting the risks of coronary heart disease and strokes. They are low in gluten but contain more phytates than other cereals. Phytates counter hormones that can lead to tumours, so protecting against some cancers. But phytates can also interfere with the absorption of minerals such as

iron, copper, magnesium and zinc, so health experts recommend that whole grains are soaked or fermented before eating. Whole oats have a low glycaemic index (GI) and so are useful in the regulation of blood sugar. Traditionally, herbalists have used oats to induce sleep. Best eaten in porridge made from pinhead oatmeal in which the whole grain kernel has been cut in half.

Nutrients
Oats contain higher levels of protein and fat than most other grains. They are rich in the B vitamins thiamine, riboflavin and B6. Useful amounts of the minerals calcium, iron, magnesium, phosphorus and potassium. Small amount of vitamin E and folic acid. Soluble fibre.

ONIONS

What to Avoid
Avoid chemically grown onions. Go for crops that have been grown in soils which have received liberal dressings of well-made compost. A healthy soil with plenty of biological activity will ensure the onions have their full complement of trace elements, vitamins and sulphur-containing compounds. If you're shopping in supermarkets go for the organically grown variety.

What to Buy
The onion is one of six hundred plants belonging to the genus *allium* – the lily family – which includes garlic, chives, scallions, shallots and leeks. They grow wild in many parts of the world, though there is evidence that they were first cultivated in Asia or India. They have been used in cooking for thousands of years, in part because their distinctive flavour blends well with bland-tasting foods, such as beans. Onions have also been used by healers to treat a range of health conditions. In Britain, onions grow best on deep, fertile soils with high levels of organic matter.

Benefits
Onions first came to the attention of researchers following a Chinese study that showed people with the highest intakes of *allium* vegetables had the lowest rates of stomach cancer.

The chemistry of onions is complex. They contain a bewildering array of sulphur-containing compounds, many of which have highly complex structures. A group known as cysteine sulphoxides are chiefly responsible for onion flavours and for the eye irritation that makes you cry when peeling them. Recent studies have revealed a particular compound which blocks the biochemical processes leading to asthma and inflammatory reactions.

Other medicinal benefits include the improvement of kidney function and resistance to bacterial infections. Onions have been found to lower blood lipids and blood pressure. Half a cup of raw onions a day is said to protect against the tendency of blood to clot and coagulate. Regular onion eating has also been shown to raise the blood level of the 'good cholesterol', HDL.

Nutrients

A rich source of carotenoids, the plant pigments that act as antioxidants. Rich in flavenoids, including quercetin, which has been shown to neutralize a number of potent carcinogens. Red and yellow onions and shallots have the highest flavenoid content of the *allium* vegetables. High in B vitamins including vitamin B6. A good source of vitamin C. A good source of trace elements, including calcium, magnesium

and potassium.

ORANGES

What to Avoid

As with many other fruits it's best to avoid non-organic samples. Oranges are among the fruits most often found to be contaminated with pesticide residues. They have so many healthy attributes that it makes no sense to undo the good work by getting a dose of contaminants along with the health-giving nutrients. Also avoid fruits which have soft spots or traces of mould.

What to Buy

Choose oranges with a smooth-textured skin, which are firm to the touch and which are heavy for their size. These are the fruits most likely to be juicy. Colour is largely immaterial. A bright orange colour is no indication that the fruit will be tastier or healthier than paler fruits – or even oranges that have patches of green or brown russetting on their skins. A bright orange colour may simply indicate that the fruit has been treated with a chemical dye.

Benefits

There are so many health benefits to a well grown orange

that it's hard to know where to start. Few other natural foods can match them for their levels of vitamin C. This vitamin has been shown to protect against many forms of cancer, including cervical, pancreatic, colorectal, bladder, lung and breast cancer. It helps combat heart disease by blocking the oxidation of LDL cholesterol which can lead to blocked arteries. It helps to reduce the severity of colds and protect the DNA in sperm from damage. Research has shown that merely taking supplements of vitamin C does not provide the protective benefits of the vitamin in oranges.

The fruit also contains a range of other health-giving nutrients. They include flavenoids – many of which are antioxidants – which protect cells from damage by free radicals. Others help prevent the spread of cancer cells. Compounds known as terpenes control the production of cholesterol and help produce the enzymes that neutralize dangerous carcinogens. A citrus oil known as limonene has been shown to shrink mammary tumours in rats.

As if this weren't enough a group of compounds known as polymethoxylated flavones – found in citrus fruit peels – has been found to lower blood cholesterol more effectively than prescription drugs and without side effects. The fibre in oranges also helps to reduce blood cholesterol while at the same time maintaining bowel regularity. Potassium helps regulate the fluid balance of cells and maintain normal heart function and blood pressure.

Nutrients
Exceptional levels of vitamin C in a form that is well utilized in the body. Other useful vitamins include vitamin A, folic acid and thiamine (vitamin B1). Good levels of dietary fibre. High levels of phytonutrients, including citrus flavanones, anthocyanins, hydroxycinnamic acids and polyphenols. Many work in combination with vitamin C. Useful levels of calcium plus dietary fibre.

PARSLEY

What to Avoid
Dried parsley flakes. Also the little pots of growing parsley you buy at supermarkets. Try planting them in a good soil, rich in organic matter, and watch them turn into strong healthy plants.

What to Buy

A native of the Mediterranean region of southern Europe, parsley has been cultivated for more than two thousand years. Originally grown for medicinal purposes, it was later used as a garnish for a range of dishes, a function it still fulfils today. Such are the nutritional benefits of the plant, it deserves to be more widely used.

Parsley thrives in a rich soil to which plenty of compost has been added. This allows the plant to take up the nutrients it needs and produce the full range of compounds which make it such a healthy food. Three main types are grown. The curly-leaved variety is best-known in Britain, but the flat-leaved Italian type is gaining in popularity. Hamburg parsley has an edible, turnip-like taproot.

Benefits

Parsley has a number of health-promoting volatile oils. One of the more important is myristicin, which has been shown to inhibit tumour formation, particularly on the lungs. Parsley's volatile oils enable the plant to protect against some types of carcinogen, such as the benzopyrenes found in cigarette smoke.

Parsley is also a rich source of antioxidants. Flavenoids in the plant – particularly lutein – help to prevent cell damage. Vitamin C, found at high levels in parsley, protects against a number of diseases, including heart disease, some cancers, diabetes and asthma. The plant's rich store of beta-carotene reduces the risk of diabetes, heart disease, asthma and arthritis. Cardiovascular health is also promoted by the high levels of folate found in parsley. Folate reduces the levels of damaging homocysteine, so reducing the risk of heart attack or stroke in some people.

Nutrients

High levels of vitamins C and K. Good source of the vitamin A precursor, beta-carotene. Rich in flavenoids, some of which act as antioxidants, while others deactivate hormones that might otherwise encourage tumour growth. Contains coumarins, compounds which help to prevent blood clots and may have anti-cancer properties. Good source of folate. Contains monoterpenes, anti-oxidants that help to reduce blood cholesterol levels and which may have anti-cancer properties. Contains polyacetylenes, compounds that may protect against cancer by blocking the formation of prostaglandins.

PHEASANTS

What to Avoid
The vast majority of pheasants and partridges are reared for game shooting. There is no industry for rearing them in large numbers for the table. Most roam free and eat a diet rich in natural foods. As a result there are no fakes of this healthy meat.

What to Buy
Game birds such as pheasants and partridges are reared to roam through woods and hedgerows. Unlike commercial poultry, which are usually confined to sheds and fed on cereals, game birds search for the seeds and insects that occur naturally in the countryside. As a result, their meat is rich in minerals and other valuable nutrients. In Britain, pheasants and partridges are principally reared for sport shooting. As part of their day-to-day management they are often fed cereals outside, but because they are unconfined these feed supplements rarely make up a large part of the diet. About half the pheasants shot in Britain are sold to game dealers for marketing in High Street shops. The endorsement of game meat by high profile chefs has led to a renewed interest in what is now considered to be a particularly healthy meat.

Benefits
Because it is generally high in the important trace element selenium, the meat of pheasants and partridges can make an important contribution to health and well-being. Selenium, which is generally low in the British diet, is involved in a number of vital metabolic functions. It can act as a powerful antioxidant. Deficiency of the element can lead to a wide range of serious conditions, including heart disease and a number of cancers. Selenium deficiency has also been linked to depression and mood swings, so inclusion of the element in the diet can greatly enhance feelings of well-being.

Nutrients
The meat of both partridges and pheasants is higher in selenium than other meats. Levels of iron are higher than in turkey and chicken. Contains far lower levels of saturated fats than red meats such as

lamb and beef. A good source of vitamin B6.

PORK

What to Avoid

Most pork is produced from pigs kept in crowded conditions inside sheds. Pigs are intelligent animals with a strong set of behavioural instincts. They are happiest when they are rooting about in pasture or woodland – turning over the ground with their snouts in search of roots, insects or acorns. Yet all too often they are kept indoors in conditions where space is limited and where they are fed on a bland, unchanging diet of pellets made from chemically-grown grain. Under these confinement conditions they often become bored and aggressive. Whatever the morality of keeping sentient animals this way, it certainly doesn't produce the best pork.

What to Buy

Find a butcher who sells pork from local farms where the animals are kept outdoors. If you can't find a butcher who can tell you this, buy your pork elsewhere. Animals that have been allowed to forage in pasture or woodland – and which have been able to supplement their basic ration with roots, pasture and beetles – will taste incomparably better than intensively farmed pork.

If you're looking for the best meat it's also worth hunting out pork produced from rare or minority breed pigs, animals like the Berkshire, the Saddleback, the Tamworth, the Middle White and the Oxford Sandy and Black. These breeds have been bred for outdoor production and will produce meat of superb flavour. It's an exceptional butcher who can supply this kind of pork, but they are around.

Farmers' markets are also good places to search. If you need to buy your pork in a supermarket insist on organically-reared meat. This will guarantee that the animal has been reared outdoors and that its feed was free of GM materials and routine pharmaceuticals like antibiotics.

Benefits

Pork is sometimes thought of as high in fat, but many cuts are relatively lean with little more total fat than beef. If the animal has been raised outdoors on pasture the fat will contain more of the healthy polyunsaturated fats than pigs reared inside. Like other red meats, pork is a good source of high quality protein and provides many vitamins including vitamin A and the B vitamins. Pork is particularly rich in folic acid, making it especially valuable for pregnant women. It also supplies iron in a readily available form.

Nutrients
Complete protein including sulphur-containing amino acids. Contains B vitamins including thiamine, riboflavin, niacin, pyridoxine, pantothenic acid and vitamin B12. Also a good source of vitamin A. A rich source of iron, it also contains useful amounts of other minerals including magnesium, phosphorus, potassium, zinc and selenium, which is deficient in many British diets.

RASPBERRIES

What to Avoid
Since raspberry canes remain productive for many years, they grow on soils that are not subject to the chemical abuse heaped on arable land. However, the most nutrient-rich fruits come from land that is regularly mulched with compost and whose mineral levels are replenished, for

example, with seaweed, rock dust or sea solids. If you don't know the full history, choose organic.

What to Buy
Wild raspberries are thought to have originated in Asia, though they later spread around the world. They are known as aggregate fruits since they are made up of small, seed-containing fruits, or drupelets, arranged around a hollow core. This structure gives them a delicate texture. With a sweet, slightly sharp taste they are, for many, a favourite fruit. In nutritional terms they are exceptionally rich in protective nutrients. They are at their best when grown on deep, rich soils with plenty of organic matter and an active microbial community.

Benefits
Raspberries are rich in an important antioxidant called ellagic acid, which belongs to a group of phytonutrients called tannins. In the body it is active in neutralizing free radicals that would otherwise cause damage to cell membranes and other structures.

Raspberries also contain a group of flavenoids called anthocyanins which give them their rich, red colour. These help to give the berries their supreme antioxidant properties, as well as protecting against certain bacterial and fungal infections. Another group of antioxidants called ellagitannins are found almost exclusively in the fruit. Raspberries are reported to have 50 per cent more antioxidant activity than strawberries and ten times more than tomatoes. They have also been shown to have anti-cancer properties and to protect against macular degeneration of the eye.

Nutrients

Rich in minerals, especially manganese, magnesium, potassium and copper. Good levels of vitamin C, vitamin B2 (riboflavin) and vitamin B3 (niacin). A rich source of ellagic acid and ellagitannins. High in dietary fibre. A good source of folate. High in anthocyanins, including quercetin.

SAUSAGES

What to Avoid

The cheapest sausages are rarely worth eating. They're likely to be the ones with the lowest meat content and the highest levels of preservatives, 'fillers' and water, so however cheap they are they will represent poor value for money.

The traditional sausage was a healthy, high-fat product containing nutritious but cheap cuts of meat. They were preserved using the natural process of lacto-fermentation which actually increased nutrient availability. Today nitrites and nitrates are commonly used as preservatives in addition to traditional salt since they enhance the colour of the cured meat. These compounds can lead to disease.

The cheapest sausages often have a meat content of less than 50 per cent, which is bulked up with rusk and water. The meat itself can include mechanically recovered meat (MRM) which is extracted from bones by a combination of high pressure and temperature. The skins or casings of cheap sausages are rarely made from the natural material, the intestine of a pig or cow. They're more likely to be made from collagen or cellulose.

What to Buy

Sausages are often used as an outlet for poor quality meat; that's why it's worth paying a bit more for a good product. It should have a meat content of at least 90 per cent. The best products can contain as much as 97 per cent meat, while the poorest may have a meat content as low as 45 per cent.

When I was a kid we always had sausages on a Saturday. That's because the local butcher made his own sausages on a Saturday morning using whatever 'trimmings' were available at the end of the week. There was no need for preservatives because people recognized this as a fresh, perishable product.

Nowadays sausages – even organic ones – need to have a good shelf life or the supermarket won't be willing to stock them. That means almost all will have some level of preservatives, unless, that is, they are made by the continental method of partially cooking the meat. Unless you know a good butcher or farm shop where they make their own, it's worth buying organic.

Benefits
Well-made sausages made from good quality meat and without too many preservatives will deliver most of the health benefits of good beef or pork. But because poor meat is so easily disguised in this product, its worth taking the time to track down ethical butchers or producers of good beef or pork

who just happen to process their own meat.

Nutrients
Pork or beef sausages will provide a complete protein including sulphur-containing amino acids. Contain B vitamins including thiamine, riboflavin, niacin, pyridoxine, pantothenic acid and vitamin B12. Also good sources of iron and zinc, with useful amounts of other minerals including magnesium, phosphorus, potassium and selenium, which is generally deficient in many British diets. They will contain relatively high levels of fat, but as long as the beef is from outdoor-reared and preferably pastured animals, the fat will be of the healthy, high value sort.

SHELLFISH

What to Avoid
Frozen or ready cooked shellfish. These are often prepared in salty water and are likely to carry an excessive amount of salt. Foods like mussels, clams and oysters are highly perishable and are quick to spoil. So only buy those you know to be fresh. Also be sure to buy only those shellfish that are in season. It's also a good idea to buy from someone who

can tell you where the fish came from.

Mussels and other shellfish can be polluted because of our unsavoury tradition of disposing of sewage in the sea around our coasts. Shellfish from partially enclosed estuaries are more likely to be contaminated than those from bays facing the open sea.

What to Buy

Crustaceans such as crabs, oysters, prawns, scampi and shrimps are best bought live, or cooked and eaten on the day of purchase. Molluscs are the other form of shellfish and include mussels, clams, oysters and scallops. Like crustaceans they quickly deteriorate and should be bought live and cooked and eaten on the day of purchase. Buy shellfish fresh from fishmongers who can tell you about their source. Some people are allergic to shellfish and should avoid them totally.

Benefits

Shellfish such as scallops, mussels, oysters, clams, shrimps, crabs and lobsters are highly valued by many traditional peoples. And with good reason. Shellfish generally deliver a wide range of health benefits. They are rich in iodine and the antioxidant selenium.

Many parts of the world have soils which are low in iodine. Unless people eat foods that are – like shellfish – rich in iodine, they are at risk of thyroid gland disorders. In the same way many soils are deficient in selenium, putting the people who live in these areas at risk from cardiovascular and other diseases.

Shellfish provide the element in a reliable form. Molluscs such as cockles, clams, oysters and mussels are a good source of iron in a readily available form. Zinc is another essential element supplied by some shellfish. It plays an important part in the functioning of the human immune system. There's evidence that some shellfish have an anti-inflammatory action. New Zealand green lipped mussels have been found to help relieve symptoms of rheumatoid arthritis.

Nutrients

Cooked shellfish is a low-fat, low-calorie source of protein with many essential minerals. All are rich in selenium and iodine. Crabmeat, lobster, mussels, oysters, prawns and scallops are good sources of zinc while mussels are rich in iron. Many shellfish are useful sources of copper, phosphorus and magnesium. Most shellfish contain useful amounts of some B vitamins including riboflavin, nicotinic acid and vitamin B12. Oysters have good levels of calcium and vitamin D, while prawns contain vitamin E. Crabmeat and mussels contain significant amounts of omega-3 fatty acids.

SPELT

What to Avoid

Little to worry about here. Spelt is generally grown without the high inputs of chemical fertilizer and pesticides used on modern wheat varieties. As a result, it's more likely to be nutrient-rich than the grain that goes into most of our bread and pastries.

What to Buy

A native of the Middle East, spelt is an ancient grain, one of the first to be used in bread-making. Though related to wheat, it has many advantages over the modern hybrids which are currently used in today's breads, cakes and pastries. The medieval sage Saint Hildegard praised it as especially suited to the weak and sick. Its gluten seems to break down more easily during fermentation, making it more digestible than modern wheats. It also offers a broader spectrum of nutrients than modern hybrid varieties.

Benefits

Spelt is a good source of vitamin B2 (riboflavin) which is essential for normal energy metabolism within cells. Riboflavin has been found to reduce the incidence of migraine headaches in sufferers. Spelt also contains good levels of Vitamin B3 (niacin), which helps reduce levels of blood cholesterol and lipoprotein (a), a compound which damages blood vessels. The fibre in spelt also helps reduce levels of total cholesterol and LDL cholesterol.

Regular servings of whole grains such as spelt have been shown to slow down vascular disease in post-menopausal women. Recent research has shown spelt and other whole grains to have far higher antioxidant properties than was once thought. Whole grains also contain a group of phytonutrients called lignans which are thought to protect against hormone-dependent cancers. Whole grains contain a battery of compounds with antioxidant properties. They include vitamin E, selenium, tocotrienols and phenolic acids.

Cholesterol-lowering compounds include polyunsaturated fatty acids, oligosaccharides, plant sterols and stanols, and saponins. It's the slow release of these substances in the gut that makes whole grains so beneficial.

Nutrients

Contains good levels of vitamin B1 (thiamine), vitamin B2 (riboflavin) and vitamin B3 (niacin). Minerals, including good levels of manganese and copper. High in anti-oxidant activity resulting from a broad range of phytonutrients. The whole grain is high in dietary fibre. Contains vitamin E.

SPINACH

What to Avoid

Spinach grown on impoverished soils will not deliver the battery of health-giving nutrients supplied by the real thing. Unless you know the grower and the way the land has been looked after, it's safer to stick to organic. If you can buy locally from a grower who knows how to manage soil for maximum fertility you're likely to get a better product.

What to Buy

For spinach to be high in minerals and antioxidants it has to be grown in soils high in organic matter. This means soils that receive regular applications of compost or which are frequently sown with cover crops and green manures. Spinach also does best on soils that are rich in lime. Acid soils low in organic matter are unlikely to produce crops rich in protective nutrients. If you're buying in supermarkets, choose organically grown crops.

Benefits

In popular wisdom spinach was considered beneficial as a rich source of iron, which helps prevent iron-deficiency anaemia. But there's evidence that the iron in spinach is not easily absorbed. Even so, it's a good source of other minerals including calcium and magnesium, which help maintain normal blood pressure and build strong bones. Oxalic acid found in spinach can interfere with calcium absorption, but the acid is neutralized during cooking. Potassium helps regulate the electrolyte balance and ensure normal heart function.

Spinach contains pyridoxine – vitamin B6 – which aids the metabolism of protein and fat, and which boosts the immune system. Folic acid protects against birth defects and some forms of cancer and heart disease. Equally important are the carotenes lutein and zeaxanthine which protect against age-related macular degeneration, and also reduce the risk of cancer and heart disease. In laboratory animals spinach has been found to lower blood cholesterol.

Nutrients

Carotenoids including leutine and zeaxanthine. Minerals including iron, magnesium, potassium, boron, manganese and cobalt. Vitamins B6 (pyridoxine), B2 (riboflavin), and C. Folic acid.

STRAWBERRIES

What to Avoid

Non-organic ones. Strawberries are very fragile fruits and are susceptible to disease, particularly during the ripening stage. This means that conventional farmers spray repeatedly to keep them free of disease. As a result strawberries are one of the foods most often found to be contaminated with pesticide residues.

Organic growers have to find alternatives to chemicals – such as spacing their plants more widely to maintain an airflow to reduce the impact of fungal disease. At their best strawberries are so filled with flavour and nutrients that it makes sense to buy only the organic ones. Avoid fruits showing any form of mould, also fruits that are not fully ripe as indicated by green or yellow areas. Once picked the fruit won't ripen any further so they won't ripen at home.

What to Buy

Apart from choosing organic, look for fruits that are fresh, ripe and free of mould. The best berries are firm and plump with a deep red colour. Healthy fruits should be shiny and have their green 'plugs' still in place. Mid-sized strawberries have better flavour than large ones. If you're buying them pre-packaged make sure the container has no visible damage and that there's no sign of condensation on the inside. Moisture in the pack could lead to deterioration.

Benefits

Ripe and freshly picked, strawberries are one of nature's healthiest foods. They're low in calories and provide – per portion – more than your daily requirement of vitamin C. As an antioxidant, vitamin C helps prevent the oxidation of LDL cholesterol which can lead to hardening of the arteries. Vitamin-C-rich foods have been shown to offer protection against some forms of rheumatoid arthritis.

Strawberries also contain a host of other antioxidants including anthocyanins and ellagitannins. This battery of phytonutrients gives strawberries powerful protective action against heart disease and cancer. The fruit's unique assembly of phenols gives it anti-inflammatory properties. In studies strawberries have regularly emerged as one of the most protective foods against cancer. Like other fruits they also combat the age-related vision defect known as macular degeneration.

Nutrients

An excellent source of vitamin C with its own unique range of powerful antioxidants. Other vitamins include folic acid, riboflavin, pantothenic acid and pyridoxine. A good source of minerals including manganese, iodine, potassium magnesium and copper. A useful source of dietary fibre. Also contains omega-3 fatty acids.

TOMATOES

What to Avoid

These include most of the tomatoes you'll find in your local superstore. Many of today's commercial tomatoes never see soil, fertile or otherwise. They are grown hydroponically in a nutrient solution. While perfect in shape and free from blemishes, the fruits lack flavour and nutrients. Sometimes the fruits are picked while they're still green and ripened in ethylene gas. This turns them red while adding nothing to the flavour. To be sure of getting real fruits choose organically grown tomatoes that have been ripened on the vine. While tomatoes will ripen in the store or at home, they'll never taste as good as freshly picked ripe tomatoes of the sort you buy in Mediterranean markets. Since this is one of the few fruits that retains many of its nutritional qualities during canning it might be best to stick with the canned version outside the summer months.

What to Buy

The starting point for nutritious tomatoes is a deep fertile soil with plenty of organic matter to hold moisture. The other key element is sunshine. Tomatoes originated in Central and South America and were introduced to Europe in the sixteenth century. In Britain the season for outdoor tomatoes is short. They ripen in September just before the winter frosts destroy them. Growing them under plastic extends the season to about three months. While there's nothing to touch a well-grown, vine-ripened tomato for taste and nutrients, for much of the year these need to be imported from sunnier climes.

Benefits

Tomatoes are one of a small number of fruits that are rich in a carotenoid called lycopene. This is a powerful anti-oxidant. It has been said that a tomato a day may make the difference between developing cancer and remaining free of the disease. Studies show that people with high blood levels of lycopene greatly reduce their risk of contracting a number of cancers. Fortunately lycopene survives cooking and processing. In fact, it may be more available for absorption in the form of canned tomatoes, tomato juice or paste. Sadly, vitamin C, which is also plentiful in ripe tomatoes, doesn't fare so well during processing.

Nutrients

Vitamin C, which helps the immune system. Carotenoids, particularly lycopene. B vitamins. Minerals including potassium, magnesium, phosphorus and calcium. Fibre.

VENISON

What to Avoid

Fortunately there are no real fakes to worry about. Though it's best to go for wild venison whenever you can get it, farmed venison remains a healthy meat. While deer farmers use some cereals in the feeding process, the bulk of the feed is still grass and forage. Whether you're going for wild or farmed venison, try to find a local source if you can.

What to Buy

There's historical evidence to suggest that venison has been consumed for far longer than other meats, including beef, pork and chicken. Human beings have hunted wild deer since the earliest times, and their domestication for food seems to have begun in the Stone Age.

Today, deer are still hunted in many parts of the world and

venison is an established part of many cuisines. In addition, farmed venison is becoming more popular. Britain, New Zealand and the United States are among the principal deer-farming countries. While the diets of wild deer are chiefly made up of vegetation, farmers frequently use some high-energy cereals during the production process.

Benefits
Though venison is rarely thought of as a health food, it has many health-promoting properties. Compared with other red meats it's relatively low in fat, and is a good source of protein, B vitamins and minerals, including iron. Venison is a particularly good source of iron in a readily available form. Iron is a key component of haemoglobin, which transports oxygen from the lungs to the cells.

It also plays an important role in enzyme systems for energy production and metabolism. As a mineral source, venison is particularly valuable to menstruating women who are at greater risk of iron deficiency than the general population. Growing children and adolescents also have an increased need of iron in a readily available form. Vitamin

B12 and vitamin B6 in venison help prevent the build up of the potentially damaging compound homocysteine, which damages blood vessels. Another B vitamin, riboflavin, plays an important part in energy metabolism and helps reduce the occurrence of migraine attacks. The B vitamin niacin greatly reduces the risk of developing osteoarthritis.

Nutrients
Good source of high-quality protein. Rich in B vitamins, particularly vitamin B2 (riboflavin), vitamin B3 (niacin), vitamin B6 (pyridoxine) and vitamin B12 (cobalamin). Minerals, particularly iron, phosphorus, selenium, zinc and copper.

WALNUTS

What to Avoid
Ready shelled and loose-packed walnuts are best avoided. Omega-3 linoleic acid, with its three double carbon bonds, is susceptible to turning rancid. So try to eat only those nuts you have shelled yourself.

What to Buy
The English walnut, one of many species of walnut, originated in India and in the region of the Caspian Sea. The

tree is highly ornamental and prized for its beauty. The popularity of walnut in the nineteenth century led to the loss of many trees. Even so, many trees still survive in old woodlands and parks. Commercially grown walnuts are chiefly confined to the United States, Turkey, China, Iran, Romania and France, where the nut is so valued that a mature tree is worth, in rental terms, as much as an acre of cultivated land. Walnuts ought to be valued because in nutrients terms they are among our finest foods.

Benefits

Walnuts are uniquely high in omega-3 essential fatty acids. This gives them many health benefits including cardiovascular protection, improved cognitive function and anti-inflammatory properties which help counter asthma, rheumatoid arthritis, eczema and psoriasis. Omega-3s help prevent erratic heart rhythms, blood clots and high cholesterol levels. In addition, monounsaturated fats in walnuts help in the lowering of LDL cholesterol, the potentially harmful form.

Walnuts have also been shown to help prevent gallstones and to raise levels of the hormone melatonin, so promoting better sleep. Walnuts contain the antioxidant compound ellagic acid, which helps prevent cancer. High levels of the minerals manganese and copper support a number of key enzyme systems in the neutralizing of potentially damaging free radicals.

Nutrients

Walnuts contain levels of omega-3 fatty acids rarely found outside marine sources. Rich in the minerals manganese and copper. Also contain iron, magnesium, phosphorus, potassium and zinc. Contain good levels of the amino acid tryptophan which can be used in the body to make vitamin B3 (niacin). Good levels of monounsaturated fatty acids. Contain the antioxidant compound ellagic acid, which supports the immune system and has anti-cancer properties.

WHEAT

What to Avoid

The vast majority of wheat-based foods should be considered fake. The deception starts on the farm where most crops are grown on soils damaged by constant treatment with chemical fertilizers and pesticides. Modern hybrid varieties are chosen for their ability to take up large amounts of chemical nitrate fertilizer and their suitability for the mechanized, high-speed Chorleywood bread process. Little effort is made to maintain the nutritional standard of the grain. In any case most of the nutrients are lost during milling, a deficiency not remedied by so-called 'enrichment' of the flour with synthetic vitamins and minerals. (See Bread, Breakfast Cereals, Spelt, above.)

What to Avoid

Most of the wheat grown in Britain is winter wheat; it is planted in the autumn for harvesting the following summer. The crop thrives in cool, temperate climates, and has been grown in the Midlands and eastern counties for centuries. Wheat is deep rooted and resistant to drought, as well as being frost hardy. It does best on rich, fertile soils with plenty of 'body', that is, heavy soils such as strong loams and clays. So long as there's plenty of organic matter in the soil, the grains it produces will be packed with nutrients.

Benefits

Though wheat has played an important part in human nutrition for thousands of years, traditional societies used it with care. They always soaked or fermented the grains before turning them into porridge, bread or gruel. This greatly improved the nutritional value by neutralizing phytic acid in the outer layer or bran. Untreated, phytic acid in wholemeal foods can block the absorption of minerals, including calcium, magnesium, iron and zinc, leading in extreme cases to severe deficiencies or even bone loss. With this proviso the B vitamins in wheat play a part in the functioning of almost every body system, including the nervous and vascular systems, the skin, vision, fertility and hearing. Similarly, minerals such as potassium, iron, magnesium and zinc play a part in most metabolic systems. The high fibre content of whole-grain wheat is believed to reduce the risk of some cancers, including colorectal and breast cancers.

Nutrients

Minerals including potassium, iron, magnesium and zinc. Selenium may be present in small amounts, depending on its level and availability in the soil. Vitamin E, a potent antioxidant which greatly reduces the risk of heart attack, cancer and diabetes. Dietary fibre. Protein of a higher value than those of other cereals. However, wheat protein is incomplete, deficient in the amino acid lysine. Rich source of omega-3 linoleic acid.

YOGHURT

What to Avoid

Low fat yoghurts – like skimmed and semi-skimmed milk – deliver fewer of the health benefits associated with whole milk. They are best avoided. So are the fruit yoghurts that are all too often laden with sugar. Strictly speaking, products made with pasteurized milk are fake, too. Many of the health benefits of fermented milk are lost following pasteurization; the improved digestion of lactose, for example. There's also evidence that even heating milk above a hundred degrees to make modern yoghurt causes damage to milk protein.

What to Buy

The origins of health-promoting yoghurt are the same as those for milk, a fertile pasture filled with herbs, as well as grasses. The fermented milk of grass-fed cows has been an important feature of the diets of some of the world's longest-living people. Needless to say the starting point was always raw, unpasteurized milk. In traditional societies milk fermentation cultures were often passed unchanged from generation to generation. Many were used as medicines, particularly in the treatment of ailments in the intestinal tract.

Benefits

The longevity of peoples in Bulgaria, Vilcabamba in Ecuador and other parts of the world has long been linked to yoghurt and other fermented milk products. Modern science has now begun to show the reasons why. Regular consumption of cultured dairy products lowers blood cholesterol levels and combats bone loss. They also improve digestion, strengthen immune systems and defend against pathogenic organisms, greatly reducing the risk of infections. Yoghurt cultured with *Lactobacillus acidophilus* combats vaginal yeast infections and protects against *Salmonella* dysentery. Cultured milk has been shown to improve the digestion of milk protein and to enhance the absorption of minerals, especially calcium and phosphorus. There's also evidence that the consumption of raw milk, fermented raw milk and other fermented foods can be of real benefit to autistic children.

Nutrients

Minerals, particularly calcium, potassium and phosphorus. Calcium helps maintain bone strength and prevent osteoporosis. Vitamin D and other fat-soluble vitamins including A, E and K. Water soluble vitamins including vitamin C, vitamin B12, riboflavin. Vitamin B12 works with folic acid in helping to prevent anaemia. Enzymes which improve the digestion of lactose in the digestive tract.

Sources

Earl Mindell, *The Food Medicine Bible*, Souvenir Press, 1994.

Sally Fallon, *Nourishing Traditions*, New Trends Publishing, 1999.

The George Mateljan Foundation. The World's Healthiest Foods http://www.whfoods.com

Dr Michael Sharon, *Complete Nutrition*, Carlton Books, 1989.

References

Chapter 1

1 W. J. Reader, *Imperial Chemical Industries: A History, Vol. 1, 1870–1926*, Oxford University Press, 1970, p. 352.
2 Ibid. pp. 154–5.
3 W. J. Reader, *Imperial Chemical Industries: A History. Vol. 2, 1926–1952*, Oxford University Press, 1975.
4 Frederick Keeble, *Fertilizers and Food Production*, Oxford University Press, 1932, p. 61.
5 Philip Conford, 'A Forum for Organic Husbandry: The *New English Weekly* and Agricultural Policy, 1939–49, *Agricultural History Review*, Vol. 46 (2), 1998, pp. 197–210.
6 Quentin Seddon, *The Silent Revolution*, BBC, pp. 21–22.
7 Colin Tudge, *So Shall We Reap*, Allen Lane Penguin, 2003, p. 197.
8 H. J. Massingham (ed.), *England and the Farmer*, Batsford, 1941, p. 50.
9 OECD Paris, *Farm Household Income, Issues and Policy Responses*, 2003.
10 Colin Tudge, op. cit., p. 197.
11 Vaclav Smil, *Enriching the Earth*, MIT Press, 2001, pp. 155–76.

Chapter 2

1 Louise Atkinson, 'You're Eating the Wrong Fruit and Veg', *Daily Mail*, 4 July 2006; http://salvestrolscience.com
2 http://laverstokepark.co.uk

3   E. Walter Russell, *Soil Conditions and Plant Growth*, Ninth Edition, Longmans, 1961, p. 183. Russell quotes figures from the long-running Broadbalk experiment at Rothamsted experimental station in Hertfordshire. A plot fertilized with organic manure contained one million earthworms to the acre weighing 200kg. Plots receiving heavy dressings of chemical fertilizer contained fewer than half the number of worms, weighing between 22kg and 45kg an acre.

4   Michael Pollan, *The Omnivore's Dilemma*, Bloomsbury, 2006.

Chapter 3

1   Weston A. Price, *Nutrition and Physical Degeneration*, Sixth Edition, Price-Pottenger Nutrition Foundation, 2004.

2   Price began his mammoth study on root canal infections in 1900. In 1915 the National Dental Association – later to become the American Dental Association – appointed him their first research director. Leading a research team of sixty, he published his findings in 1923. They appeared in two volumes – *Dental Infections Oral and Systemic*, and *Dental Infections and Degenerative Diseases*. The first volume is currently published by the Price-Pottenger Nutrition Foundation.

3   Rex Harrill, *Using a Refractometer to Test the Quality of Fruits and Vegetables*, Pineknoll Publishing, 1994.

4   Sally Fallon, *Nourishing Traditions*, New Trends Publishing, 2001, pp. 40–5.

5   Peter Crawford, *The Living Isles – A Natural History of Britain and Ireland*, BBC, 1985, p. 64.

6   Douglas Palmer (ed.), *The Illustrated Encyclopedia of Dinosaurs and Prehistoric Animals*, Marshall Publishing, 1988, p. 279.

7   An unusually large race of red deer still occupies forest land in the west of Ireland. Known as the giant red stags of Connemara, they were reintroduced by an estate owner following the shooting of the original deer during the famines of the 1840s. The introduced stags have astonished deer experts by growing to an immense size. One of the reasons for their size – and the dimensions of their antlers – is thought to be the underlying limestone, which supplies large amounts of calcium via vegetation. Duff Hart-Davis, 'The Antler Heroes', *Daily Telegraph*, 14 May, 2005.

Chapter 4

1 M. Fields, *Proceedings of the Society of Experimental Biology and Medicine*, 1984, Vol. 175, pp. 530–7.
2 Surgeon Captain T. L. Cleave, *The Saccharine Disease*, John Wright, 1974.
3 Dr Walter Yellowlees, 'Ill Fares the Land', in *Soil, Food and Health*, Wholefood Trust, 1989, pp. 15–42.
4 Originally published by Faber, the book was later republished by the McCarrison Society. R. McCarrison, *Nutrition and Health*, Westbury Press, 1982.
5 Sulphonamide – a drug developed in the 1930s from the red dye prontosil – was found to have powerful anti-microbial properties, particularly against streptococcus bacteria. The discovery was made in 1933 by the German chemist Gerhard Domagk, director of research for the company Bayer. Using derivatives of sulphonamide, chemists went on to develop treatments for hypertension, diabetes, heart failure, glaucoma, thyrotoxicosis, malaria and leprosy. See James Le Fanu, *The Rise and Fall of Modern Medicine*, Little Brown, 1999, pp. 210–5.
6 James Le Fanu, op. cit., p. 210.
7 *Cancer Trends in England and Wales 1950–1999*, Office for National Statistics, 2005.
8 *Coronary Heart Disease Statistics 2005*, British Heart Foundation, June 2005.
9 L. J. Melton et al., 'Bone Density and Fracture Risk in Men', *Journal of Bone Mineral Research*, 1998, Vol. 13, p. 1915; L. J. Melton, E. A. Chrischilles and C. Cooper, et al., 'Perspective: How Many Women Have Osteoporosis?', *Journal of Bone Mineral Research*, 1992, Vol. 7, p. 1005.
10 *Compendium of Health Statistics*, 16th Edition, 2004–5, Office for Health Economics.

Chapter 5

1 Andre Voisin, *Soil, Grass and Cancer*, New York: Philosophical Library, 1959.
2 Max B. Lurie, *Resistance to Tuberculosis: Experimental Studies in Native and Acquired Defensive Mechanisms*, Harvard University Press, 1964.

3 Helen Fullerton, *Bovine Tuberculosis: A Nutritional Solution*, Farming and Livestock Concern UK, 2002.

4 David Thomas, 'A Study on the Mineral Depletion of the Foods Available to Us as a Nation Over the Period 1940 to 1991[prime], *Nutrition and Health*, 2003, Vol. 17, pp. 85–115.

5 Tom Stockdale, 'Coronary Heart Disease: A New Perspective', *Nutrition and Health*, 2004, Vol. 18, pp. 73–5. Stockdale argues that a marginal deficiency in selenium over many years causes coronary heart disease. He links the continuing high UK incidence of the disease to the switch from Canadian hard wheats to European wheats by the country's flour millers . From the late nineteenth century selenium-rich Canadian wheat used to produce the standard white loaf protected UK consumers from deficiency diseases. But since the ending of Canadian wheat imports in the 1980s, a considerable proportion of the UK population has suffered from one or more symptoms of selenium deficiency, while those who were already marginally deficient are now severely affected. This last group are subject to a range of conditions including obesity, late onset diabetes, ADHD and depression.

6 M. P. Rayman, 'The Argument for Increasing Selenium Intake', *Proceedings of the Nutrition Society*, Vol. 61, pp. 203–15.

7 Colin Tudge, *So Shall We Reap*, Allen Lane, 2003, pp. 108–9.

8 Nigel Hawkes, 'Vitamin Boost for Young Criminals Cuts Offence Rate', *The Times*, 26 June, 2002.

9 Jane Seymour, 'Hungry For a New Revolution', *New Scientist*, 30 March, 1996.

10 *Diet, Nutrition and the Prevention of Chronic Diseases*, Report of the Joint WHO/FAO Expert Consultation, April, 2002.

11 Andre Voisin, op. cit., 1959.

12 Institute of Grassland and Environmental Research, North Wyke. Experimental results presented at an Associate's Day, 2006.

Chapter 6

1 Pesticide Residues Committee, *Annual Report 2003.* http//www.pesticides.gov.uk

2 Caroline Cox, 'Herbicide Factsheet: Glyphosate (Roundup)', *Journal of Pesticide Reform*, 1998, Vol. 18, No. 3, pp. 3–17.

3 W. S. Pease et al., 'Preventing Pesticide-Related Illness in California Agriculture: Strategies and Priorities', *Environmental Health Policy*

Program Report, Berkeley, CA, 1993, University of California School of Public Health Policy Seminar.

4 California Environmental Protection Agency, Department of Pesticide Regulation, Case Reports Received by the California Pesticide Illness Surveillance Program in Which Health Effects were Attributed to Glyphosate, 1998, Unpublished Report, Sacramento, CA, cited in Caroline Cox, op. cit.

5 California Environmental Protection Agency, Department of Pesticide Regulation, Worker Health and Safety Branch. Case Reports received by the California Pesticide Illness Surveillance Program in which health effects were attributed to exposure to malathion, alone or in combination, 2003, Unpublished Database, cited in Caroline Cox, 'Insecticide Factsheet: Malathion', *Journal of Pesticide Reform*, 2003, Vol. 23, No. 4, pp. 10–15.

6 Ibid.

7 G. Cabello et al., 'A Rat Mammary Tumor Model Induced by the Organophosphorous Pesticides Parathion and Malathion, Possibly Through Acetylcholinesterase Inhibition', *Environmental Health Perspectives*, 2001, 109, pp. 471–9.

8 Vyvyan Howard, 'Synergistic Effects of Chemical Mixtures – Can We Rely on Traditional Toxicology?', *The Ecologist*, 1997, Vol. 27, No. 5, pp. 192–5.

9 Ontario College of Family Physicians, Review of Research on the Effects of Pesticides on Human Health, 2004. http//www.ocfp.on.ca

10 Albert Howard, 'Soil Fertility', in H. J. Massingham (ed.), *England and the Farmer*, Batsford, 1941.

11 Graham Harvey, *The Forgiveness of Nature*, Jonathan Cape, 2001.

12 Michael Pollan, *The Omnivore's Dilemma*, Bloomsbury, 2006, pp. 47–8.

13 Vandana Shiva, 'Globalization and the War against Farmers and the Land', in Norman Wirzba (ed.), *The Essential Agrarian Reader*, Kentucky University Press, 2003.

14 The comparison was made in a conversation between Mr Furuno and a group of mono-crop rice growers from Texas. The conversation is reported by North Dakota organic farmer Frederick Kirschenmann, who is also director of the Leopold Center at Iowa State University. See: Frederick Kirschenmann, 'The Current State of Agriculture: Does It Have a Future?' in Norman Wirzba, op. cit.

15 Marc Bonfils studied and travelled in Africa, researching traditional tribal agriculture in his hunt for methods that worked with nature rather than against it. He was greatly influenced by the

work of Japanese farmer Masanobu Fukuoka, and has adapted many of his natural farming methods to European conditions. See Mark Moodie, *The Harmonious Wheatsmith*, available from eco-logic books, 19 Maple Grove, Bath, BA2 3AF. http//www.ecologic books.com. Bonfils himself authored a number of works including *Culture Du Ble d'Hiver*, available from Las Encantadas, B. P. 217, F-11300, Limoux, France.

16 William C. Edgar, *The Story of a Grain of Wheat*, George Newnes, 1902, pp. 13–14.

17 Sally Fallon, *Nourishing Traditions*, New Trends Publishing, 1999, p. 24.

18 Sally Fallon, 'Dirty Secrets of the Food Processing Industry', *Wise Traditions in Food, Farming and the Healing Arts*, Fall, 2001. www.westonprice.org

19 'Why Kelloggs saw red over labelling scheme', *Guardian*, 28 December 2006.

20 Gene Logsdon, 'All Flesh is Grass', in Norman Wirzba (ed.), *The Essential Agrarian Reader*, University Press of Kentucky, 2003, pp. 154–70.

Chapter 7

1 Arthur Hollins, *The Farmer, the Plough and the Devil*, Ashgrove Press, 1984.

2 C. A. Daley et al., 'A Literature Review of the Value Added Nutrients Found in Grass-fed Beef Products', *Nutrition Journal*, June 2006. http://csuchico:edu/agr/grassfedbeef/health-benefits

3 Ibid.

4 Ibid.

5 F. M. Whittington and J. D. Wood, 'Effect of Pasture Type on Lamb Product Quality', from *Eating Biodiversity: An Investigation of the Links Between Quality Food Production and Biodiversity Protection*, a report from Bristol University, 2006.

6 Newman Turner, *Fertility Farming*, Faber and Faber, 1951, pp. 67–8.

7 Robert H. Elliot, *The Clifton Park System of Farming*, Faber and Faber, 1898, p. 139.

8 C. Ip et al., 'Conjugated Linoleic Acid: A Powerful Anti-Carcinogen from Animal Fat Sources', *Cancer*, 1994, Vol. 74 (3 suppl.), pp. 1050–4.

9 T. R. Dhiman et al., 'Conjugated Linoleic Acid Content of Milk from Cows Fed Different Diets', *Journal of Dairy Science*, 1999, Vol. 82 (10), pp. 2146–56.

10 Richard Manning, *Grassland: The History, Biology, Politics, and Promise of the American Prairie*, Penguin Books USA, 1995, p. 127.

11 S. K. Duckett et al., 'Effects of Time of Feed on Beef Nutrient Composition' *Journal of Animal Science*, 1993, Vol. 71 (8), pp. 2079–88.

12 T. A. Dolecek et al., 'Dietary Polyunsaturated Fatty Acids and Mortality in the Multiple Risk Factor Intervention Trial (MRFIT)', *World Review of Nutrition and Dietetics*, 1991, Vol. 66, pp. 205–16.

13 English Beef and Lamb Executive, 'Latest Finisher Costings Give CAP Reform Hope', Briefing Note No. 04/14, September 2004.

14 Artemis P. Simopoulos, 'n-3 Fatty Acids and Human Health: Defining Strategies for Public Policy', *Lipids*, 2001, Vol. 36, Supplement, pp. S83–89.

15 Associate Parliamentary Food and Health Forum, Evidence Given to Joint Meeting on Diet and Behaviour, 21 January 2003. http//www.fhf.org.uk

16 C. Iribarren et al., 'Dietary Intake of Omega-3, Omega-6 Fatty Acids and Fish: Relationship with Hostility in Young Adults – The CARDIA Study', *European Journal of Clinical Nutrition*, 2004, Vol. 58, No. 1.

17 D. S. Siscovick et al., 'Dietary Intake and Cell Membrane Levels of Long-Chain n-3 Polyunsaturated Fatty Acids and the Risk of Primary Cardiac Arrest', *Journal of the American Medical Association*, 1995, Vol. 274 (17), pp. 1363–7.

18 A. P. Simopolous and Jo Robinson, *The Omega Diet*, HarperCollins, 1999.

19 D. P. Rose et al., 'Influence of Diets Containing Eicosapentaenoic or Docosahexaenoic Acid on Growth and Metastasis of Breast Cancer Cells in Nude Mice', *Journal of the National Cancer Institute*, 1995, Vol. 87 (8), pp. 587–92.

20 James Le Fanu, op. cit., pp. 348–9.

21 Sally Fallon and Mary G. Enig, 'It's the Beef – Myths and Truths about Beef', *Wise Traditions in Food, Farming and the Healing Arts*, Weston A. Price Foundation, Spring 2000.

22 Michael Pollan, *The Omnivore's Dilemma*, Bloomsbury, 2006, pp. 125–9.

23 Joel Salatin, 'Forgiveness farming', *Acres USA*, December 2006, Vol. 36, No. 12, pp. 16–21.

Chapter 8

1 Colin Tudge, op. cit., p. 190.
2 Charles Darwin, *The Formation of Vegetable Mould Through the Action of Worms, with Observations on Their Habits,* John Murray, 1881, p. 148.
3 Elaine Ingham, 'The Soil Foodweb: Its Importance in Ecosystem Health,' A Report from the Department of Botany and Plant Pathology, Cordley Hall 2082, Oregon State University, Corvallis. http//www.soilfoodweb.com
4 David Pimental et al., 'Environmental, Energetic and Economic Comparisons of Organic and Conventional Farming', *Bioscience,* July 2005, Vol. 55, No. 7, pp. 573–82.
5 The research results are summarized in John Reeves' *The Roots of Health,* available from Eastleigh, Greenfield Close, Joys Green, Lydbrook, Gloucestershire, GL17 9RD.
6 James Caird, *English Agriculture in 1850–51,* Frank Cass, Kelly Reprints of Economic Classics, 1967, pp. 457–8.
7 Tom Stockdale, 'Coronary Heart Disease – A New Perspective', *Nutrition and Health,* 2004, Vol. 18, pp. 73–5.

Chapter 9

1 Uffe Ravnskov, *The Cholesterol Myths,* New Trends Publishing, Washington, DC, 2000.
2 James Le Fanu, *The Rise and Fall of Modern Medicine,* Abacus, 1999, p. 149.
3 Mary Enig, *Know Your Fats,* Bethesda Press, Silver Spring, 2000, cited in Ron Schmid, *The Untold Story of Milk,* New Trends Publishing, Washington DC, 2003, p. 169.
4 Charles Sanford Porter, *Milk Diet as a Remedy for Chronic Disease,* Long Beach, California, 1905.
5 Sally Fallon, *Nourishing Traditions,* New Trends Publishing, Washington D. C., 1999, pp. 34–5.
6 J. R. Crewe, 'Raw Milk Cures Many Diseases', *Certified Milk Magazine,* January, 1929, pp. 3–6.
7 Jo Robinson, *Why Grassfed is Best,* Vashon Island Press, Vashon, Washington, 2000, p. 22.
8 T. R. Dhiman et al., 'Conjugated Linoleic Acid Content of Milk from Cows Fed Different Diets', *Journal of Dairy Science,* 1999, Vol. 82 (10), pp. 2146–56.

9   H. Timmen and S. Patton, 'Milk Fat Globules: Fatty Acid Composition, Size and In Vivo Regulation of Fat Liquidity', *Lipids*, 1988, Vol. 23, pp. 685–9.

10   Marius Collomb et al., 'Correlation Between Fatty Acids in Cows' Milk Produced in Lowlands, Mountains and Highlands of Switzerland and Botanical Composition of the Fodder', *International Dairy Journal*, 2002, Vol. 12, pp. 661–8.

11   Chin et al., 'Dietary Sources of Conjugated Dienic Isomers of Linoleic Acid, a Newly Recognised Class of Antocarcinogens', *Journal of Food Composition and Analysis*, 1992, Vol. 5, pp. 185–97.

12   J. H. Nielsen and T. Lund-Nielsen, 'Healthier Organic Livestock Products: Anti-oxidants in Organic and Conventionally Produced Milk', *Book of Abstracts. First Annual Congress of the EU Project Quality Low Input Food and the Soil Association Annual Conference, Newcastle, 6–9 January 2005.*

13   J. Robertson and C. Fanning, *Omega-3 Polyunsaturated Fatty Acids in Organic and Conventional Milk*, University of Aberdeen, 2004.

14   C. F. Garland et al., 'Can Colon Cancer Incidence and Death Rates be Reduced with Calcium and Vitamin D?' *American Journal of Clinical Nutrition*, 1991, Vol. 54, p. 193S.

15   J. L. Outwater et al., 'Dairy Products and Breast Cancer: The IGF-1, Oestrogen and bGH Hypothesis', *Medical Hypothesis*, 1997, Vol. 48, pp. 453–61.

16   Jonathan Long, 'Effective Control Strategy Keeps Mastitis Bills Down', *Farmers Weekly*, 21 October 2005.

17   Julian Mellentin, 'Omega Factor', Dairymen, Supplement to *The Grocer*, 10 September, 2005.

18   Using Fatty Acids for Enhancing Classroom Achievement, Report of Durham Educational Authority, Jan. 2004. http://durhamtrial.org.uk

19   R. J. Dewhurst et al., 'Forage Breeding and Management to Increase the Beneficial Fatty Acid Content of Ruminant Products', *Proceedings of the Nutrition Society*, 2003, Vol. 62, pp. 329–36.

20   Dairy Supply Chain Margins 2003–04, Milk Development Council, August 2004.

21   A Campaign for Real Milk. A Project of the Weston A. Price Foundation. http//www.realmilk.com

22   Ron Schmid, *The Untold Story of Milk*, New Trends Publishing, 2003, pp. 367–8.

23   A. J. Hosier, 'Open-Air Dairying', *Journal of the Farmers' Club*, Part 6, November 1927.

Chapter 10

1 Masanobu Fukuoka, *The One-Straw Revolution*, Other India Press, 1992, p. 2.
2 Department for Environment, Food and Rural Affairs, 2004 Harvest: Final Estimates of Cereal Production United Kingdom, 14 January 2005.
3 Masanobu Fukuoka, op. cit., pp. 65–6.
4 Newman Turner, *Fertility Farming*, Faber and Faber, 1951, pp. 17–18.
5 Department for Environment, Food and Rural Affairs, 'UK Farming in Context', Climate Change and Agriculture in the United Kingdom, 2000.
6 George Henderson, *The Farming Ladder*, Faber and Faber, 1944.
7 The present-day figure depends on the basis of the conversion. According to E. H. Net Economic History Services, using Gross Domestic Product as the basis of the conversion the 2002 equivalent is around £497,000. On the basis of change in the Retail Price Index, the 2002 figure becomes £128,000. http://eh.net/hmit/ukcompare/
8 This is on the basis of the change in average earnings. See E. H. Net Economic History Services http://eh.net/hmit/ ukcompare/
9 Colin Tudge, *So Shall We Reap*, Allen Lane, 2003, p. 83.
10 H. J. Massingham, *The Wisdom of the Fields*, Collins, 1945, p. 138.
11 Feeding the Fifty Million, A Report of the Rural Reconstruction Association Research Committee, Hollis and Carter, 1955, p. 95.
12 The estates were the Hiam Estates, a 7,000-acre holding in the Fens; Mr Rex Paterson's 11,000-acre estate in Hampshire; and Messrs. Parker's 30,000 acres in Norfolk, Lincolnshire and Leicestershire. The financial outputs of the three holdings were £220,600, £200,000 and £500,000, indicating a fall in output per acre as the size of holding increased. The figures were published in the 'Peterborough' column of the *Daily Telegraph* on the 5 June and 15 June, 1943. George Henderson, op. cit., p. 166.
13 Masanobu Fukuoka, op. cit., p. 91.

Chapter 11

1 Colin Tudge, op. cit., p. 264.
2 Jules Pretty, 'The Real Costs of Modern Farming', *Resurgence*, March/April 2001.

3   Ibid.
4   'Danish Pesticide Use Reduction Programme', Report of Pesticide Action Network Europe, June 2005.
5   Joanna Blythman, *Shopped — The Shocking Power of British Supermarkets*, Harper Perennial, 2004, p. 16.
6   Alison Smith and Paul Watkiss, 'The Validity of Food Miles as an Indicator of Sustainable Development', Report for Defra by AEA Technology plc, July 2005.
7   J. N. Pretty et al., 'Farm Costs and Food Miles: An Assessment of the Full Cost of the UK Weekly Food Basket', *Food Policy*, Vol. 30, No. 1, February 2005, pp. 1–19.

Chapter 12

1   Joanna Blythman, *Shopped – The Shocking Power of British Supermarkets*, Harper Perennial, 2004, p. 50.
2   Benjamin Newell, David Lagnado and David Shanks, *Straight Choices: The Psychology of Decision Making*, Psychology Press, 2007.
3   Matt Rudd, 'Locavores: the new food fad', The *Sunday Times*, 1 July 2007.
4   Katie Austin, 'Independent spirit', *Evening Standard*, London, 18 April 2007.

Chapter 13

1   Sally Fallon, *Nourishing Traditions*, New Trends Publishing, Washington DC, 1999, p. 34.
2   Edward Howell, *Enzyme Nutrition: The Food Enzyme Concept*, Avery, New York, 1985, pp. 100–1.
3   Peter King, *Traditional Cattle Breeds*, Farming Books and Videos, 2004, p. 17.
4   http://rbst.org.uk
5   Jim Worthington, *Natural Poultry-Keeping*, Crosby Lockwood, 1970, p. x.
6   Joel Salatin, 'Pastured Poultry: The Polyface Farm Model', The Weston A. Price Foundation, 11 August 2002, http://weston-aprice.org
7   Sally Fallon, op. cit., p. 452.

8 Jen Allbritton, 'Wheaty Indiscretions', Weston A Price Foundation, http://www.westonaprice.org

9 National Farmers' Retail and Markets Association, personal communication. http://www.farma.org.uk

10 'Local Food Costs Less at Farmers' Markets', South West Local Food Partnership, March 2002.

11 http://www.seedsofhealth.co.uk

12 Jonathan Riley, 'Organic Sales Rise by 22 per cent', *Farmers Weekly*, 7 September, 2007.

Acknowledgements

Special thanks to Margaret Adams, Jim and Kay Barnard, Malcolm Bole, Brian Castle, Mark Draper, Sally Fallon, Neil Hopkins, Danny Goodwin Jones, Martin Lane, David Marsh, Robert Plumb, John Reeves, Lyn Searby, David Thomas, Richard Vincent, Peter Wallace, David Henry Wilson, Walter Yellowlees and, not least, my wife Annie, whose support and encouragement has been, as ever, amazing.

Index

Entries in this index refer to the main text. Don't forget to look up individual foods in the alphabetical directory of Which Foods to Buy (pp.359–412) – entries contain information on nutrient content and their benefits to our health.

C

The directory has been compiled with thanks to *The Organic Directory 2006*,
The Guardian Food Directory, Rick Stein's *UK Directory of Produce*,
www.countrymanmagazine.co.uk, www.thefoody.com, www.bigbarn.co.uk,
www.farmersmarkets.net and www.organic-store.co.uk